60p

Essential
Neonatal
Medicine

ERYMU

Essential Neonatal Medicine

4th Edition

Malcolm I Levene MD, FRCP, FRCPCH, FMedSc
Professor of Paediatrics and Child Health
Leeds General Infirmary
School of Medicine
Leeds, UK

David I Tudehope AM, MBBS, MRACP, FRACP
Director of Neonatology
Mater Mothers' Hospital
South Brisbane, Queensland
Australia
and
Professor of Paediatrics and Child Health
University of Queensland
Australia

Sunil K Sinha MD, PhD, FRCP, FRCPCH, FIAP
Professor of Paediatrics and Neonatal Medicine
University of Durham
and
The James Cook University Hospital
Middlesbrough, UK

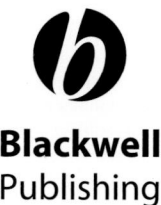

Blackwell
Publishing

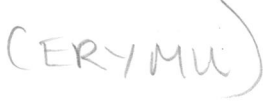

207   GSTM   (CERYMU)

First published 1987
Second edition 1993
Third edition 2000
Fourth edition 2008

1   2008
Library of Congress Cataloging-in-Publication Data

Levene, Malcolm I.
Essential neonatal medicine/Malcolm I. Levene, David I. Tudehope, Sunil K. Sinha. – 4th ed.
  p. ; cm.
  Rev. ed. of.: Essentials of neonatal medicine/Malcolm I. Levene, David I. Tudehope, M. John Thearle. 3rd ed. 2000.
  Includes bibliographical references and index.
  ISBN 978-1-4051-5710-0
1. Neonatology. I. Tudehope, David I. II. Sinha, Sunil K., M.D., Ph.D. III. Levene, Malcolm I. Essentials of neonatal medicine. IV. Title.
[DNLM: 1. Infant, Newborn, Diseases. 2. Neonatology. WS 421 L657e 2008]

RJ251.L48 2008
618.92′01–dc22

                                                                                2007031923

ISBN: 978-1-4051-5710-0

A catalogue record for this title is available from the British Library

Set in Palatino 9pt/12pt by Newgen Imaging Systems (P) Ltd, Chennai, India
Printed and bound in Singapore by Markono Print Media Pte Ltd

Commissioning Editor: Vicki Donald
Development Editors: Hayley Salter & Fiona Pattison
Production Controller: Debbie Wyer

For further information on Blackwell Publishing, visit our website:
http://www.blackwellpublishing.com

The publisher's policy is to use permanent paper from mills that operate a sustainable forestry policy, and which has been manufactured from pulp processed using acid-free and elementary chlorine-free practices. Furthermore, the publisher ensures that the text paper and cover board used have met acceptable environmental accreditation standards.

Contents

Preface to the fourth edition

Neonatal medicine continues to make rapid developments. In the eight years since the last edition was published there have been major advances in new technologies for neonatal respiratory support; advances in fetal medicine resulting in the delivery of more babies that would have died in utero and the attendant ethical and medical problems posed by these infants; hypothermia for brain protection; and further advances in neonatal surgery. In addition, parental expectations have risen and the increase in legal challenges to adverse outcomes that are perceived to be due to questionable care has made the practice of neonatal medicine more challenging. In the last 40 years our speciality has changed from being a "miracle of medical science against nature" to being one with routine expectations that very preterm infants will survive intact.

This fourth edition has tried to meet these challenges. With John Thearle's retirement we have taken on a new co-author, Professor Sunil Sinha, which has added to the authoritative nature of the book. Our goal has been to summarise complicated and often controversial management, and extract the "best evidence" currently available. Where best evidence is not clear we have used our combined experience to suggest the most effective management for our patients.

This book is intended for trainee clinicians (doctors, nurses and midwives), and we have deliberately reduced the references to a minimum to avoid it becoming a large textbook of neonatology. We hope that it will serve the next generation of neonatal clinicians well.

Malcolm Levene
David Tudehope
Sunil Sinha

Preface to the first edition

There has been an explosion of knowledge over the last decade in fetal physiology, antenatal management and neonatal intensive care. This has brought with it confusion concerning novel methods of treatment and procedures as well as the application of new techniques for investigating and monitoring high-risk neonates. The original idea for this book was conceived in Brisbane, and a *Primer of Neonatal Medicine* was produced with Australian conditions in mind. We have now entirely rewritten the book, and it is the result of cooperation between Australian and British neonatologists with, we hope, an international perspective.

We are aware of the need for a short book on neonatal medicine which gives more background discussion and is less dogmatic than other works currently available. We have written this book to give more basic information concerning physiology, development and a perspective to treatment which will be of value equally to neonatal nurses, paediatricians in training, medical students and midwives. Whilst collaborating on a project such as this we are constantly aware of the variety of ways for managing the same condition. This is inevitable in any rapidly growing acute speciality, and we make no apologies for describing alternative methods of treatment where appropriate. Too rigid an approach will be to the detriment of our patients!

A detailed account of all neonatal disorders is not possible but common problems and their management are outlined giving an overall perspective of neonatology. Attention has been given to rare medical and surgical conditions where early diagnosis and treatment may be lifesaving. It is easy to be carried away with the excitement of neonatal intensive care and forget the parents sitting at the cotside. Our approach is to care for the parents as well as their baby, and we have included two chapters on parent–infant attachment as well as death and dying. The final chapter deals with practical procedures and gives an outline of the commonly performed techniques used in the care of the high-risk newborn. We have also provided an up-to-date neonatal Pharmacopoeia as well as useful tables and charts for normal age-related ranges.

Malcolm I. Levene
David I. Tudehope
M. John Thearle

Acknowledgements

During the preparation of this book help and advice have been freely given by many colleagues, both medical and nursing. We are particularly grateful to Dr Henry Halliday and colleagues for permitting us to publish diagrams in Chapter 30 on procedures. We also thank Dr Tim Milward and Dr John Parsons for allowing us to publish their illustrations.

We are indebted to Karen Lynch (née Brierly), a former neonatal unit sister, for drawing a number of most helpful and clear diagrams of practical procedures; and to the Medical Graphics department at the Mater Misericordiae Public Hospitals for so generously giving their time to prepare high-quality photographs and diagrams.

1 Perinatal epidemiology and audit

Conception, embryonic and fetal development, parturition, and subsequent neonatal growth and development form a continuum. Obstetricians and neonatologists, however, have arbitrarily divided this continuum into rigid categories, which are used to audit standards of care during the perinatal and subsequent periods. Unfortunately, international agreement regarding some of the terminology is lacking; the definitions within this developmental continuum given here are those used in the UK and Australia.

Definitions (see also Fig. 1.1)

A live birth is one in which the infant shows signs of life (breathing, heartbeat or spontaneous movement) after its complete expulsion from the mother, irrespective of the gestational age or birthweight.

A stillbirth, or fetal death, is defined as an infant expelled from the birth canal at or after 24 weeks of pregnancy who shows no signs of life and has no heartbeat.

In Australia, stillbirth is defined as an infant born at or after 20 weeks' gestation and/or weighing ≥400 g with no signs of life. As the definition varies from country to country, comparisons of figures may be misleading. The stillbirth rate is expressed as the number of infants born dead at or after 24 weeks (or ≥20 weeks in some countries) per 1000 live births and stillbirths.

Gestational age This is calculated from the first day of the last normal menstrual period to the date of birth, and is expressed in completed weeks.

Term delivery occurs when the infant is born at or after 37 weeks' and before 42 weeks' gestation.

Preterm delivery occurs if the infant is born after less than 37 weeks' gestation. In the UK and Australia, 6–9% of infants are born preterm.

Post-term delivery occurs if the infant is born at or after 42 completed weeks of gestation. Approximately 1% of infants are born post-term.

Low birthweight (LBW) refers to any infant who weighs less than 2500 g at birth. In the UK and Australia, approximately 6% of live births are LBW. These infants are either born too early (preterm), or have grown inadequately in the uterus and are classed as 'small for gestational age'. Some LBW infants may be both preterm and small for gestational age.

Very low birthweight (VLBW) infants are those who weigh less than 1500 g at birth. Approximately 1–1.5% of liveborn infants are VLBW.

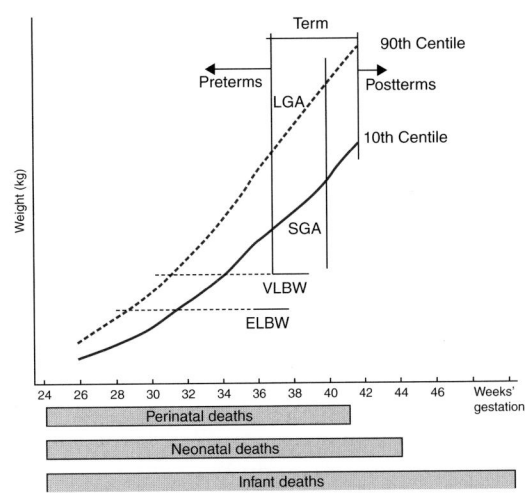

Figure 1.1 Definitions of terminology used in perinatal care (n.b. LGA: Large for Gestational Age).

Extremely low birthweight (ELBW) infants are those who weigh less than 1000 g at birth. This category accounts for approximately 0.7% of all births.

Small for gestational age (SGA). This term is generally synonymous with the fetus who has suffered intrauterine growth restriction (IUGR). Diagnosis depends on accurate assessment of gestational age (see p. 78) and plotting of weight on an appropriate growth chart. There is no international consensus on the definition of SGA, which varies from less than the 10th, 5th or 3rd percentiles, or more than two standard deviations below the mean birthweight. Accordingly, incidence figures will vary. In the UK SGA is defined as a baby weighing below the 10th centile for gestational age. Asymmetrical SGA refers to a baby whose weight is below the 10th centile, but whose head is above the 10th centile. This usually indicates late-onset intrauterine growth restriction (p. 84).

Changing trends

In order to make comparisons of death rates between years and across countries, some audit rates are widely used, but unfortunately the definitions may vary (see above).

Perinatal mortality rate (PMR)

$$PMR = \frac{\text{Number of stillbirths and neonatal deaths}}{\text{Number of stillbirths and live births}} \times 1000 \quad (1.1)$$

For international comparisons, the rate refers to all births of at least 1000 g birthweight or, when birthweight is unavailable, of at least 28 weeks' gestation, and neonatal deaths occurring within 7 days of birth – as recommended by the World Health Organization (WHO).

For Australian national statistics, the PMR refers to all births ≥500 g birthweight or ≥22 weeks' gestation, and the neonatal period is up to day 28.

For the UK, the PMR refers to stillbirths ≥24 weeks and neonatal deaths in the first 7 days of life.

For Australian states, PMR refers to all births ≥400 g birthweight or ≥20 weeks' gestation, and the neonatal period is up to day 28.

Neonatal death rate in the UK and Australia refers to the number of deaths within 28 days of birth of any child who had evidence of life after birth. Birthweight and/or gestational age criteria apply as for PMR.

Neonatal death is death occurring within 28 days of birth in an infant whose birthweight was at least 500 g or, if the weight was not known, an infant born after at least 22 weeks' gestation.

Postneonatal death rate (or late infant deaths) refers to the number of deaths of liveborn infants dying after 28 days but before 1 year of age per 1000 live births.

Infant death is death occurring within 1 year of birth in a liveborn infant whose birthweight was at least 500 g, or at least 22 weeks' gestation if the birthweight was not known. This category includes neonatal deaths as defined above.

Infant mortality rate (IMR) *(per 1000 live births)*

$$IMR = \frac{\text{Number of neonatal deaths and postneonatal deaths}}{\text{Total live births}} \times 1000 \quad (1.2)$$

Factors affecting perinatal death rates

Perinatal deaths relate to a wide variety of causes, sometimes arising as a result of maternal illness or problems of the fetus or newborn. In both the UK and Australia in 2004 the PMR was 8.2 per 1000 live births, comprising 67% fetal deaths and 33% neonatal deaths (Fig. 1.2). The highest risk groups were mothers aged <20 and ≥40 years, with PMRs of 12.0 per 1000 births. Social class is also an important factor. In the UK, there is almost a 100% difference in PMR between women in socioeconomic class I (professional groups) and those in class V (unskilled occupations).

The sex of the fetus or infant is also important. In Australia in 1993–95, the male perinatal death rate was 8.6 per 1000, as compared with 7.4 per 1000 for females. Maturity is of course an important factor in the PMR: about half of all deaths occur in babies who weigh less and of this group more than half weigh less than 1000 g. For twins the PMR is 4.3 times higher than for singletons. For higher order multiples it is nine times greater.

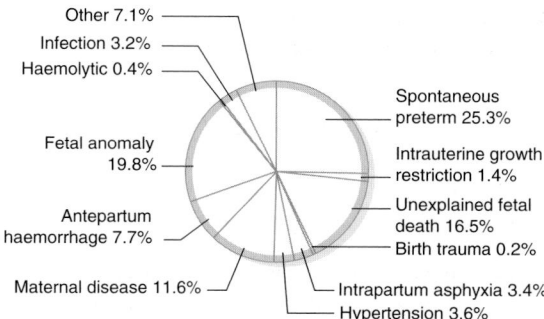

Figure 1.2 Causes of perinatal death, Queensland 1996. These proportions are similar to those in many parts of the UK.

Classification of perinatal deaths

It is difficult for doctors to agree on the cause of death in a diverse group of patients. Epidemiologists, obstetricians, neonatologists and pathologists may analyse deaths differently and report inconsistent rates. A traditional method for classifying perinatal deaths is based on the main maternal conditions or major obstetric antecedents.

The most reliable cause of death is obtained by an experienced perinatal pathologist conducting an autopsy examination, but even following such examination the precise cause of death may be undetermined, particularly when the infant dies before birth (see Fig. 1.2). For this reason, classification systems have been devised to identify the pathological processes occurring in the mother. A useful system is shown in Table 1.1.

The Perinatal Society of Australia and New Zealand (PSANZ) have developed the PSANZ Perinatal Death Classification (PSANZ-PDC) to identify the single most important factor leading to the chain of events resulting in a perinatal death, and the PSANZ-Neonatal Death Classification (PSANZ-NDC) to identify the single most important factor in the neonatal period that causes a death (Chan *et al*. 2004)

The role of the Coroner

Most jurisdictions have a Coroners Act that requires all reportable deaths to be reported to the Coroner. Usually a stillborn child is not reportable.

Table 1.1 Cause of perinatal death, Whitfield classification

1	*Spontaneous preterm*
	Multiple pregnancy
	Previous bleeding
	Previous spontaneous rupture of membranes
	Incompetent cervix
	Other
	Idiopathic
2	*IUGR*
3	*Unexplained IUFD*
4	*Birth trauma*
5	*Intrapartum asphyxia*
6	*Hypertension*
	Pre-eclampsia
	Renal
	Essential hypertension
7	*Maternal disease*
8	*Antepartum haemorrhage*
	Placental abruption
	Placenta praevia
	Undetermined origin
9	*Fetal abnormality*
	Chromosomal
	CNS
	CVS
	Renal
	Multiple malformations
	Metabolic errors
	Other
10	*Haemolytic disease*
	Rhesus incompatibility
	Other fetomaternal blood group incompatibility
	Haemoglobinopathy of α-thalassaemia
11	*Infection*
12	*Other*

Prevention of perinatal mortality and LBW

Despite not knowing the exact causes of perinatal mortality and LBW, the implementation of preventative measures can make substantial progress towards improving the outcome of pregnancy, as evidenced by the situation in developed countries compared with developing countries. The factors that are known to reduce perinatal mortality and LBW include improvement in maternal health and education, reduction in unplanned pregnancy, and provision of prenatal care in a comprehensive and coordinated manner.

References

Chan A, King JF, Flenady V *et al.* Classification of perinatal deaths: development of the Australian and New Zealand classifications. *J Paediatr Child Health* 2004;**40**:340–347.

Perinatal Statistics, Queensland 1996. Brisbane: Queensland Health, 1998.

Whitfield CR, Smith NC, Cockburn F, Gibson AAM. Perinatally related wastage – a proposed classification of primary obstetric factors. *Br J Obstet Gynaec* 1986; **93**:694–703.

Further reading

Avery GB, Fletcher MA, MacDonald MG (eds). *Neonatology: Pathophysiology and Management of the Newborn*, 4th edn. Philadelphia: Lippincott-Raven, 1994.

Day P, Lancaster P, Huang J. *Australia's Mothers and Babies 1995*. Sydney: AIHW National Perinatal Statistics Unit, 1997.

Office for National Statistics. *Series* DH3 (29) *Mortality Statistics. Childhood, Infant and Perinatal*. London: The Stationery Office, 1996.

World Health Organization. *International Statistical Classification of Diseases and Related Health Problems*, 1, 10th revision. Geneva: WHO, 1992.

CHAPTER 2

2 Fetal physiology, assessment of fetal wellbeing and adaptation to extrauterine life

Perinatology is a term used to describe the study of diseases involving the fetus and newborn infant. This involves the clinical disciplines of fetal medicine and neonatology. The obstetrician must have a thorough knowledge of pregnancy and its effects on the mother and fetus, as well as fetal development and physiology. He or she must also have an understanding of fetal adaptation to the extrauterine environment. The neonatologist specializes in the medical care of the newborn infant but must have a thorough understanding of fetal development and physiology. This chapter briefly reviews some aspects of fetal assessment and physiology to provide the paediatrician and neonatal nurse with a better understanding of events leading to normal fetal-to-neonatal adaptation and adverse consequences arising from failure to do so.

Placental function

The placenta is a fetal organ that has two major functions: transport and metabolism. The trophoblast of the placenta acts as a barrier to prevent the maternal immune system from reacting against 'foreign' fetal antigens. Rejection does not occur because the trophoblastic cells appear to be non-antigenic.

The uterus is supplied by maternal blood from the uterine arteries, which dilate throughout pregnancy, increasing fetoplacental blood supply 10-fold by term. Maternal blood bathes the inter-villous space and is separated from fetal blood by the chorionic plate. Transport of nutrients and toxins occurs at this level. Oxygenated fetal blood in the capillaries of the chorionic plate leaves the placenta via the umbilical cord to the fetus (Fig. 2.1).

Transport

The placenta transports nutrients from the mother to the fetus, and waste products in the other direction. This occurs in a number of different ways, including simple diffusion for small molecules and, for larger molecules, active transport, which is an energy-requiring carrier-mediated process.

The placenta also acts as a 'lung' and is responsible for gaseous exchange of O_2 and CO_2 as well as maintenance of acid–base status.

Metabolism

The placenta is metabolically active and produces hormones, including human chorionic gonadotrophin (HCG), human placental lactogen (HPL) and human chorionic thyrotrophin (HCT). It also detoxifies drugs and metabolites.

Oestriol cannot be produced by the placenta alone because the latter cannot hydroxylate pregnenolone. This is done by the fetal liver and adrenal glands. The metabolites are then sulphated by the placenta to form oestrogens, one of which is oestriol.

Because of its metabolic activity, the placenta has very high energy demands and consumes over 50% of the total oxygen and glucose transported across it.

Fetal function

The placenta is an essential organ for maintaining fetal homeostasis but the fetus is capable of performing a variety of physiological functions.
1 The fetal liver is responsible for the production of albumin, coagulation factors and red blood cells.

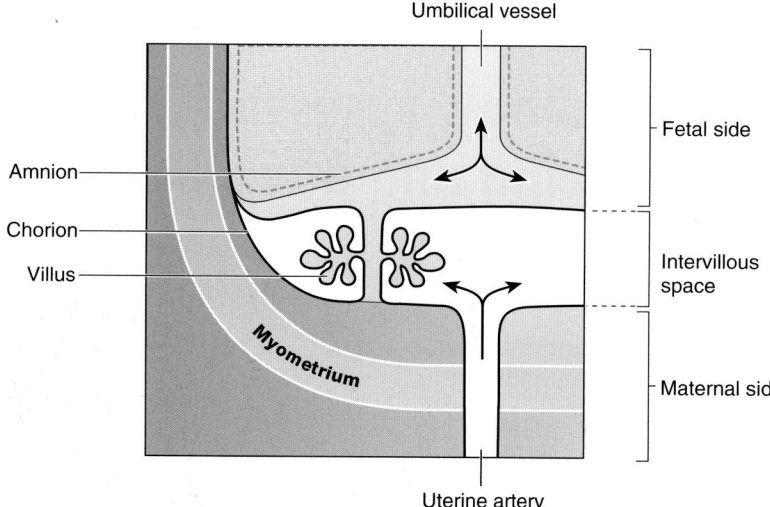

Figure 2.1 Diagram of placental structures showing blood perfusion.

2 The fetal kidney excretes urine, which contributes to amniotic fluid.

3 Fetal endocrine organs produce thyroid hormones, corticosteroids, mineralocorticoids, parathormone and insulin from 12 weeks' gestation.

4 Some immunoglobulins are produced by the fetus from the end of the first trimester.

5 The fetus breathes from about 11 weeks' gestation, but this is irregular until 20 weeks. It is not until 36 weeks that the fetus breathes regularly for 55–90% of the time. One purpose of fetal breathing is to promote an intermittent tracheal flux of fetal lung fluid into the amniotic fluid. This explains why fetal lung maturity can be assessed by measuring the lecithin/sphingomyelin (L/S) ratio on amniotic fluid (see p. 95). With ultrasound techniques, fetal breathing *in utero* can be observed (see p. 10).

Fetal circulation

The fetal circulation consists of two umbilical arteries bringing deoxygenated blood to the placenta, and a single umbilical vein carrying oxygenated blood back to the heart. The aorta of the fetus divides into the common iliac arteries and then the internal and external iliac arteries. The umbilical arteries are branches of the internal iliacs. The umbilical vein drains into the portal sinus and thence bypasses the liver via the ductus venosus to reach the inferior vena cava (Fig. 2.2).

The fetal circulation is quite different from the neonatal circulation. Deoxygenated blood is carried via the two umbilical arteries to the placenta, where it is oxygenated as it comes into close apposition with maternal blood in the intervillous spaces. Oxygenated fetal blood is carried in the umbilical vein, where it bypasses the liver via the ductus venosus. The blood then passes into the inferior vena cava and right atrium of the heart (Fig. 2.3). At atrial level much of the blood is shunted across the foramen ovale from the right atrium to the left. Oxygenated blood is pumped by the right ventricle into the pulmonary artery, but the majority bypasses the lungs via the ductus arteriosus to flow into the aorta. Only 7% of the combined ventricular output of blood passes into the lungs. The right ventricle is the dominant ventricle, ejecting 66% of the combined ventricular output.

In summary there are three shunts:

1 The ductus venosus bypasses blood away from the liver.

2 The foramen ovale shunts blood from the right atrium to the left atrium, bypassing the lungs.

3 The ductus arteriosus shunts blood from the pulmonary artery to the aorta.

The last two shunts can only function because of the very high fetal pulmonary vascular resistance and high pulmonary artery pressure that is characteristic of fetal circulation.

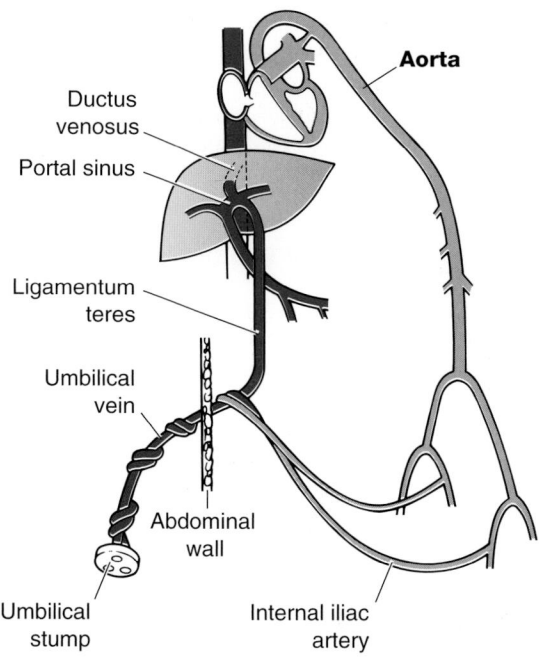

Figure 2.2 Schematic diagram of the vessels comprising the fetal circulation.

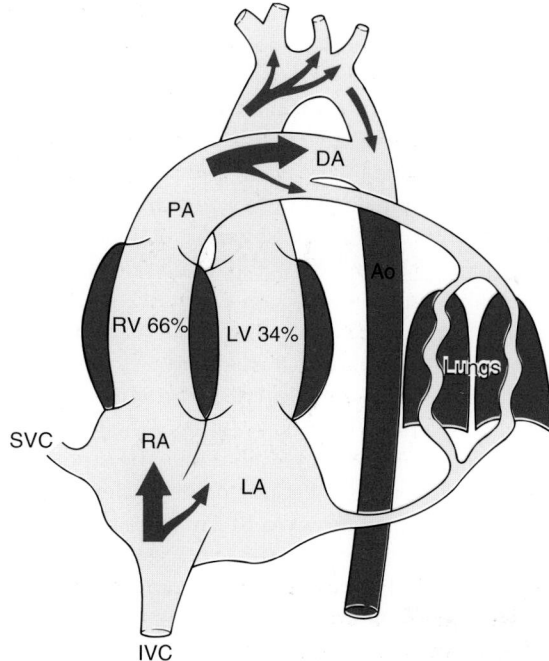

Figure 2.3 Diagram of the fetal circulation through the heart and lungs, showing the direction of flow through the foramen ovale and ductus arteriosus (DA). The percentages refer to the proportion of the cardiac output from each ventricle. The size of the arrow represents the proportion of flow. IVC, inferior vena cava; SVC, superior vena cava; RA, right atrium, LA, left atrium; RV, right ventricle; LV, left ventricle; PA, pulmonary artery; Ao, aorta. (After Rudolph & Heymann 1970.)

Umbilical vessels

Usually there are two umbilical arteries and one umbilical vein. Approximately 1% of babies have only one umbilical artery, and this may be associated with growth retardation and congenital malformations, especially of the renal tract. Chromosomal anomalies are also more common in infants with a single umbilical artery. An ultrasound assessment of renal anatomy is desirable in infants born with a single umbilical artery if this is associated with any other abnormality, and chromosomal analysis is undertaken where multiple anomalies are present.

Cardiovascular adaptations required for extrauterine life

While the fetus is breathing *in utero* the lungs are filled with fluid, but at the time of birth the baby generates enormous negative pressures of approximately 60–90 cmH$_2$O and fills the lungs with air. With the first two or three breaths much of the fetal lung fluid is expelled. The remainder is absorbed into pulmonary lymphatics and capillaries over the first 6–12 h. Sometimes these clearance mechanisms fail, or else there is too much fluid to start with and the baby develops symptoms. This condition is known as transient tachypnoea of the newborn (see p. 94) or retained fetal lung fluid. The stimulus for the first breath is not known with certainty, but is probably due to the bombardment of the baby with physical stimuli, such as cutaneous and thermal changes. It is also due in part to emptying of the lungs of fluid.

With the first few breaths the arterial oxygen tension (P_ao$_2$) increases from the fetal level of 2–3.5 kPa (15–25 mmHg) to the newborn level of 9–13 kPa (60–90 mmHg). This relative hyperoxia results in closure of the ductus arteriosus: this is functionally closed by 10–15 h, but not anatomically closed until 4–7 days. There is a marked fall in pulmonary vascular resistance shortly after birth, so that pulmonary blood flow increases. Because of the decrease in pulmonary blood pressure, there is a drop in pressure on the right side of the heart, and consequently no further shunting of blood from right to left atrium across the foramen ovale. The latter takes some time to close, and in 10% it remains patent through life. After birth there is a marked decrease in blood flow in the inferior vena cava, and the ductus venosus closes in response to this. A vestigial remnant of the ductus venosus – the ligamentum teres – remains throughout life. The umbilical vessels take longer to become obliterated and may still be cannulated for up to 10 days after birth.

Many factors may interfere with these changes at birth. If the baby has suffered from severe birth asphyxia or has respiratory distress syndrome, blood may continue to be shunted through fetal channels. A clinical syndrome of 'persistent pulmonary hypertension of the newborn' (PPHN), in which pulmonary pressures remain elevated, is well recognized (p. 189). A similar clinical picture can arise in situations where pulmonary pressure is normal but systemic pressure is decreased, such as in systemic hypotension due to any cause, because the net direction of blood flow (shunting through the fetal channels) depends on the gradient of blood pressure between pulmonary circuit and systemic circulation.

Assessment of fetal wellbeing

Assessment of fetal wellbeing is an integral part of the management of pregnant mothers. It includes assessment of the fetoplacental unit and fetal maturity, diagnosis of fetal abnormality, monitoring of fetal growth and evaluating wellbeing in the third trimester, as well as monitoring in labour (Fig. 2.4).

Assessment of maturity

Clinical assessment
Clinical assessment of maturity depends on the measurement of fundal height. This is most accurate in the first 10 weeks of pregnancy but can be very unreliable in later pregnancy or in obese women. Fetal quickening can help in dating the duration of pregnancy: in primiparous women

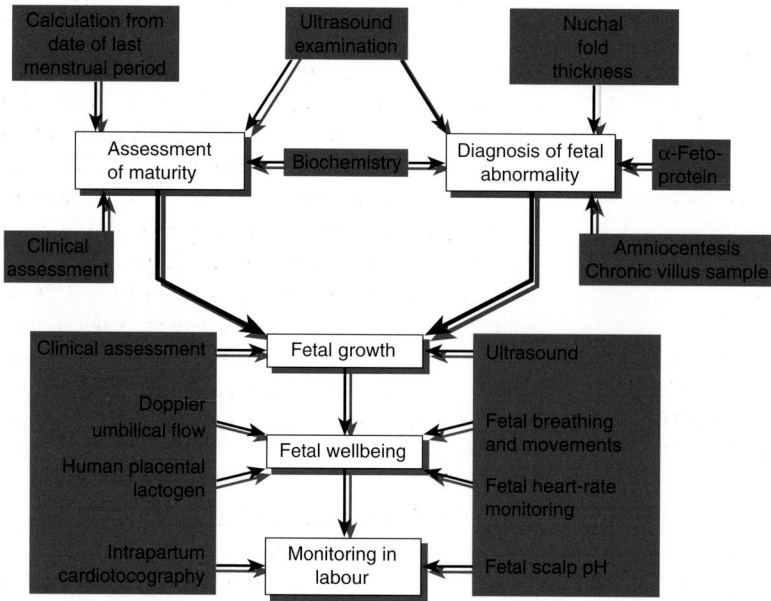

Figure 2.4 A plan for the assessment of fetal wellbeing. See text for description.

movements are first felt at about 20–21 weeks, and in multiparous women at approximately 18 weeks.

Ultrasound

Early ultrasound measurement of fetal size is the most reliable way to estimate the duration of pregnancy and is considered to be even more reliable than calculation from the date of the last menstrual period. There are a number of ultrasonic measurements that correlate well with gestational age in the first trimester. These include crown–rump length (may be technically a difficult measurement to make), biparietal diameter (BPD) and femur length. The BPD measurement between 12 and 18 weeks' gestation appears to be among the best of all methods for assessing the duration of pregnancy.

Fetal radiography

Radiography of the fetus is now rarely used as a method of establishing maturity. The talus ossifies at approximately 26 weeks, and the lower femoral epiphysis appears at 37 weeks, but there is considerable variation, and unnecessary exposure to radiation makes this method redundant.

Diagnosis of congenital abnormality

Maternal blood screening

Abnormally elevated α-fetoprotein (AFP) levels are associated with open neural tube disorders and are used as a screening test in early pregnancy. Low levels of AFP correlate with increased risk of trisomy 21, and this in conjunction with other biochemical markers in the mother's blood, such as unconjugated oestriol or beta human chorionic gonadotrophins (the triple test), can be used to screen for this condition. The test can be used to give a high or low risk for Down syndrome but does not give a definitive diagnosis. Some units now use a quadruple marker screening with inhibin, which is mainly produced from the placenta.

Ultrasound

Ultrasound examination of the fetus for congenital abnormalities is now highly developed and is offered as a routine procedure in many centres. Major malformations of the central nervous system, bowel, heart, genitourinary system and limbs should be detected and can be diagnosed in specialized centres early enough to consider termination of pregnancy. Down syndrome can often be detected by measurement of nuchal lucency and thickness.

Fetal magnetic resonance imaging (MRI) is now feasible and can be used in specific clinical or anatomical situations. The large field of view, excellent soft tissue contrast and multiple planes of construction make MRI an appealing imaging modality to supplement the weaknesses of ultrasound in cases such as maternal obesity and oligohydramnios, but unlike ultrasound MRI cannot be used for routine screening.

Amniocentesis

Amniotic cell culture or fluid analysis is valuable for the diagnosis of a variety of fetal abnormalities. Cells can be cultured for chromosome analysis or to study enzyme activity. Measurement of the optical density in amniotic fluid at 450 nm will detect haemolysis occurring as a result of rhesus haemolytic disease (see p. 196). Decisions regarding early delivery or intrauterine transfusion can be made on the basis of serial amniocentesis measurements.

Chorionic villus sampling

Chorionic villus sampling (CVS) involves the transcervical or transabdominal passage of a needle or cannula into the chorionic surface of the placenta at 9–11 weeks' gestation to withdraw a small sample of tissue into a syringe. Because of the 1% risk of abortion related to the procedure, the test is reserved for detection of genetic or chromosomal abnormalities in at-risk pregnancies, rather than as a mere screening test. There is concern that CVS may cause damage to the developing embryo and it is less commonly performed than previously.

Fetal blood sampling (cordocentesis)

Fetal blood sampling is an ultrasound-guided technique for sampling blood from the umbilical cord to assist in the diagnosis of chromosome abnormality, intrauterine infection, coagulation disturbance, haemolytic disease or fetal compromise.

Fetal growth

Clinical assessment

Monitoring uterine size is a time-honoured clinical method of assessing fetal growth. Unfortunately, up to 50% of growth-restricted infants are not detected clinically.

Ultrasound

Serial estimates of BPD, head circumference, abdominal circumference and head-to-abdomen ratios are widely used to monitor fetal growth. In fetuses suffering intrauterine growth retardation, head growth is usually the last to slow down. In recent years, estimating fetal weight by ultrasound has become a major focus of assessment for critical obstetric and neonatal decision-making that influences the timing of delivery in order to avoid fetal jeopardy.

Fetal wellbeing

Biochemical assessment

Assessment of fetal wellbeing by biochemical surveillance has now ceased in most centres as its sensitivity and specificity are very poor. Consistent unrecordably low levels of oestriols suggest either placental sulphatase deficiency or adrenal hypoplasia (see p. 171).

Ultrasound imaging and Doppler flow velocity analysis

The location of the placenta can be confidently established by ultrasound, and with the use of colour Doppler the fetal vessels can be identified near the cervix permitting the identification of cord presentation. Doppler flow velocity waveforms of the umbilical artery are now used as a major determinant of fetal wellbeing. In fetuses who show growth restriction, abnormal Doppler waveforms are a reliable prognostic feature. Reversed flow velocity during diastole is an ominous sign and is associated with the risk of imminent fetal demise. The significance of absent diastolic flow velocity is uncertain. Recently, Doppler measurement of peak systolic blood flow velocity in the middle cerebral artery (MCA) has become a part of the assessment of fetal anaemia and isoimmunization (see Chapter 18).

Alterations in amniotic fluid volume, both excessive (polyhydramnios) and reduced (oligohydramnios), are often associated with adverse fetal otcome. This is easily recognizable and can be quantified by measurement of the maximum pool size of fluid.

The measurement of amniotic fluid is often combined with non-stress testing, movement counts and breathing (see below) for an index of fetal wellbeing.

Fetal breathing movements

These can be assessed by ultrasound and show marked variability. Abnormalities include gasping-type respiration, extreme irregularity of breathing in a term fetus and complete cessation of breathing. This technique has not yet been fully evaluated and its practical value is limited.

Antepartum monitoring or non-stress test (NST)

The response of the fetal heart trace to naturally occurring Braxton Hicks contractions or fetal movements provides information on fetal health during the third trimester. The fetal heart trace is classified as reactive or non-reactive, depending on whether there is a minimum of two accelerations of 15 bpm or more, lasting at least 15 s, in response to fetal movements over a 20-min observation period.

Monitoring in labour

Intrapartum monitoring

Continuous electronic monitoring of the fetal heart rate can be performed non-invasively with a cardiotocograph (CTG) strapped to the abdominal wall, or invasively with a fetal scalp electrode inserted after the membranes have ruptured. The trace allows observation of four features:

1 *Baseline heart rate* – defined as 110–160 bpm.
2 *Beat-to-beat variability*. This is normally ≥5 bpm between contractions. Abnormal variability is <5 bpm for ≥90 min.

3 *Fetal heart decelerations* (Fig. 2.5):

(a) *Early*. Slowing of the fetal heart rate (FHR) early in the onset of a contraction with return to baseline by the end of the contraction.

(b) *Late*. Repetitive, periodic slowing of FHR with onset at middle to end of the contraction reaching nadir >20 s after peak of contraction and ending after the contraction.

(c) *Variable*. Variable, intermittent, periodic slowing of FHR with rapid onset and recovery.

(d) Prolonged. Abrupt fall in FHR to below baseline lasting at least 60–90 s. These are pathological if they last >3 min.

4 *Fetal heart accelerations*. These are normal and reassuring. There are transient increases in FHR of >15 bpm lasting 15 s or more. The significance of absent accelerations as a single feature is not known.

The interpretation of the CTG has been agreed by critical examination of best evidence (Anon 2001) as:

1 *Normal:* a CTG trace where all four features fall into a reassuring category.

2 *Suspicious:* a CTG trace with one non-reassuring feature, but all three others are reassuring.

3 *Pathological:* a CTG trace with two or more non-reassuring features.

Despite the widespread use of fetal heart rate monitoring for over 20 years it has not been shown to reduce morbidity in term infants. It has, however, increased the rate of delivery by caesarean section. There is no evidence that routine fetal heart rate monitoring in the low-risk fetus improves outcome. Careful monitoring with intermittent auscultation in these cases seems to be as reliable.

Fetal scalp pH

This technique should be used in conjunction with intrapartum cardiotocograph monitoring. In the presence of abnormal fetal heart rate patterns, fetal scalp pH measurement may be helpful. Clinical decisions are made on the severity of the blood acidosis:

≥7.25	No action, continue to monitor fetus electronically
7.21–7.24	Repeat pH within 30 min
≤7.20	Deliver urgently

Fetal pulse oximetry

The feasibility of using pulse oximetry to measure fetal oxygen saturation during labour has been investigated from time to time, but the sensitivity of the technique for detecting poor outcome is low and there is no evidence that pulse oximetry is superior to current methods of fetal surveillance.

Fetal electrocardiogram (ECG)

It has been suggested that relative changes in fetal ECG waveforms may help to discriminate patterns of fetal heart rate, but this approach remains a research tool. There is no evidence to suggest that changes in P–R or R–R interval is discriminatory for fetal hypoxia, but the use of S-T waveform analysis seems to offer the most significant advances in intrapartum monitoring.

Fetal distress

Fetal distress is a commonly used clinical term, although there are difficulties with its definition. Fetal distress usually means a stressed fetus showing signs of compromise due to lack of oxygen or undernutrition. It may also be used to describe an investigatory finding, such as failure of head growth on serial biparietal ultrasound examinations.

As used here, the term describes the 'at-risk' fetus. Fetal distress may be related to the following basic underlying causes:

1 *Maternal:* hypotension, hypertension, diabetes mellitus, cardiovascular disease, anaemia, malnutrition and dehydration.

2 *Uterine:* hypertonia, usually due to excessive use of Syntocinon.

3 *Placental:* premature separation, vascular degeneration.

4 *Umbilical:* prolapse, knot or cord around fetal neck.

The features of fetal distress are:

1 reduction in fetal movements (this has a weak correlation with adverse outcome);

2 passage of thick meconium into the amniotic fluid;

3 fetal scalp pH <7.20;

4 fetal heart rate abnormality as defined above.

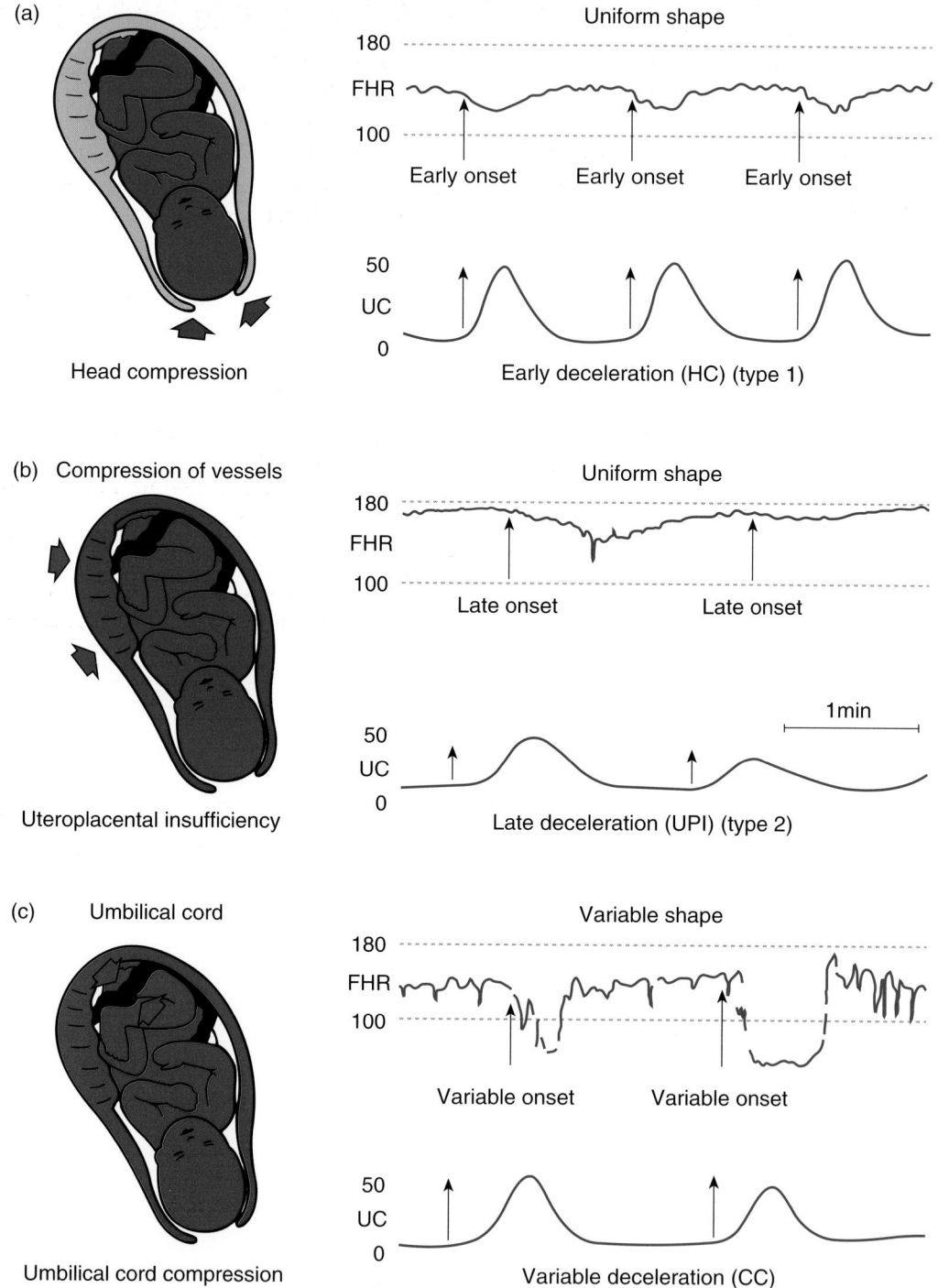

Figure 2.5 Commonly recognized variations in fetal heart rate recordings. (Reproduced with permission from Hon *et al*. 1975.)

PRACTICE POINT

- Maladaptation is often a sign of serious underlying problem such as cardiac, respiratory, neurological or infectious disorder.

- Never assume that the baby is in primary apnoea; appropriate resuscitation measures should be started immediately.

- Respiratory maladaptation may involve respiratory distress syndrome (RDS) in a preterm infant, and transient tachypnoea or pneumonia in a term infant.

- Circulatory maladaptation may result from as well as lead to PPHN.

- If a newborn baby fails to respond to an appropriately performed resuscitation consider an underlying neurological problem.

References

Anon. *Electronic Fetal Monitoring. Evidence-based Clinical Guidelines Number 8.* Royal College of Obstetricians and Gynaecologists, 2001, London.

Hon EH, Zanini B, Cabal LA. *An Introduction to Neonatal Heart Rate Monitoring.* University of California, Los Angeles Press, 1975, Los Angeles.

Further reading

Leone TA, Finer NN. Foetal adaptation at birth. *Curr Paediatr* 2006;**16**:373–378.

Kiserud T. Physiology of fetal circulation. *Semin Fetal Neonat Med* 2005;**10**:493–503.

Sinha SK, Donn SM. Fetal-to-neonatal maladaptation. *Semin Fetal Neonat Med* 2006;**11**:166–174.

Rudolph AM, Heymann MA. Circulatory changes during growth in the fetal lamb. *Circ. Res* 1970; **26(3)**: 289–299.

CHAPTER 3

3 Neonatal depression at birth and resuscitation of the newborn

Perinatal asphyxia is the most frequent and serious preventable problem of the fetus and newborn infant. Severe perinatal asphyxia may lead to significant problems after birth, with major long-term sequelae such as mental retardation, cerebral palsy, blindness and epilepsy. Good perinatal care can minimize fetal and neonatal hypoxia.

Neonatal depression at birth (Apgar score ≤6 at 1 min) occurs in about 14% of all births, and so an expert in neonatal resuscitation must be available within 2 min of being called for all births. Perinatal asphyxia remains a major source of neonatal morbidity in developed countries, and ranks with perinatal infection as the cause of at least two-thirds of neonatal mortality in developing countries. Owing to problems with definition, reported incidences in full-term neonates vary from 2 to 4/1000 live births, even more so for very low birthweight (VLBW) infants, with rates of up to 60%.

Fetal responses during labour

Every contraction during labour may cause relative hypoxia and hypoperfusion, a condition that can be considered as mild asphyxia. During these episodes the fetus has a repertoire of responses that protects him or her from injury (Table 3.1). Only if these responses become overwhelmed does the fetus suffer injury. These reflexes are designed to maintain function in vital organs such as the brain and myocardium. In addition, episodes of fetal bradycardia may occur during contractions. These are part of the 'diving seal reflex' and are normal, although episodes of fetal bradycardia may be mistaken for fetal distress. Anaerobic metabolism may also occur during transient periods of asphyxia, and is again a normal physiological adaptation.

Immediate effects of perinatal asphyxia

Acute asphyxia is usually an intrapartum event: birth liberates the fetus from a hostile environment and adequate resuscitation may restore the infant to a normal physiological state. The asphyxiated baby follows a predictable sequence of reactions, and both the respiratory and cardiovascular systems are directly involved.

Respiratory activity

Initially there is a stage of increased respiratory activity, which is followed by a period of apnoea (primary apnoea). This is then followed by a series of rhythmical gasps, which eventually become less frequent until secondary (or terminal) apnoea occurs. Spontaneous recovery can only occur if the baby is rescued before the secondary apnoea phase. Once terminal apnoea has occurred, active

Table 3.1 Responses of the normal fetus to transient episodes of 'asphyxia' in labour

Redirection of blood flow towards:
  brain
  myocardium
  adrenals

and away from:
  skin
  bowel
  muscles

'Diving seal reflex' comprising:
  bradycardia
  increased blood pressure

Episodes of anaerobic metabolism resulting in metabolic acidosis resuscitation is required to save the baby's life. The precise time at which terminal apnoea occurs in the human fetus or newborn during birth is not known for obvious reasons. Sometimes this can precede delivery.

Cardiovascular activity

Heart rate changes occur simultaneously with the respiratory changes described above. Initially, there is a rise in heart rate, followed by a decline until the onset of primary apnoea. This fall is probably mediated by vagal stimulation. Transient rises in heart rate and blood pressure occur at the time when gasps develop, but heart rate and blood pressure fall again when secondary apnoea develops. This is due to myocardial anoxia, and without resuscitation the fetus/newborn dies. The pulmonary vascular resistance increases dramatically with the stage of secondary apnoea, and the newborn circulation generally tends to revert to a fetal state. Figure 3.1 summarizes these changes in graphical form.

A baby with primary apnoea will appear blue with some tone and reflex activity and the heart rate will be accelerating. The baby will usually recover spontaneously, but this can be accelerated by physical stimulation.

In contrast, the baby with secondary (or terminal) apnoea has passed his or her last gasp and will not recover without vigorous resuscitation. In this case the baby is white or intensely cyanosed, unresponsive and flaccid; the heart rate is less than 100 bpm and perfusion is poor.

Unfortunately, in the delivery room one often cannot distinguish between primary and secondary apnoea, so that energetic resuscitation of all apnoeic infants should be undertaken on the assumption that all these infants have secondary apnoea.

After resuscitation it can usually be determined whether the apnoea was primary or secondary. Babies with primary apnoea have a rapidly accelerating heart rate, and will either show a few gasps or start to breathe normally. In contrast, babies with secondary apnoea will show some initial rise in heart rate in response to ventilation, start to gasp some time after and then continue to do so for some time before normal, regular breaths ensue.

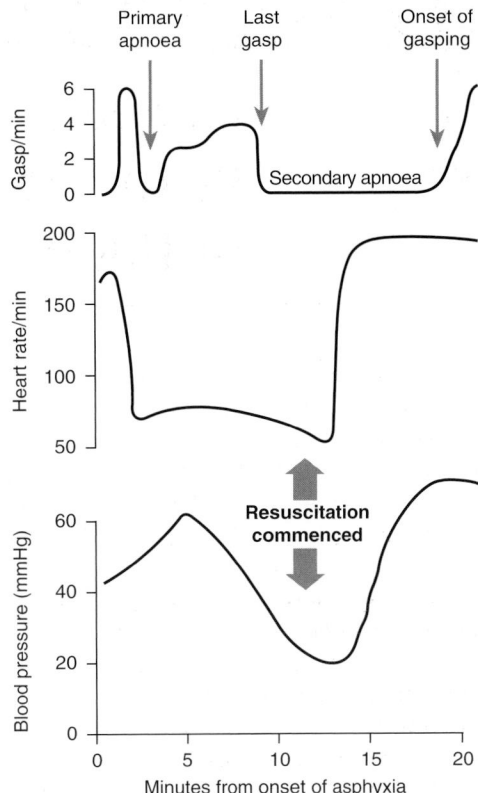

Figure 3.1 The physiological effect of acute asphyxia and the response to resuscitation. (Redrawn from Dawes 1968, with permission.)

Assessment of the infant at birth

Traditionally Apgar scores (Table 3.2) have been used to assess a baby's condition at birth, at 1 min and at 5 min. Unfortunately the Apgar score has limited prognostic significance (see p. 21): many infants can be resuscitated despite an Apgar score of 0 at birth, and may sustain no long-term neurological damage.

In view of the subjective nature of the Apgar score and poor reproducibility it is considered more appropriate to describe the infant's condition in terms of

1 Heart rate (>100, <100 but slow, very slow or absent).
2 Breathing effort (present, absent or ineffective).
3 Central colour (pink, blue or white).
4 Muscle tone (good, decreased or very floppy).

Table 3.2 The Apgar score

Sign	0	1	2
Heart rate	Absent	< 100/min	> 100/min
Respiratory effort	Absent	Weak cry	Strong cry
Muscle tone	Limp	Some flexion	Good flexion
Reflex irritability (suctioning pharynx)	No response	Some motion	Cry
Colour	Pale. Overall cyanosis	Centrally pink, periphery blue	Pink

Generally babies in secondary apnoea will have a heart rate (HR) <100, show absence of breathing, and appear blue or even white and very floppy (and will therefore have Apgar scores of 0–3. Persisting poor condition, especially by 10 min despite good resuscitation, is a poor prognostic sign.

What is asphyxia?

Virginia Apgar introduced the scoring system that now bears her name in an attempt to describe the condition of the infant shortly after birth. Although she did not intend it to refer to asphyxia, it has nevertheless become widely used for that purpose, and in many centres asphyxia is defined (incorrectly) on the basis of a low Apgar score alone. Using this criterion (an Apgar score of 3 or less at 5 min), the incidence of asphyxia is 3–9/1000 full-term infants (Nelson & Ellenberg 1981; Ergander *et al.* 1983). If asphyxia is defined as the requirement for intermittent positive-pressure ventilation for more than 1 min, then 5/1000 full-term infants had this condition (MacDonald *et al.* 1980).

The terms 'birth asphyxia' and 'perinatal asphyxia' were previously loosely used to describe depression at birth, but because of the potential medicolegal implications stringent criteria must now be satisfied for their use.

The essential characteristics of the newborn's response to asphyxia of a potentially harmful degree are:
1 apgar score 0–3 at >5 min;
2 neonatal neurological sequelae (early onset encephalopathy characterized by hypotonia, seizures, coma);

3 evidence of multiorgan system dysfunction in the immediate neonatal period (additional evidence of hypoxic-ischaemic injury to other organs such as the kidneys, heart and liver);
4 umbilical cord arterial pH <7.0; and
5 umbilical cord arterial base deficit ≥16 mmol/L.

To state objectively that there was a likelihood of a prolonged acute hypoxic-ischaemic event in labour causing permanent brain injury to a previously healthy fetus in labour, one also needs:
1 Evidence of a major 'sentinel' hypoxic event, e.g. a ruptured uterus, antepartum haemorrhage, cord prolapse or amniotic fluid embolism; i.e. something that significantly changes normal fetal oxygenation in labour.
2 Evidence of possible fetal compromise ('distress') from the time of the sentinel event, e.g. major changes in the fetal heart rate and/or fetal acidosis on fetal blood sampling.
3 Evidence that encephalopathy is not due to other causes, such as infection, metabolic diseases and intracranial problems (e.g. intracerebral haemorrhage or congenital brain malformation).

Assuming that there was evidence of intrapartum asphyxia (causation), to prove that acute asphyxial brain damage was preventable (liability) one needs to show that
1 it could reasonably be detected;
2 an unnecessary delay then occurred; and
3 there was another mechanism of delivery that could reasonably have been achieved in a very much shorter time without major risk to the mother.

Communication between clinicians caring for the woman and those caring for the neonate is best served by replacing the term 'fetal distress' with 'non-reassuring fetal status', followed by a further description of findings, for example, repetitive variable decelerations, fetal bradycardia or biophysical profile score of >2.

Fetal responses to hypoxia

Most perinatal hypoxic-ischaemic cerebral injury (90% of cases) originates antepartum, with only a small but highly controversial component being solely attributed to intrapartum events. The fetus has highly efficient protective reflexes to combat hypoxia and hypoperfusion, which are active antepartum but particularly so during labour.

Perinatal asphyxia

Causes of perinatal asphyxia

The most common clinical settings associated with hypoxic-ischaemic injury are listed in Table 3.3.

Prevention of perinatal asphyxia

The prevention of perinatal asphyxia involves the following:

1 recognition of high-risk pregnancies;
2 accurate assessment of gestation;
3 assessment of fetoplacental function, e.g. Doppler ultrasound, fetal movements;
4 assessment of pulmonary maturity (see p. 95) and the use of antenatal steroids;
5 intrapartum fetal heart rate monitoring;
6 treatment of fetal distress *in utero*;
7 ensuring that a trained person is available to resuscitate the infant if necessary. This should be done before the infant is born to give the trained person time to read the notes, check the equipment and, if possible, introduce him- or herself to the parents.

Communication with the paediatrician during labour or prior to delivery by caesarean section is the key to a successful resuscitation.

A person experienced in neonatal resuscitation should be present at the following types of delivery:

- *High-risk pregnancy* – rhesus isoimmunization, moderate to severe pre-eclampsia, growth-restricted fetus, insulin-dependent diabetic, antepartum haemorrhage, prolonged rupture of the membranes.
- *Abnormal labour* – fetal distress, deep transverse arrest, cephalopelvic disproportion.
- *Abnormal delivery* – emergency caesarean section, moderate or heavy meconium staining of liquor, prolapsed cord, vacuum, mid- or high forceps, rotation forceps.

Table 3.3 Major causes of neonatal depression in delivery room

Cause	Major effect	Examples
Drugs	Respiratory depression	Anaesthetics, narcotics, $MgSO_4$, tranquilizers
Uteroplacental failure	Hypoxia, acidosis	PET, IUGR, placenta praevia, tetanic contractions
Haemorrhage	Hypovolaemia/shock	Abruptio placentae, fetomaternal transfusion
Developmental anomalies	Cardiac, pulmonary insufficiency	Congenital heart disease, diaphragmatic hernia
Oligohydramnios	Pulmonary insufficiency	Potter's syndrome, PROM
Physical/mechanical	Interruption of blood supply	Prolapsed cord, breech with head entrapment
Severe immaturity	Pulmonary insufficiency	RDS, inadequate respiratory effort
Post-maturity	Meconium passage, placental deterioration	Meconium aspiration syndrome, persistent pulmonary hypertension of newborn
Environmental	Hypothermia	Unplanned home birth
Iatrogenic	Hypoxia, vagal stimulation, excessive ventilation	Pulmonary air leak, intubation of oesophagus/bronchus, apnoea/bradycardia
Extrinsic pulmonary compression	Pulmonary insufficiency	Pleural effusion, pulmonary hypoplasia
Precipitate delivery, abnormal presentation	Birth trauma	Intracranial haemorrhage
Premature, prolonged rupture of membranes	Perinatal infection, chorioamnionitis, pneumonia	

PET, Pre-eclamptic toxaemia; UUGR, Intrauterine growth retardation; PROM, Prolonged rupture of membrane.

- *Abnormal presentation* – breech, face, brow, compound, shoulder.
- *Abnormal gestation* – preterm delivery.
- *Abnormal fetus* – hydramnios, known abnormality, past history of serious abnormality, multiple births.

Preparation of equipment is of the utmost importance prior to a successful resuscitation. The nursery personnel should be notified and the necessary equipment prepared. If the mother has had a significant antepartum haemorrhage, or if a severely rhesus-immunized infant is expected, fresh O-negative blood should be easily obtainable. The history of analgesics and sedatives administered to the mother should be obtained. When preparing for an asphyxiated infant, it is appropriate always to expect the worst possible situation so that all equipment will be ready.

Resuscitation equipment should include: oxygen supply and pressure-limited T-piece/mask circuit or bag-valve mask ventilation, oropharyngeal (Guedel) airways, laryngoscope, suction apparatus for pharynx, stomach and endotracheal tube, meconium aspirator, overhead radiant warmer, sterile warm towels, endotracheal tubes of the appropriate size, a stopwatch and drugs (sodium bicarbonate, 1/10 000 adrenaline, 10% glucose).

Routine resuscitation of a non-asphyxiated infant should consist of:
1 Dry and wrap the baby and give to mother.
2 Assess condition clinically at 1 and 5 min and intervene if (rarely) necessary.
Figure 3.2. summarizes neonatal resuscitation.

Suctioning of the airway

The commonest reason for a floppy baby to fail to establish regular breathing is airway blockage due to the tongue dropping back and the posterior pharyngeal wall flopping forwards (best treated by jaw thrust or two-person airway control, or use of an oropharyngeal airway). Sometimes, however, failure to establish adequate breathing movement in the newborn is due to obstruction of the airway with mucus, blood, meconium or amniotic fluid. The baby should then receive pharyngeal suction under direct vision with a large-bore suction catheter (size 12 or larger) or a paediatric Yankauer sucker.

If there has been moderate or heavy meconium staining of the liquor and the baby is floppy, the pharynx should be suctioned under laryngoscopic vision

Resuscitation of the infant with moderate depression (see Fig. 3.2 for a summary algorithm)

If a baby does not breathe at birth, the airway should be opened by putting the head in a neutral position and the baby should be given five 2–3-s inflation breaths at a pressure of 30 cmH$_2$O. The heart rate should increase (or chest movement should be seen by the fourth or fifth breath). If neither happens assume that the airway is not open (reposition and consider use of jaw thrust or oropharyngeal airway). After reassessment if the baby is responding, ventilation at lower pressure may be necessary for a while until the baby is breathing spontaneously (reassessing every 30 s).

Ventilation

All medical, midwifery and nursing staff who work in a delivery suite should be proficient in providing assisted ventilation with either a pressure-regulated T-piece/mask circuit or bag-valve-mask. A soft, well-fitting face mask (Bennett or Laerdal type) should be selected, of the appropriate size for the baby's face. This should fit snugly around the bridge of the nose and chin, and not obstruct the nares or protrude over the orbits or the lower jaw. The jaw should be held forward as the operator ventilates at a rate of about 30 breaths/min. The chest should be watched for adequate inflation. Heart rate and colour should be continuously reassessed. The T-piece circuits have a set blow-off pressure whereas the bags use a spring relief valve. Transiently the latter can reach fairly high pressures if the bag is squeezed very quickly. If air entry is unsatisfactory, a two-handed jaw thrust may be needed or a pharyngeal airway may need to be inserted. It should be possible to ventilate all infants adequately until more experienced help arrives (see Chapter 30 for a more detailed description).

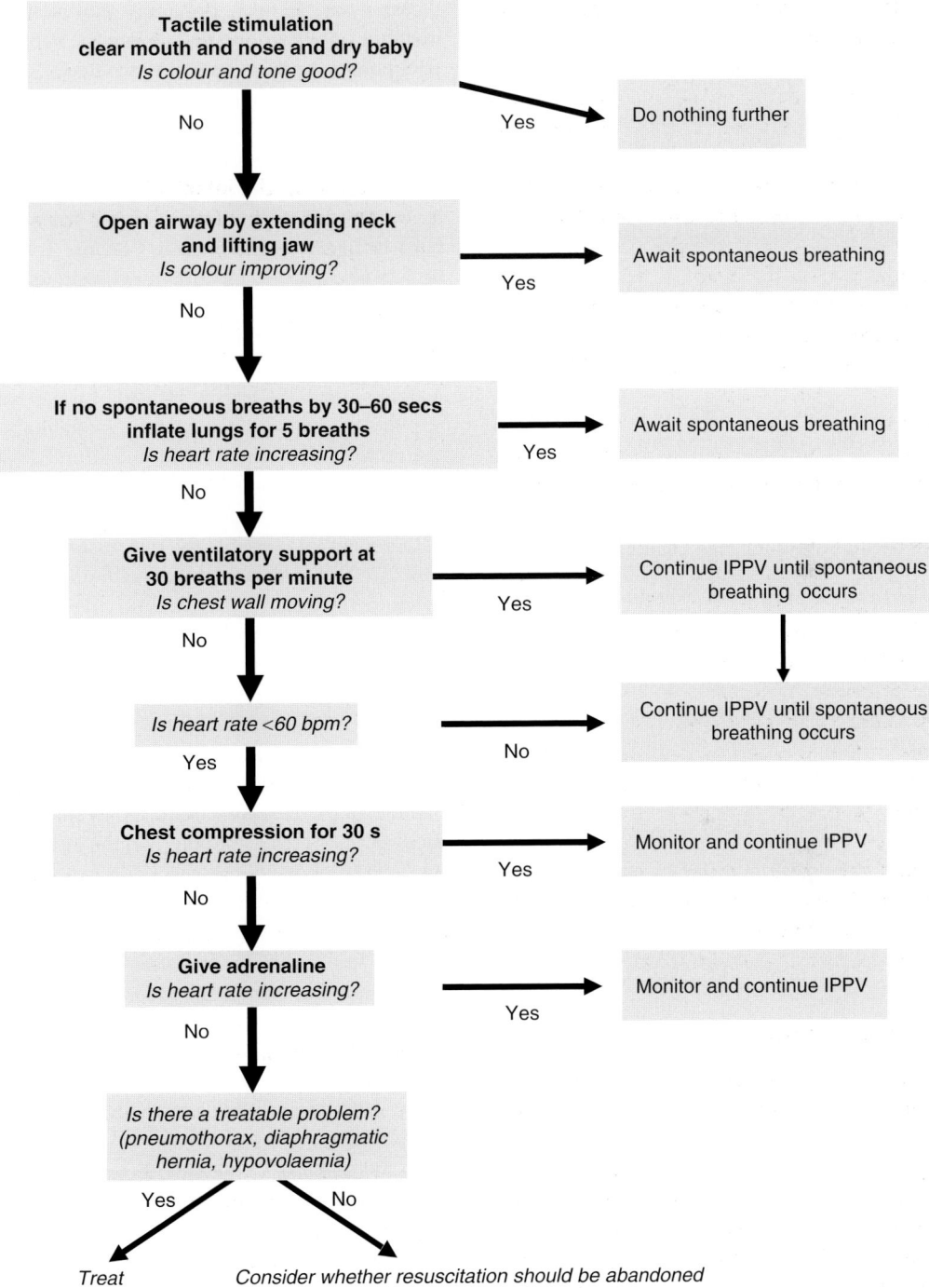

Figure 3.2 A flow chart for resuscitation (IPPV, Intermittent positive pressure ventilation).

Intubation and positive-pressure ventilation (see Chapter 30)

Intubation and positive-pressure ventilation will be infrequently required if good basic airway skills are employed. It may be done electively for conditions such as prematurity (often to deliver surfactant) or diaphragmatic hernia, or during the course of a prolonged resuscitation to stabilize the airway. If there is any doubt about the tube being in the trachea this can be quickly confirmed by using a colour-change capnograph in the circuit. Intubation should be orotracheal with a suitable tube (usually 3.5 mm for a term baby). A suitable infant laryngoscope is necessary, with as wide a blade as possible to improve the view of the larynx (such as an Oxford rather than a Wisconsin blade).

External cardiac massage (see Chapter 30)

If the baby has a heart rate less than 60/min in spite of adequate ventilation, the baby requires external cardiac massage. Both hands are placed around the infant's chest with the fingertips on the back and the thumbs touching over the sternum (one finger breadth below the internipple line), and the thumbs are pressed down at a rate of 80–100/min. The heart massage should be interspersed with ventilation so that there are three compressions for each breath.

In summary, the priorities in neonatal resuscitation are described in the order 'ABC':

A *Airway* – first establish an adequate airway
B *Breathing* – then institute appropriate ventilation
C *Circulation* – then ensure adequate circulation.

Drugs required in resuscitation

Drugs are rarely used but include the following:
1 Sodium bicarbonate (8.4%) is given as a slow dilute intravenous infusion in a dose of 1–2 mmol/kg for severe metabolic acidosis when the baby has not responded to oxygenation and ventilation (see also Chapter 11). This is best given via an umbilical venous catheter (1 mL is equivalent to 1 mmol of 8.4% sodium bicarbonate).

Bicarbonate should only be administered for metabolic acidosis and only when the baby is being adequately ventilated and oxygenated.
2 Adrenaline (epinephrine; 1 in 10 000) in a dose of 0.1 mL/kg into the umbilical vein. It may also be effective if given via an endotracheal tube (0.3 ml/kg) but there is no trial evidence of this.
3. As a result of the physiological stresses on the baby he or she may be hypoglycaemic. If blood can be obtained from an umbilical venous catheter (UVC) direct near bedside testing is available. Otherwise 10% dextrose may be given at a dose of 2.5–5 mL/kg (0.25–0.5 g/kg).
4. Naloxone. This is only indicated when the baby appears to have respiratory depression as a result of maternal opiate administration within 3 h prior to delivery. Small doses of naloxone (40-μg ampoule of 'Neonatal' naloxone) provides only transient antagonism of respiratory depression and a full dose (200 μg) intramuscularly should be given if naloxone is indicated. Intramuscular use is preferred to intravenous use except if the baby is shocked with poor tissue perfusion. Never use naloxone without suspicion of neonatal opiate depression. Do not give naloxone to the baby of an opiate-dependent mother as this may cause acute and severe withdrawal symptoms in the baby.

If drugs are genuinely required despite good cardiorespiratory resuscitation then the outlook is very likely to be poor.

Sequelae of birth asphyxia

The sequelae of birth asphyxia may be divided into early and late.

Early sequelae
Early sequelae may involve any organ system:
1 *Metabolic:*
 (a) metabolic acidosis (infants respond with tachypnoea, which may mimic respiratory distress syndrome (RDS));
 (b) inappropriate antidiuretic hormone secretion (see p. 236).
2 *Respiratory:*
 (a) RDS – acidosis/hypoxia in the perinatal period increases the severity of RDS, or if surfactant

production was already only marginal it may even cause RDS;

(b) transient tachypnoea of the newborn – retained fetal lung fluid worsened by birth asphyxia;

(c) aspiration of meconium antenatally may lead to meconium aspiration syndrome (p. 102).

3 *Cardiac:*

(a) myocardial ischaemia, often with tricuspid insufficiency and congestive heart failure due to a severe hypoxic-ischaemic insult to the myocardium. Characteristically changes may be seen on the electrocardiogram (ECG), which include flat or inverted T waves, ST segment depression, abnormal Q waves, and sometimes complete bundle branch block. Real-time echocardiography may show a poorly contracting myocardium. Cardiac enzymes (especially troponin T) are raised;

(b) persistent pulmonary hypertension (persistence of fetal circulation);

(c) patency of ductus arteriosus.

4 *Central nervous system:* hypoxic–ischaemic encephalopathy (see below).

5 *Renal impairment* (see p. 240): the kidney is very vulnerable to hypoxic-ischaemic insults, and either glomerular or tubular function (or both) may be affected. In its most extreme form acute anuria occurs, but more commonly the baby is oliguric (passes <1 mL of urine/kg/h). Up to 20% of asphyxiated full-term infants develop significant renal compromise and almost all will demonstrate oliguria, proteinuria, haematuria and elevated creatinine levels.

6 *Haematological:* disseminated intravascular coagulation (see p. 204) or other problems with prolonged bleeding may occur.

7 *Gastrointestinal:* necrotizing enterocolitis (p. 254) may occur in these babies.

Late sequelae

The long-term outlook depends on the severity of the asphyxia. There have been few good studies giving clear indications for prognosis. The clinical severity of hypoxic-ischaemic encephalopathy is a better predictor of long-term outcome than Apgar scores or cord blood arterial pH.

Hypoxic-ischaemic encephalopathy

Clinical features

Asphyxia is the simultaneous combination of hypoxia and ischaemia, and the clinical neurological syndrome associated with this is referred to as hypoxic-ischaemic encephalopathy (HIE).

After the initial resuscitation, the infant may be flaccid, hypotonic and unresponsive. The clinical signs characteristically progress over the first 12–24 h, and then gradually improve in all but the most severe cases.

The severity of the HIE syndrome is ascribed retrospectively to one of three grades: mild, moderate or severe (Table 3.4).

Grade I includes increasing irritability with some degree of hypotonia, together with poor sucking, which recovers completely by 3 days of age. These infants often appear to be 'hyperalert', a state in which they seem hungry but feed poorly and respond vigorously to minimal stimuli. Other causes of irritability, such as hypoglycaemia and infection, must be excluded.

Grade II includes more marked abnormalities of tone, with marked lethargy and usually a lack of interest in feeding. Seizures often develop between 12 and 24 h but are not severe. These infants classically show a differential increase in tone, in the neck extensors more than in the neck flexors, and leg tone is greater than that in the arms. Improvement in these symptoms over the first week of life is essential before allocation to this group.

Grade III describes the most severely affected infants. They may initially breathe normally but rapidly

Table 3.4 A scheme for the clinical severity of hypoxic–ischaemic encephalopathy (Levene *et al.* 1985)

Grade I (mild)	Grade II (moderate)	Grade III (severe)
Irritability	Lethargy	Coma
Hyperalert	Seizures	Prolonged seizures
Mild hypotonia	Marked abnormalities of tone	Severe hypotonia
Poor sucking	Requirement for tube feeding	Failure to maintain spontaneous respiration

become comatose, requiring ventilatory support. At this time they are profoundly hypotonic and often have multiple seizures, which are frequent and difficult to control. They are often areflexic. Fatalities occur predominantly in this group, and there may be no improvement prior to death.

Management of encephalopathy

Treatment is largely directed towards complications. General measures include
1 adequate tissue oxygenation;
2 maintenance of environmental temperature (avoiding hyperthermia);
3 treatment of possible infection;
4 correction of coagulation disturbances;
5 correction of electrolyte imbalance; and
6 avoidance of hypoglycaemia.
   Specific complications include:
1 intracranial haemorrhage;
2 hypotension;
3 seizures;
4 cerebral oedema.

Intracranial haemorrhage is uncommon in full-term asphyxiated babies, and subdural collection is the most (common) important finding as observed on scran. This may be suspected on ultrasound examination if there is midline shift, but computed tomography (CT) and magnetic resonance imaging (MRI) are the most sensitive investigations for this.

Hypotension may lead to further cerebral hypoperfusion, and low systemic blood pressure must be rapidly recognized and effectively treated with volume and/or inotropic support. The latter may be guided by echocardiographic assessment. Continuous intravascular blood pressure monitoring is the most reliable measurement method.

Seizures are common and may be subtle, at least in their early stages. Their recognition and treatment are fully discussed in Chapter 19.

Treatment aimed at minimizing cerebral oedema, including fluid restriction (less than usual requirement) is traditional in birth asphyxia, but there is very little data to prove its beneficial effects. There are no valid reasons for recommending dexamethasone treatment, which in fact has been shown to be associated with poor neurodevelopmental outcome in such cases. Mannitol 20% 1 g/kg has been shown

to be effective in lowering intracranial pressure (ICP) in infants known to have intracranial hypertension (Levene & Evans 1985); it can be used if there is clinical evidence of raised ICP (bulging fontanelle or acute deterioration in neurological condition), but its effects are short lived.

Cerebral neuroprotection

It is now recognized that the immature brain is remarkably resistant to the effects of acute brain injury such as hypoxic-ischaemic insult (asphyxia). The acute asphyxial insult may cause some initial neuronal injury, but sets in train a process of abnormal biochemical events that leads to delayed neuronal death, which may occur over days rather than hours. There is no one single route to neuronal death, but rather a whole series of pathways, which may be interconnected. These involve damage to the cerebral vasculature (in part mediated by macrophages), free radical generation, excessive calcium entry due to glutamate neurotransmitter overstimulation, and apoptosis. Apoptosis is 'programmed cell death', a normal function of any cell that does not receive survival signs from adjacent cells. This process is energy requiring and is different from neuronal necrosis. Apoptosis is a normal process in the developing brain, but insults such as asphyxia may exacerbate the process, leading to delayed neuronal loss. Table 3.5 summarizes mechanisms of neural loss to assist the reader in understanding the background to the potential therapies.

Hypothermia is the most promising technique to protect the mature brain following severe perinatal asphyxia. To date two randomized control trials have shown benefit from cooling the baby's brain within 6 h of delivery to 33.5°C for a total of 72 h compared with a group nursed normothermically. Hypothermia also appears to be a relatively safe technique and is beginning to be used outside controlled trials. Because of ongoing uncertainty about its efficacy and safety it is recommended that: (i) hypothermia is used only in experienced centres, after ascertaining by means of a 20-min cerebral function monitoring (CFM) trace that the brain is significantly compromised; and (ii) that all babies are logged into a national or international database for follow-up purposes.

Prognosis

The severity of HIE is the best clinical guide to prognosis (Levene *et al.* 1986). Babies with mild encephalopathy have an excellent prognosis; those with moderate encephalopathy have a 25% risk of serious sequelae, including cerebral palsy and mental retardation. Severe encephalopathy has a poor prognosis, with 80% of infants dying or surviving to be severely handicapped, but about 20% of such infants may survive without significant disability.

As well as cerebral palsy, mental retardation, epilepsy, deafness, blindness, microcephaly or hydrocephaly may all occur as sequelae to perinatal asphyxia. Minor handicaps such as specific learning difficulties, behavioural problems and clumsiness may not manifest until many years after birth.

The best predictive indicators of outcome following perinatal asphyxia are:

1 Electroencephalography (EEG) or CFM. Very abnormal EEG/CFM traces 6 h after birth indicate a 70% risk of adverse outcome (death or severe disability). The most abnormal traces in mature babies include an isoelectric or very low voltage signal and burst suppression (Fig. 3.3).

2 Doppler assessment of cerebral haemodynamics. Doppler assessment of the anterior or middle cerebral arteries has also been found to be a good predictor of a bad outcome, but is only reliable at 24 h after birth. A Pourcelot Resistance Index (PRI) of <0.5 on Doppler assessment accurately predicts adverse outcome (Gray *et al.* 1993).

3 MRI. The change that best predicts a bad outcome is abnormality in signal intensity in the posterior limb of the internal capsule (PLIC) and basal ganglia (Fig 3.4) with sensitivity 90%, specificity 100% and positive predictive value of 100% (Aida *et al.* 1998).

Table 3.5 Mechanism of neural loss

	Primary intracellular insult	Reactive reperfusion	Secondary delayed response
Na/H$_2$O flux/ neural instability	+++	−	−
Calcium influx	+++	+	+
Glutamate receptor	+++	−	+
Free radical	++	−	++
Macrophage	++	++	+
Apoptosis	−	−	+++

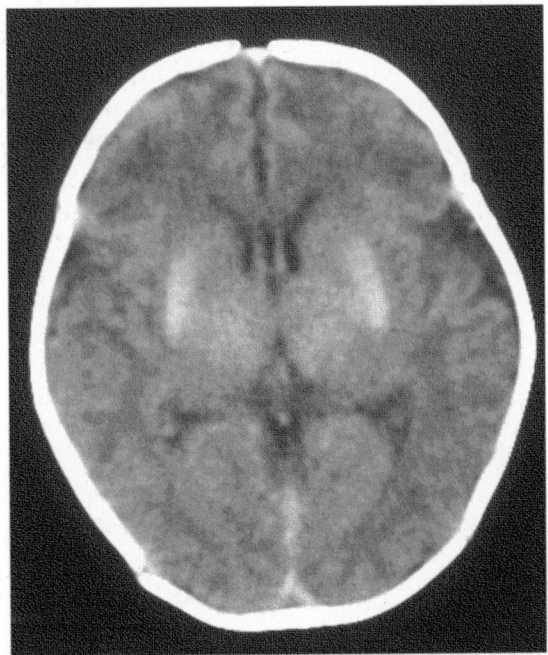

Figure 3.4 Abnormality in the thalamic nuclei in a term baby indicating a poor prognosis following intrapartum asphyxia.

Figure 3.3 Abnormal CFM trace in a severely asphyxiated baby showing low voltage activity and seizure activity (arrows).

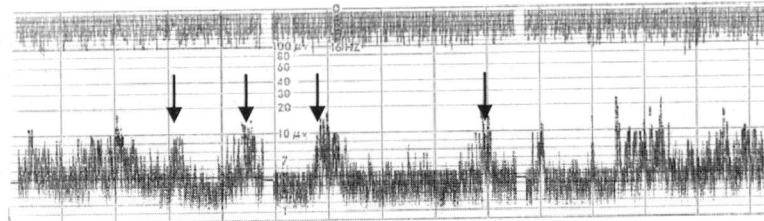

When to stop resuscitation

As mentioned above, babies born apparently dead can be resuscitated and survive without significant neurodevelopmental sequelae. Vigorous resuscitation should be attempted on all infants who were believed to be alive immediately prior to delivery. Yeo and Tudehope (1994) reported that all infants who have Apgar scores of 0 at 1 and 5 min, who survive with the aid of vigorous resuscitation, either subsequently die (80%) or are moderately to severely disabled.

Most recent published data (Haddad *et al.* 2000; Patel & Beeby 2004) suggest that if there is no cardiac output after 10 min, resuscitation should be abandoned.

Ergander *et al.* (1983) have shown that, in surviving infants who did not breathe for more than 20 min, about two-thirds were without major handicap. There are other possible reasons apart from asphyxia for a delay in establishing spontaneous respiration; we advise that if there is doubt as to whether to continue resuscitation, and if a senior experienced doctor is not available, the baby should be taken to the neonatal unit for further care until more detailed assessment by a consultant can be undertaken.

'Brain death' cannot be diagnosed in the neonatal period. A condition referred to as 'irreversible brain injury' is a better concept because in many cases those babies with massive brain insult likely to cause permanent and major brain damage can be detected within the first 24 h of life. In practice a severely abnormal EEG/CFM at 6 h, together with a repeat EEG/CFM and abnormal Doppler at 24 h, will predict an adverse outcome, which can be described to parents as representing 'irreversible brain damage'.

References

Aida N, Nishimura G, Hachiya Y. MR imaging of perinatal brain damage: comparison of clinical outcome with initial and follow-up MR findings. *Am J Neuroradiol* 1998;**19**:1909–1921.

Apgar V. A proposal for a new method of evaluation of the newborn infant. *Curr Res Anesthesia Analgesia* 1953;**32**:253–267.

Dawes G. *Fetal and Neonatal Physiology*. Chicago: Year Book Publishers, 1968.

Ergander U, Eriksson M, Zetterstrom R. Severe neonatal asphyxia. Incidence and prediction of outcome in the Stockholm area. *Acta Paediatr Scand* 1983;**72**:321–325.

Gray PH, Tudehope DI, Masel JP *et al.* Perinatal hypoxic-ischaemic brain injury. Prediction of outcome. *Dev Med Child Neurol* 1993;**35**:965–973.

Haddad B, Mercer BM, Livingston JC *et al.* Outcome after successful resuscitation of babies born with Apgar scores of 0 at both 1 and 5 minutes. *Am J Obstet Gynecol* 2000;**182**:1210–1214.

Levene MI, Evans DH. Medical management of raised intracranial pressure after severe birth asphyxia. *Arch Dis Childhood*, 1985;**60**:12–16.

Levene MI, Kornberg J, Williams T. The incidence and severity of post-asphyxial encephalopathy in full-term infants. *Early Hum Dev* 1985;**11**:21–26.

Levene MI, Bennett MJ, Punt J (eds). *Fetal and Neonatal Neurology and Neurosurgery*. Edinburgh: Churchill Livingstone, 1986.

MacDonald HM, Mulligan JC, Allen AC, Taylor PM. Neonatal asphyxia. I. Relationship of obstetric and neonatal complications to neonatal mortality in 38,405 consecutive deliveries. *J Pediatr* 1980;**96**:898–902.

Nelson KB, Ellenberg JK. Apgar scores as predictors of chronic neurological disability. *Pediatrics* 1981;**68**:35–44.

Patel H, Beeby PJ. Resuscitation beyond 10 minutes of term babies born without signs of life. *J Pediatr Child Health* 2004;**40**:136–138.

Yeo CL, Tudehope DI. Outcome of resuscitated apparently stillborn infants: a ten year review. *J Paediatr Child Health* 1994;**30**:129–133.

Further reading

Levene MI, Chervenak FC (eds). *Fetal and Neonatal Neurology and Neurosurgery*, 3rd edn. Edinburgh: Churchill Livingstone, 2001.

Volpe JJ. *Neurology of the Newborn*, 4th edn. Philadelphia: WB Saunders, 2001.

4 Examination of the newborn

Clinical examination

The newborn infant is examined by a variety of people. The birth attendant will notice major congenital abnormalities, and the mother will closely scrutinize the baby for congenital defects, birthmarks, etc. Consequently, most obvious defects will be detected shortly after birth. It has been said that the newborn physical examination is the most valuable screening test performed at any time during life, because the early detection of various occult abnormalities (congenital heart disease, hip dislocation, cataracts, etc.) may allow early and effective treatment before morbidity occurs.

Measurement

It is important to ensure that the infant is kept warm during the examination and that appropriate hand-washing is done to avoid cross-infection.

The baby should be measured and the results recorded.

1 Birthweight (naked) is measured to the nearest 10 g.

2 Head circumference is recorded as the maximum occipitofrontal circumference. A number of measurements should be made and only the maximum or mean of the largest two measurements is recorded. A non-stretchable tape measure should be used for this purpose, and the measurement recorded to the nearest millimetre.

3 *Length.* The crown–heel measurement is recorded; this is reliable only if performed on a neonatal measuring board (e.g. Harpenden neonatometer). This requires two people: one to secure the infant's head at the top of the board and a second to extend the legs so that the foot board firmly touches the infant's soles. An average of three measurements should be made and the value recorded to the nearest millimetre.

All these measurements should be plotted on standard charts appropriate to the infant's gestational age and sex.

Physical examination

Clinical examination of the newborn must be carried out in a regular sequence so that items are not forgotten. A useful approach is the 'head to toe' technique. Whenever possible the infant should be examined in the presence of at least one parent. For a meaningful examination to be made it is essential to review the maternal history, method of delivery and difficulties at birth.

The physical examination can be considered under the headings below, and normal variations are discussed in the appropriate sections. The following descriptions include various common congenital abnormalities.

General appearance
Facies

There is a wide range of recognizable patterns of abnormalities based on facial features. These are well described by Jones (2005). Many are rare, but chromosomal disorders such as trisomies 21, 18 and 13 should be recognized (see p. 151). In addition, the following are often obvious: fetal alcohol syndrome (see Fig. 14.2, p. 145), Crouzon syndrome (Fig. 4.1), Treacher–Collins syndrome (Fig. 4.2) and Potter's syndrome (see Fig. 22.2, p. 238).

Colour

The infant should be uniformly pink, but acrocyanosis (blueness of the hands and feet) is not abnormal. Generalized cyanosis, pallor, jaundice, plethora,

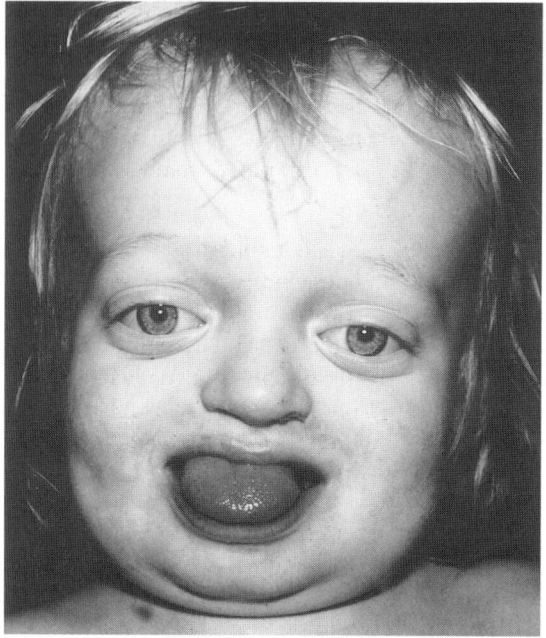

Figure 4.1 Crouzon syndrome.

bruises and petechial haemorrhages are abnormal and should be recorded and investigated further.

Posture

Note the infant's posture and range of spontaneous movements observed during the examination. In the term infant the normal position is one with the hips abducted and partially flexed, the knees flexed, and the arms adducted and flexed at the elbow. Limited movement, exaggerated or asymmetrical movements, hypotonia or stiffness must be recorded.

Cry

This should be vigorous and sustained after stimulation, but it should be possible to console the infant by cuddling. A cry that is weak, high-pitched or hoarse is abnormal.

Skin appearance

This varies with gestation, and mild peeling in mature babies is not abnormal. Abnormal appearances, pigmentation and naevi are described in Chapter 24. African and Asian babies may show little generalized pigmentation at birth, except for the genitalia.

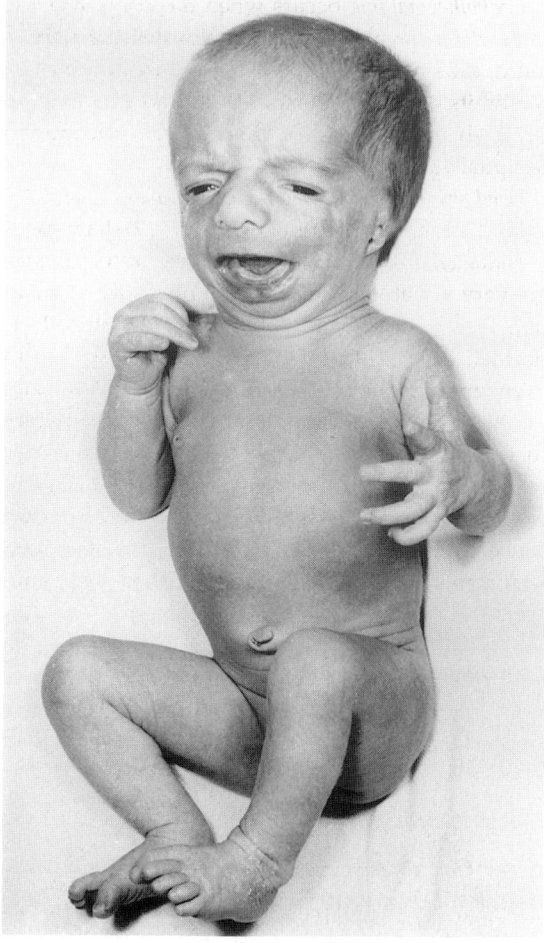

Figure 4.2 Treacher–Collins syndrome.

Shape

Moulding and caput succedaneum (oedematous thickening of the scalp due to passage through the vagina) is normal in newly born infants and disappears within 2–3 days.

Plagiocephaly (parallelogram head) is usually seen as a flattening of the occipital region on one side. It is thought to be due to the position the infant has been lying in *in utero* and has no pathological significance. It usually improves with age. Plagiocephaly seen in older infants suggests limitation of neck rotation on the same side as the occipital flattening.

Scaphocephaly (long head with flattened temporoparietal regions) occurs commonly in premature infants and becomes less obvious with age.

Cephalhaematoma occurs when bleeding over the outer surface of a skull bone elevates the periosteum, causing a soft fluctuant swelling confined to the limits of the bone (Fig. 4.3). It may be bilateral, but only crosses the midline in the uncommon occipital variety.

Head size should be measured, and hydrocephaly (see p. 211) and microcephaly (see p. 212) diagnosed.

Fontanelles. The anterior and posterior fontanelles are very variable in size and are normally soft and flat. Visible pulsation of the anterior fontanelle is normal. Bulging of the fontanelle may be due to raised intracranial pressure and is always abnormal.

Craniosynostosis. This term refers to premature fusion of one or more of the skull bones. Any bones may be affected, but the sagittal suture is most commonly involved. Facial bones may be affected and cause dysmorphism, such as is seen in Crouzon syndrome (Fig. 4.1). On examination of the head, the anterior fontanelle is usually small and the suture is ridged on palpation. Craniosynostosis causes abnormal head growth; if the sagittal suture is involved, the head becomes scaphocephalic. If this condition is suspected, X-ray will often confirm the synostosis, but computed tomography (CT) scanning may be necessary.

Craniotabes (ping-pong ball skull) refers to the softening of the skull bones, and with pressure the skull may be momentarily indented before springing out again. It is more common in preterm infants but also occurs in full-term babies. It usually has no significance, but congenital rickets and, more rarely, osteogenesis imperfecta or congenital hypophosphatasia may cause it.

Eyes (see also Chapter 20)
Site

The position of the eyes in relation to the nasal bridge should be noted. If they are too far apart, this is referred to as hypertelorism; if too close together, hypotelorism. These conditions are usually part of a more generalized syndrome.

Conjunctiva

This is usually clear, but subconjunctival haemorrhages are not uncommon in otherwise normal infants.

Conjunctivitis is a serious symptom and infection (e.g. gonococcus, chlamydia; see p. 70) must be excluded. Excessive lacrimation may be associated with a blocked nasolacrimal duct.

Cornea and iris

The cornea should be clear and a red reflex elicited. The pupils should constrict to light both directly and consensually.

Eyelids

Mild lid oedema may be present following a long labour, particularly in a face or brow presentation.

Ears
Shape

There is a wide familial variation.

Preauricular skin tags or sinuses are common. The tags should not be tied off if large or multiple, and

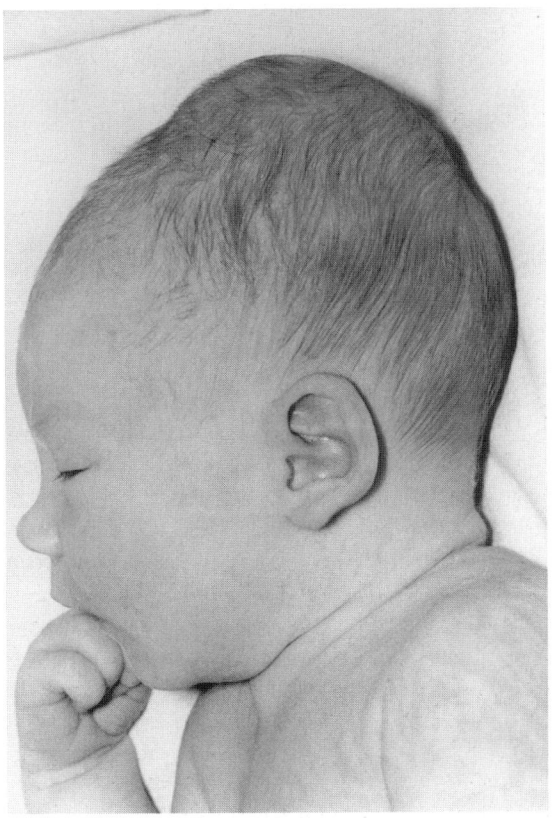

Figure 4.3 Cephalhaematoma of the left parietal bone.

the opinion of a plastic surgeon should be sought. Ear malformation may be part of Treacher–Collins syndrome (Fig. 4.2).

Position
The top of the pinna should be at or above a horizontal line from the inner and outer canthi. Low-set ears are seen in a variety of conditions, including Potter's syndrome (see p. 238).

Nose
Patency
Choanal atresia is excluded by gently passing a feeding catheter through both nostrils. Atresias may be bilateral or, more commonly, unilateral, and may be membranous or bony.

Mouth
Lips
There is wide familial variation. Unilateral or bilateral cleft lip is a common congenital abnormality (1/1000 births). An absent philtrum (groove in the upper lip) and thin vermillion border (red part of the upper lip) are seen in *fetal alcohol syndrome* (see Fig. 14.2, p. 145).

Palate
Epstein's pearls (small inclusion cysts in the midline of the hard palate) are normal and eventually disappear.

Cleft palate. Use a torch to examine the mouth for cleft palate, bifid uvula or high arched palate. A submucous cleft palate can only be diagnosed by inserting the little finger into the mouth to feel for a mucous membrane-covered bony cleft.

Tongue
If the tongue is large and protruding consider hypothyroidism (see p. 168), Down syndrome (usually accompanied by a small mouth; see p. 151) and Beckwith–Wiedemann syndrome (see p. 159). Tongue tie is due to a short frenulum. It should not be cut, and rarely causes speech problems.

Jaw
Micrognathia (small underdeveloped jaw) is seen in Pierre Robin syndrome (see p. 246) and associated with cleft palate and cyanotic spells due to tongue prolapse.

Teeth
Natal teeth, mostly lower incisors, are not uncommon and if loose are best removed to prevent aspiration.

Mucous membranes
White patches suggest candidiasis, which needs to be distinguished from milk curd.

Ranulas are bluish-white mucous gland retention cysts on the floor of the mouth and usually require no treatment.

Saliva
Drooling or excessive saliva suggests an inability to swallow. Oesophageal atresia, or more rarely a neuromuscular disorder, should be excluded.

Neck
Sternomastoid tumour. Check for a full range of neck movements. Limitation of lateral rotation (turning) suggests shortening of the sternomastoid muscle due to haemorrhage. Sternomastoid tumour occurs in the middle third of that muscle and is best treated with physiotherapy.

Turner syndrome (see p. 151) and *Down syndrome* (see p. 151) are associated with redundant skin at the back of the neck. A low hairline is seen in Turner syndrome.

Klippel–Feil syndrome is associated with a short neck with limited movement. It is a rare condition.

Cystic hygroma. Swelling of the side of the neck, which usually transilluminates brilliantly (Fig. 4.4). Branchial clefts may give rise to a branchial cyst, a branchial sinus or branchial fistula.

Goitre may be present at birth and is always in the midline.

Chest
Shape
The chest should be symmetrical in shape and move equally on respiration.

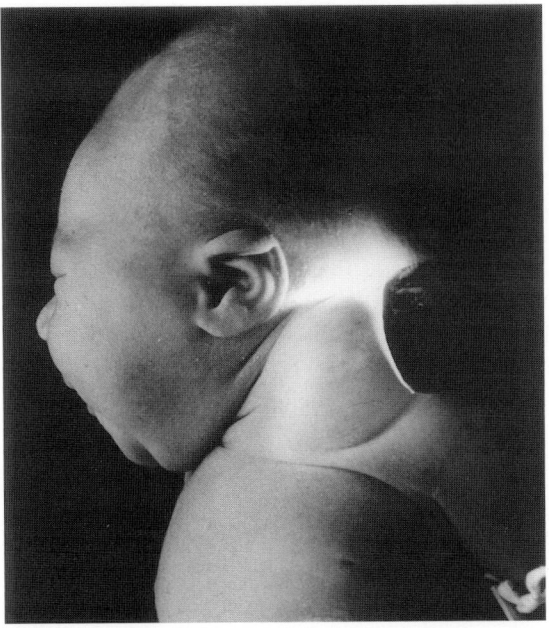

Figure 4.4 Cystic hygroma of the neck (transilluminated).

Respiratory distress of any cause will result in sternal and intercostal recession.

Size
A small chest occurs in infants with hypoplastic lungs and in a variety of rare syndromes.

Breast
Engorgement occurs commonly in both sexes and is due to an oestrogen effect. 'Milk' may be secreted from the nipple and this is not abnormal. Palpation and expression of the engorged breast should be discouraged in order to prevent infection.

Supernumerary nipples are a common finding.

Lungs
Respiratory distress. The features of respiratory distress are tachypnoea (normal respiratory rate in the newborn is 30–60 breaths/min), retraction, cyanosis, grunting and flaring of the alae nasi. Chest retractions (sternal, substernal, intercostal or subcostal) suggest pulmonary disease.

Stridor (see p. 127) indicates upper airway obstruction. An inspiratory stridor implies extrathoracic obstruction, whereas expiratory stridor implies intrathoracic obstruction. Other signs of upper airway obstruction include suprasternal retraction, croupy cough and a hoarse cry.

Breath sounds should be symmetrical (if unilateral, suspect pneumothorax or diaphragmatic hernia). Auscultate with the diaphragm of the stethoscope for symmetry, air entry and adventitial breath sounds. Crepitations may be normal in the first hours of life.

Cardiovascular disease
Pulses
The normal heart rate varies between 90 and 160/min. The cause of tachycardia and bradycardia is discussed in Chapter 12. The radial and femoral pulses should be palpable. Generally reduced peripheral pulses suggest hypoplastic left heart or cardiogenic shock (see p. 186), and absent femorals suggest coarctation of the aorta (see p. 186). Collapsing or bounding pulses are a feature of delayed closure of the ductus arteriosus (see p. 188).

Apex beat
This should be localized to the fourth intercostal space in the midclavicular line. The left ventricular impulse, palpated at the apex, and the right ventricular impulse, palpable at the lower left sternal edge, are recorded as normal or, if increased, as +, ++ or +++.

A right-sided heart suspected on auscultation may be primary or due to left-sided pneumothorax, left diaphragmatic hernia or true dextrocardia.

Auscultation
A triple or gallop rhythm is always abnormal. Systolic murmurs may be normal in the first 24 h of life. Congenital heart disease is discussed in Chapter 17. Auscultation of a heart murmur in systole is ascribed as $\frac{1}{6} \rightarrow \frac{5}{6}$ according to intensity, site of maximal intensity and radiation.

Abdomen
Distension suggests an *intestinal obstruction* or intra-abdominal mass. A scaphoid abdomen suggests diaphragmatic hernia. A lax abdominal wall with much redundant skin is seen in the 'prune-belly' syndrome. *Divarication* of the rectus muscles

may produce a bulge in the abdominal wall between the medial edges of the rectus muscles. No treatment is required and the condition disappears with age.

Liver

This is normally palpable up to 1 cm below the right costal margin. Hepatomegaly may be due to lung hyperinflation, cardiac failure, sepsis, hepatitis, intrauterine infection or haemolysis.

Spleen

The tip can be palpated in about a quarter of normal infants. Splenomegaly suggests infection (prenatal or postnatal) or haemolysis.

Kidney

May be palpable normally, particularly if the baby is relaxed. Moderate kidney enlargement may be due to hydronephrosis, dysplastic or cystic kidneys or rarely a Wilms tumour. An adrenal mass (e.g. haemorrhage or neuroblastoma) may be very difficult clinically to distinguish from a renal mass. Massive kidney enlargement occurs in bladder neck obstruction or cystic disease.

Anus

This should be checked to be patent and normally situated. Imperforate anus is usually associated with a fistula into the vagina or bladder (in males).

Umbilicus

Vessels

Normally two thick-walled arteries and a thin-walled vein are seen. One to two per cent of infants have a single umbilical artery, and other congenital malformations may rarely be present in conjunction with this. If a single umbilical artery is found and the fetus has had a normal prenatal anomaly scan, no further investigations are required. If an anomaly scan has not be done, then a renal ultrasound on the baby should be undertaken to exclude an anomaly.

Colour

The umbilicus is normally translucent because of Wharton's jelly. Green coloration occurs due to meconium staining, or yellow staining due to hyperbilirubinaemia.

Stump

The cord usually separates by 10 days, leaving a yellow or greenish eschar. Reddening of the skin around the umbilicus is abnormal and suggests significant infection. Discharge and cellulitis are also signs of infection. Discharge of urine or meconium from the stump suggests a patent urachus or patent omphalomesenteric duct, respectively. Exomphalos and gastroschisis are discussed in Chapter 23.

Umbilical granulomata are caused by excessive granulation tissue at the umbilical stump. They look like small red swellings resembling a strawberry, and are best treated by the application of a silver nitrate stick on one or two occasions.

Umbilical hernia of the healed umbilicus is particularly common in black babies or those born prematurely, and usually develops in the first month or so of life. A small hernia requires no treatment, and spontaneous regression by 6–18 months is the most usual outcome.

Genitalia

Ambiguous genitalia are discussed in Chapter 16.

Testes

The testes are present in the scrotum in 98% of full-term male infants. Failure to descend by 6 weeks is abnormal.

Ectopic testicles or arrest in the line of normal descent should also be referred for surgical opinion.

Penis and urethra

The foreskin in infants is not retractable and must not be forced. The urethral meatus normally opens at the tip of the glans penis.

Hypospadias occurs if the meatus opens abnormally on the ventral surface of the penis, and is most commonly glandular.

Epispadias occurs when the urethra opens on the dorsal surface of the penis.

Scrotum

A hydrocoele may be present at birth, and transilluminates brilliantly. It may extend upwards along the spermatic cord. Most disappear spontaneously during the first year of life and require no treatment other than reassurance.

Inguinal hernia rarely presents at birth but is common in infants who have been born prematurely due to a patent processus vaginalis. The scrotal swelling can usually be reduced. Surgery is required in all cases to prevent incarceration or strangulation of the hernia.

Testicular torsion. A swollen, tender or red scrotum suggests either strangulated inguinal hernia or testicular torsion. Both require an urgent surgical opinion.

Pink nappies

Occasionally, urates may react with the urine in the newborn period, leaving a pinkish-red stain on the napkin that may be confused with haematuria. The condition is usually self-limiting and only occurs in the first few weeks of life.

Hymen

Hymenal skin tags are common in the newborn female infant and are associated with a protrusion of redundant vaginal mucosa. No specific treatment is required and the condition usually regresses spontaneously in the first few weeks of life.

Hydrometrocolpos describes a bulging imperforate hymen, caused by the accumulation of vaginal secretions.

Vagina and vulva

The size of the labia majora depends on gestational age, but by term they should completely cover the labia minora.

Labial fusion occurs in the adrenogenital syndrome, and labial adhesions are also not uncommonly seen in otherwise normal infants.

Mucoid vaginal discharge occurs in most mature female infants shortly after birth. It is white and thick and may continue for 2–3 weeks.

Vaginal bleeding may occur in normal infants.

Clitoris

This is variable in size. If large, consider adrenogenital syndrome (see p. 169), a maternal progesterone effect or an intersex state (see p. 174).

Extremities

Feet

Mild postural deformities may be present, but if the ankle joint can be passively moved through the entire range of normal movements no treatment is necessary. Abnormalities include talipes equinovarus, talipes calcaneovalgus and metatarsus varus (see Chapter 21).

Hips

The hips should be carefully examined to detect a dislocated or dislocatable hip (see p. 232). This is left to the end of the examination as it usually causes the baby to become upset.

Arms

The range of normal movements should be passively tested. The fingers and palms should be examined for abnormalities. A single palmar crease may be present in Down syndrome.

Clinodactyly is a lateral curvature of the fifth finger and may be part of more generalized abnormalities.

Brachial plexus injury. Spontaneous arm movement should be observed: if abnormal, brachial plexus injury (see p. 37) or bony fractures may be present.

Neurological examination

The neurological evaluation is an essential part of the examination of the newborn, but is often poorly performed and recorded. The *behavioural state* of the infant will severely affect the neurological signs elicited. Ideally, the baby should have been fed 1 h previously; he or she needs to be fully exposed, at least in the initial phase of the examination, and warmed with a radiant heat warmer. The state needs to be recorded using Brazelton's classification (Brazelton 1973).

State I: Quiet sleep.

State II: Active sleep.

State III: Semi-wakefulness.

State IV: Awake, alert and cooperative.

State V: Awake, fussing and uncooperative.

State VI: Crying.

The assessment consists of the observation, examination and recording of the following.

Level of consciousness Assess whether the baby's behavioural state varies through the examination. Does he or she arouse if asleep? Is he or she consoled by cuddling when aroused? Consolability is an important normal feature in mature babies. When alert does the baby fix and follow a bright object with his or her eyes?

Posture The posture of a baby will depend on the gestational age (see 'Assessment of maturity', p. 78). A *hypotonic* baby will tend to be in the 'frog position' with reduced spontaneous movement. A *hypertonic* baby may be in a state of predominant flexion or extension. A baby with cerebral irritation may have extensor posturing with arching of the back, opisthotonus, scissoring of the legs, and thumbs tightly adducted in the cortical position.

Movements The quality and quantity of spontaneous movements are observed and described. Absence or reduction of movements may occur in one limb only, two limbs on the same side of the body, or both legs. The absence of spontaneous movements is often suggestive of a 'sick baby' and very rarely a sign of a paralysed baby. Observe the quality of movements; are they smooth (normal) or jerky? Note any abnormal movements such as tremors, jitteriness or convulsions. Tremulousness or jitteriness must be distinguished from convulsions (see Chapter 20).

Assessment of tone Limb tone is assessed by posture and the amount of resistance to passive movement. In the evaluation of tone a comparison is made between the two sides of the body and between the upper and the lower limbs. The head must be fixed in the midline to prevent eliciting a tonic neck response. *Hip adductor* tone is assessed by the hip adductor angle with the legs passively abducted. *Head or neck tone* is assessed with the arms held in traction and by observing the head control when the baby is held in a sitting position.

Truncal tone is assessed with the baby held in ventral suspension.

Primitive reflexes Primitive reflexes generally first appear at about 32 weeks' gestation but are not well developed until 36 weeks and not readily repeatable until term. In a sick or neurologically depressed term infant the primitive reflexes may be absent. These reflexes usually start to disappear or integrate by 6 weeks and should have disappeared completely by 12 weeks in the term infant. The persistence of primitive reflexes beyond 12 weeks after birth in the term infant, especially when associated with hypertonia, hyperreflexia and sustained ankle clonus, might suggest developing cerebral palsy. These reflexes may reappear in elderly patients who have sustained a cerebral insult. Primitive reflexes may be used to demonstrate:

- asymmetry of function;
- gestational age of baby;
- abnormal neurological function.

Only a few reflexes need to be assessed by the examiner, but they must be used consistently and their interpretation fully understood. The reflexes recommended are:

1 *Moro reflex* – elicited by placing one hand under the infant's shoulders and the other under his head and then suddenly dropping the head by several centimetres. A full response consists of abduction and extension of the arms, followed by adduction and flexion (Fig. 4.5). An asymmetry would suggest a brachial plexus palsy or a bone injury.

2 *Palmar grasp* – elicited by applying pressure to the palm of the hand, resulting in flexion of the fingers and a firm grasp of the object. If traction is then applied the infant should lift his or her head off the bed so that head lag can be assessed.

3 *Tonic neck reflex* – elicited by turning the head to one side and consisting of extensor and increased tone in the arm and leg on that side. The opposite side often shows a flexion response. This is not always demonstrable at birth, but is pathological or obligatory if the infant cannot 'break' the posture after a few seconds.

4 *Stepping reflex* – the infant is held upright and, as his or her weight is applied to the foot in contact with the bed, that leg extends while the other leg flexes;

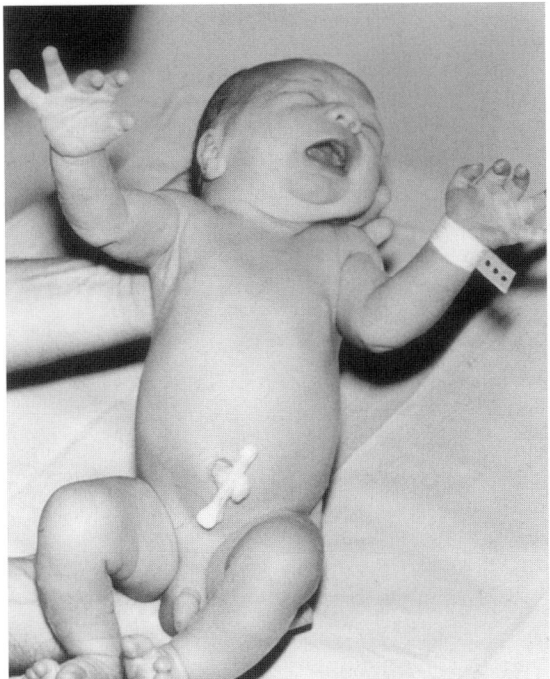

Figure 4.5 Eliciting the Moro reflex.

5 *Suck and gag.* These reflexes should be present in some form from 35 weeks' gestation and fully developed by term. It it is always abnormal when absent after this age.

6 *Check also the rooting reflex* – as the cheek is touched the head turns to the stimulus and mouthing movements commence.

Deep tendon jerks are traditionally noted but are rarely informative. Loss of deep reflexes commonly occurs in neurologically abnormal babies, who will show other signs of abnormality. The knee, biceps, ankle and hip adductor jerks are elicited by tapping the appropriate tendons with the fingers. Asymmetrical responses, or overactive or absent jerks may be significant. Ankle clonus is usually a feature of hyperreflexia and may be demonstrated by pressing the thumbs, with a rapid, abrupt movement, against the distal part of the soles of the feet. Up to six beats of clonus may be normal, but sustained ankle clonus suggests neurological impairment.

Cranial nerves. The examination of the cranial nerves may be difficult in the newborn (Table 4.1).

Table 4.1 Cranial nerves

I Impossible to test

II The term infant, when in the right behavioural state, can fixate and follow through about 60°. No conclusions can be drawn if this is not demonstrable

III, IV and VI A fixed squint may suggest a nerve lesion. Asymmetric or non-reacting pupils are abnormal

V Absent corneal reflex and rooting reflexes are abnormal

VII Facial nerve palsies are common following birth, and facial asymmetry on crying or sucking should be looked for

VII The demonstration of a startle response to a loud noise is a crude test of auditory function. An absent response is not diagnostic of a hearing deficit. Brain stem-evoked responses to auditory stimuli provide a definitive test of auditory function. Conventional audiometric testing can be misleading in the newborn infant

IX, X and XII These are usually examined together. Infants with lesions of these nerves generally exhibit features of gross bulbar palsy with absent gag, suck and swallow reflexes and palatal insufficiency. They cannot swallow their secretions and have obstructive apnoea

XI The sternomastoid muscle is visualized with the head extended and the infant lying in the supine position. The strength of the muscle is determined by the infant's attempts to right the head

Assessment of maturity

An accurate estimate of gestational age is necessary in the management of the ill or premature infant. An obstetric estimate of the duration of pregnancy may be inaccurate for a number of reasons, and assessment of gestational age should be part of the routine examination of any infant in whom this is in doubt. Gestational age is assessed on both physical and neurological criteria. The New Ballard Score (NBS) (Ballard *et al.* 1991) has been shown to be a valid, accurate assessment tool (see Chapter 8).

References

Ballard JL, Khoury JC, Wedig K *et al.* New Ballard Score, expanded to include extremely premature infants. *J Pediatr* 1991;**119**:417–423.

Brazelton TB. *Neonatal Behavioural Assessment Scale.* Clinics in Developmental Medicine, no. 50. London: SIMP, 1973.

Jones KL. (ed.) *Smith's Recognizable Patterns of Human Malformation*, 6th edn. Philadelphia: Elsevier, 2005.

Internet resources

Fuloria M, Kreiter S. The newborn examination: part I. Emergencies and common abnormalities involving the skin, head, neck, chest, and respiratory and cardiovascular systems. *American Family Physician* 2002;**65** (http://www.aafp.org/afp/20020101/61.html).

Auckland District Health Board. Examination of the newborn (http://www.adhb.govt.nz/newborn/Education/Teaching/5thYearsNewbornExam.htm).

5 Birth injury

Injuries may be sustained either during labour or at delivery, and may occur despite skilled obstetric care.

The decreased incidence in birth trauma over recent years has been attributed to changing trends in obstetric management, such as caesarean section instead of difficult vaginal delivery. Despite the falling incidence, birth injury is still a cause for concern to the obstetrician and neonatal paediatrician. Parents sometimes attribute birth injury to obstetric mismanagement, and this may result in litigation. Unfortunately, such events encourage the practice of defensive obstetrics, and a high caesarean section rate may be a consequence of this.

Illingworth (1985) maintained that it may be inappropriate to ascribe a child's so-called 'brain damage' solely to labour or delivery without considering other causative factors. 'Brain damage' can occur without difficult labour or perinatal hypoxia, and despite caesarean section. It is simplistic to relate brain damage to single factors such as breech delivery or hypoxia at birth without considering the many interacting prenatal, perinatal and postnatal factors.

Table 5.1 lists the major causes of birth injury and their incidence.

Risk factors for birth injury

The effect of changing patterns of obstetric practice on birth-associated mechanical injuries is difficult to evaluate. However, a number of risk factors for birth injury have been identified (Tables 5.2 and 5.3). Specific birth injuries are detailed below.

Soft tissue injuries

Erythema, abrasions and lacerations
These are seen following forceps and vacuum delivery, episiotomy, uterine incision at caesarean

Table 5.1 The commoner types of birth injury and their incidence

Cephalhaematoma	1:100
Congenital brachial palsy	1:1000 [0.5–2 per thousand (Volpe 2000)]
Facial nerve palsy	1:500
Bony (non-skull) fracture	1:1000
Skull fractures	Rare
Subaponeurotic haemorrhage	1:1250
Major subdural haemorrhage	1:50 000
Spinal cord injuries	Very rare

section, cephalopelvic disproportion and scalp electrode monitoring (Fig. 5.1).

Traumatic cyanosis (traumatic petechiae)
Traumatic petechiae occur over the head, neck and upper chest following a difficult delivery. They often occur with breech presentation and in infants born with the umbilical cord tightly around the neck. They may be related to a sudden increase in intrathoracic pressure during passage of the chest through the birth canal. These petechiae usually fade within 2–3 days and require no treatment other than parental reassurance. Traumatic petechiae must be clearly distinguished from generalized petechiae associated with coagulation disturbances.

Ecchymoses (bruising)
Bruising may be seen with traumatic deliveries, precipitate labour, preterm infants, poorly controlled deliveries or abnormal presentations (e.g. face, brow, breech).

Subcutaneous fat necrosis
This term is applied to well-demarcated indurated areas in the skin occurring where pressure has been

Table 5.2 Risk factors for birth injury

Fetal condition
Prematurity
Small for gestational age
Multiple pregnancy
Fetal distress
Malpresentation
Breech presentation (see Table 5.3)
Brow, face, compound presentation
Malposition
Occipitoposterior arrest
Deep transverse arrest
Cephalopelvic disproportion
Macrosomia, e.g. infant of diabetic mother, hydrops
    fetalis
Macrocephaly
Contracted pelvis:
    Shoulder dystocia
    Severe moulding
    Unengaged head
Prolonged labour
Delay–cervix fully dilated
Delay–cervix not fully dilated
Precipitate labour
Maternal factors
Nulliparity
Short stature
Obesity
Inexperienced accoucheur

Table 5.3 Injuries more likely to occur in infants delivered by breech

Haemorrhage
Subdural tears due to tentorial rupture (see p. 215)
Rupture of intra-abdominal viscus (usually liver or
    kidney)
Occipital osteodiastasis with cerebellar haemorrhage

Orthopaedic
Dislocation: shoulder, cervical vertebrae, hip, knee
Fracture: clavicle, humerus, femur; damage to sternomastoid muscle

Neurological
Asphyxia secondary to cord prolapse
Cervical plexus injury: Erb's or Klumpke's paralysis
Facial nerve palsy

Soft tissue injury
Extensive bruising, particularly genitals

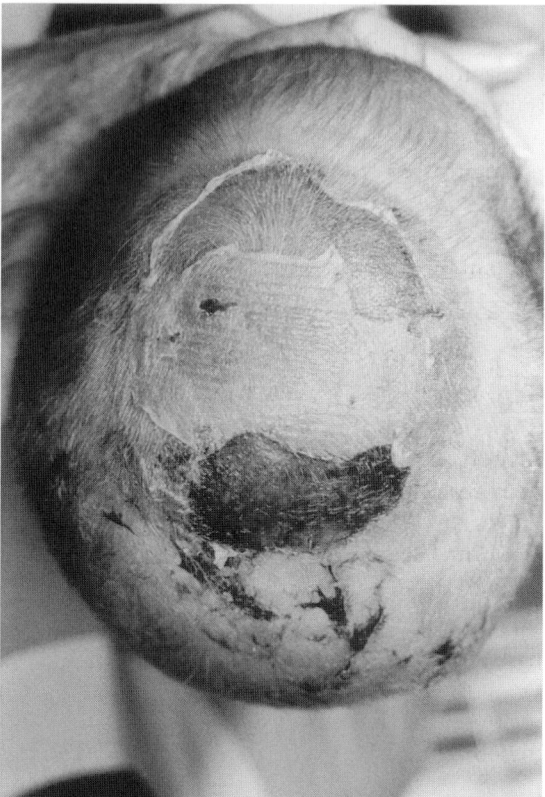

Figure 5.1 Scalp lacerations and bruising following vacuum delivery.

applied (e.g. forceps blades on the face). No treatment is required.

Sternomastoid tumour
See p. 28.

Injuries to the head

Caput succedaneum
See p. 26.

Cephalhaematoma (see Fig. 4.3)
This occurs in about 1% of newborn infants and is due to bleeding between the periosteum and the cranial bones (usually parietal, less commonly occipital) as a result of shearing or tearing of communicating veins during delivery. The extent of the swelling is limited by the underlying skull bone and does not cross suture lines. It is due to buffeting

of the fetal skull against the maternal pelvis, which is seen especially in prolonged labour. It may also occur following a forceps or vacuum delivery. Subperiosteal bleeding is slow and may not appear until the second day of life. Enlargement may occur during the first week and the swelling may persist for several weeks. This edge may be confused with a depressed fracture of the skull.

Complications associated with a cephalhaematoma may include
1 an underlying linear skull fracture;
2 jaundice due to resorption of the blood;
3 calcification at its edge, which may occur some weeks later during the resorption process; this should not be confused with a depressed skull fracture;
4 intracranial haemorrhage may rarely be associated with cephalhaematoma.

Subaponeurotic haemorrhage (subgaleal haemorrhage)

On rare occasions haemorrhage may occur beneath the aponeurotic sheet joining the two portions of the occipitofrontalis muscle of the scalp. It is seen particularly in black infants. It may be the consequence of trauma during delivery, especially with vacuum extraction, or may indicate the presence of a coagulation defect. The scalp becomes fluctuant and enlarges rapidly with a marked drop in haemoglobin. The severity of blood loss may be underestimated, and ensuing shock may be life-threatening. Affected babies require rapid diagnosis and appropriate transfusion with volume expanders and/or blood.

Skull fractures

Generally linear fractures require no specific treatment. Depressed fractures are usually associated with forceps application or head compression produced by the maternal sacral promontory. Large fractures may be associated with cerebral contusion, and neurosurgical consultation may be necessary. Depression of the skull may remain for many months after birth.

Intracranial haemorrhages

See Chapter 19.

Peripheral nerve injuries

Nerve injuries in the newborn infant may be due to stretching, compression, twisting, hyperextension or separation of the nervous tissue. They may be classified pathologically as
• *neuropraxia* (swelling of the nerve);
• *axonotmesis* (complete peripheral degeneration with total recovery);
• *neurotmesis* (complete division of all structures).

Electromyography and nerve conduction studies can distinguish a neuropraxia from a neurotmesis. The following nerve injuries occur in the newborn.

Facial nerve palsy (Fig. 5.2)

This may be due to an upper or lower motor neuron lesion, but clinical distinction between these is difficult. Lower motor neuron facial palsy usually occurs due to oblique application of the forceps blade. The nerve may also be damaged by prolonged pressure on the maternal sacral promontory. Upper motor neuron lesions are much less common and are due to brain injury or nuclear agenesis (Möbius syndrome).

The lesion is recognized clinically by an inability to close the eye and a lack of lower lip depression on crying. These are seen on the affected side. This must be distinguished from 'asymmetrical crying facies' caused by an absence of the depressor anguli oris muscle. In this condition eye closure is normal but there is failure of the mouth to move downwards and outwards on the affected side when the infant cries. Asymmetry usually remains into adult life but becomes less obvious with time. It is commonly seen in other members of the family as well.

In most cases complete recovery occurs; only rarely is permanent facial palsy seen. If the eye cannot be closed, patching and 1% methylcellulose (artificial tears) eyedrops should be used to prevent corneal damage.

Congenital brachial plexus palsy

The majority of babies with this condition are thought to have sustained birth trauma, but some cases cannot be explained in this way and a prenatal causation has been proposed for these. Trauma to the brachial plexus may be due to excessive lateral flexion, rotation or traction upon the neck. Such

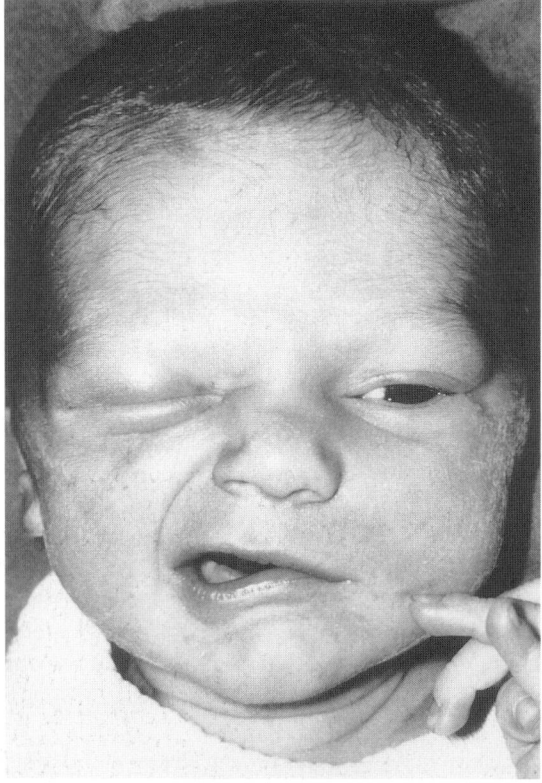

Figure 5.2 Left-sided facial palsy.

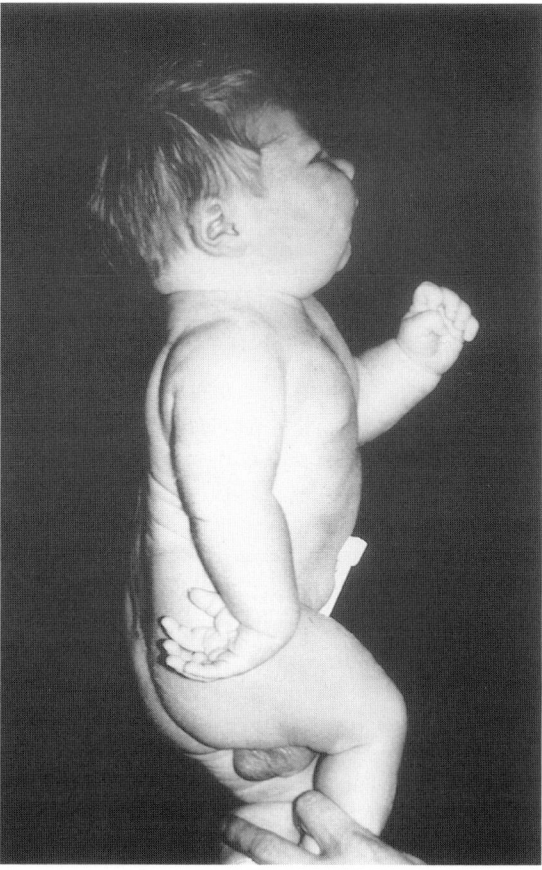

Figure 5.3 Right-sided Erb's palsy showing the typical 'waiter's tip' position of the hand.

trauma may be seen with normal delivery, with impacted shoulders or during delivery of the after-coming head of a breech. Shoulder dystocia occurred in 64% of one large series (Evans-Jones *et al.* 2003).

Three types of brachial plexus injury can be described:

Erb's palsy (upper brachial plexus palsy) (Fig. 5.3). In this lesion the fifth and sixth cervical nerve roots are injured and the arm will be held in adduction, with the elbow extended and the forearm pronated with the wrist flexed. This is traditionally known as the 'waiter's tip' position.

Klumpke's paralysis (lower brachial plexus palsy). In this uncommon lesion the seventh and eighth cervical and first thoracic segment nerve roots are injured: this involves the small muscles of the hand, with localized wrist drop and flaccid paralysis of the hand. The grasp reflex will be absent.

Total paralysis of the arm. Where all trunks of the brachial plexus have been damaged there will be complete paralysis of the arm, with flaccidity and sensory, trophic and circulatory changes. Spinal injury should be suspected when paralysis is bilateral.

Mild injuries recover within a few days, and more severe lesions can be expected to recover spontaneously in 2–4 months. Full recovery occurs in 50% of affected babies, and partial recovery in another 48%. Absence of recovery is very rare.

Management is expectant with supportive physiotherapy in all cases. The role of surgery is controversial, but is not indicated before 6 months of age and only in babies who show no improvement in function of shoulder or elbow.

Radial nerve injury

Rarely radial nerve paralysis may result from fracture of the humerus, as may occur when there is difficulty in delivering the arm during breech extraction. The use of the 'deltoid region' as a site for intramuscular injection (now usually avoided) has resulted in radial nerve injury, because the deltoid muscle of the newborn infant is so small that correct localization of the needle point is difficult. It may also be seen following repeated brachial artery sampling of arterial blood.

Sciatic nerve injury

Misplacement of the needle tip during intramuscular injection into the buttock region carries with it a risk of injuring the sciatic nerve.

Phrenic nerve injury

This is caused by injury to cervical nerve roots C3, C4 and C5, and is generally associated with brachial plexus palsy. As the newborn infant predominantly breathes with the diaphragm rather than the intercostal muscles there is often severe respiratory distress, especially when the lesion is bilateral. The clinical diagnosis is confirmed by chest X-ray, which shows an elevated hemidiaphragm, and X-ray or ultrasound screening shows an immobile diaphragm.

Recurrent laryngeal nerve

This is a rare cause of laryngeal stridor and may be due to birth injury associated with excessive lateral traction of the neck. Occasionally trauma to the recurrent laryngeal nerve occurs during cardiac surgery. The diagnosis is made by laryngoscopy, and treatment is expectant.

Spinal cord injury

This is rare and usually associated with difficult breech deliveries involving internal version and breech extraction; rarely it may occur with shoulder dystocia. The injury is due to stretching of the cervical spinal cord. There are three modes of clinical presentation:
1 poor condition from birth, respiratory depression, shock and hypothermia, death;
2 normal at birth but later develops respiratory depression, paralysed legs and urinary retention;

3 paralysis from birth, and the extent of the paresis depends on the spinal level involved.

The investigation of choice is spinal magnetic resonance imaging (MRI). Neurosurgical decompression is necessary for a large haematoma in the spinal canal. Somatosensory potentials may help to localize the level of the spinal injury.

Injury to the spinal cord is also reported as a complication of hypoxic-ischaemic insult and as the result of embolic infarction associated with placement of an umbilical catheter in the descending aorta

Bone and joint injuries

Traumatic fractures of bones are frequently associated with the classic signs of fracture, such as swelling, avoidance of movement, deformity and crepitus. Fractures of the upper limb bones may be suspected by an asymmetrical Moro reflex or failure spontaneously to move one arm.

Clavicle

This is the bone most frequently fractured during the birth process. It may be associated with impacted shoulders, especially in the infant of a diabetic mother or a difficult breech delivery. Specific treatment is not required.

Humerus

Fracture of the humerus generally involves the upper third of the shaft and there is usually considerable deformity. Radial nerve injury sometimes also occurs. Treatment consists of an immobilizing plastic backslab or immobilization with a binder to the chest.

Femur

Fracture of the femur occurs rarely during breech extraction, either vaginally or at caesarean section. It occurs predominantly in the breech with extended legs as flexion occurs. Treatment consists of immobilization in a plaster case, gallows traction or cutaneous traction, and a Thomas splint.

Multiple or unusual fractures

When these occur, osteogenesis imperfecta or non-accidental injury should be suspected.

Dislocation of joints and separation of epiphyses

These are difficult to diagnose and require specialized treatment.

Organ injuries

Liver and spleen

Subcapsular haematoma of the liver can occur after a breech extraction or following external cardiac massage. It may also result from 'atraumatic' vertex deliveries. Rupture of the liver or spleen is more likely to occur where there is hepatosplenomegaly (rhesus haemolytic disease, diabetic mother).

Adrenals

Adrenal haemorrhages may occur with breech extraction, although they are usually a postmortem finding and are unsuspected in live infants. They are more commonly associated with overwhelming bacterial infection and disseminated intravascular coagulopathy.

Kidneys

Ruptured kidneys may occur very rarely during delivery in breech preterm infants.

Testicles

Testicular bruising and haemorrhage are commonly seen in breech presentations. No treatment is necessary.

Injuries sustained in the neonatal unit

An increasing number and range of traumatic lesions are due to iatrogenic insults sustained in the modern neonatal intensive care unit. These lesions predominantly occur in preterm infants and relate to the invasive procedures and technology necessary to salvage increasingly small infants (see Table 5.4).

References

Evans-Jones G, Kay SPJ, Weindling AM *et al.* Congenital brachial palsy: incidence, causes, and outcome in the United Kingdom and Republic of Ireland. *Arch Dis Child Fetal Neonatal Ed* 2003;**88**:F185–189.

Illingworth RS. A paediatrician asks why it is called birth injury? *Brit J Obstet Gynaecol* 1985;**92**:122–130.

Volpe JJ *Neurology of the Newborn*, 4th edn. Philadelphia: W.B. Saunders, 2000.

Further reading

Fanaroff AA, Martin RH, Walsh MC (eds) *Neonatal-Perinatal Medicine: Diseases of the Fetus and Infant*, 8th edn. Philadelphia: Elsevier, 2006.

Levene MI, Chervenak FA (eds) *Fetal and Neonatal Neurology and Neurosurgery*, 4th edn. Edinburgh: Elsevier, 2008.

Internet resources

Hyman-Newman Institute for Neurology and Neurosurgery. Brachial plexus injury (http://nyneuro-surgery.org/brachial_injury.htm).

Table 5.4 Iatrogenic disease occurring in newborn infants

Skin lesions
Fetal scalp electrode lacerations
Transcutaneous Po_2 monitor burns
Calcified heel nodules from heel-stick venepuncture
Chemical burns from skin antiseptics
Extravasation lesions due to leakage of intravenous solutions
Oxygen toxicity, retinopathy of prematurity (see p. 228)
Bronchopulmonary dysplasia (see p. 107)
Hearing deficits
Antibiotics
Incubator noise
Cardiac failure from patent ductus arteriosus
Necrotizing enterocolitis (see p. 254)
Rickets (see p. 165)
Digit damage, nerve palsies, nasal deformities, oral deformities and bowel disturbance from catheters, tubes and needles
Premature thelarche
Postural deformities
Scaphocephaly
Narrow arched grooved palate
External rotation of hips and feet

6 Infant feeding and nutrition

The ideal food for healthy full-term infants is breast milk (p. 44). If the baby is born growth restricted, the volume of milk required is higher than for a normally grown baby of the same weight (see below). Premature infants have different nutritional requirements than full-term infants and need to be fed either directly into the bowel or intravenously (p. 54). Infant feeding and nutrition will be discussed under the following headings:

1 specific nutritional requirements;
2 breastfeeding;
3 formula feeding;
4 feeding the preterm infant
5 total parenteral nutrition
6 common feeding disorders;
7 specialized feeding regimens.

Specific nutritional requirements

Fluids

Water is the major constituent of infants but its proportion varies with maturity (Fig. 6.1). Newborn infants, especially preterm ones, have a higher percentage of total body water than children and adults, but the proportion decreases with age as ability to conserve water increases. For this reason, the daily requirement of the newborn is relatively higher than that of older children, and that of the premature infant is higher still. Mechanisms for conserving water are often poorly developed in immature infants, and their requirements depend on conceptual age, postnatal age and environment.

A healthy breastfed infant will consume as much fluid as is required, given ready access to the breast. Healthy bottle-fed infants will also 'know' how much fluid they need and should be allowed to consume milk when they want it, to the volume that satisfies them. Unfortunately, many mothers feel that their baby should take all his or her milk at every feed, and overfeeding may become a problem. In addition, ill or premature babies need to be given their requirements as they cannot be relied upon to take what they need. For these reasons, recommended feeding schedules have been devised (Table 6.1). These fluid requirements will be maintained up to 3 months of age, and then slowly reduced to 100 mL/kg by the age of 1 year.

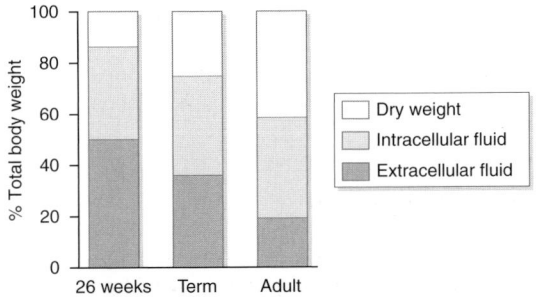

Figure. 6.1 Total body water and Extracellular fluid expressed as percentages of body weight. (Redrawn from Dear 1984, with permission.)

Table 6.1 Recommended feeding schedules (fluid volume mL/kg according to day of life)

	Day of life						
	1	2	3	4	5	6	7
Term infant	30	60	90	120	130	140	150
Preterm infant	60	80	100	120	140	160	160–180
'Sick' pre-term infant	60	70	80	90	100	110	120

Add 20 mL/kg for open radiant heat source incubator and for phototherapy.

Infants who have suffered intrauterine growth restriction should be fed to an expected weight as if they had grown normally *in utero*. This is usually a figure halfway between the 50th centile weight for gestational age and their actual weight. Ill preterm infants, particularly those with lung disease, may tolerate fluids poorly and develop worsening lung disease, patency of ductus arteriosus and oedema. Some very immature infants may lose large amounts of water through their kidneys or skin. In such cases a significantly higher fluid intake may be required.

For these reasons, recommended feeding schedules are of little value in sick infants: the fluid intake must be tailored to the infant's requirements and his or her state of hydration. Clinical assessment of hydration is made by skin turgor, fontanelle tension, moistness of the mucous membranes and urine output. In practice, clinical methods for assessing fluid requirements are unreliable: laboratory investigations are more helpful. Serum sodium, potassium, creatinine, osmolality and haemoglobin (haematocrit) should be measured daily. In addition, urinary osmolality or specific gravity (SG) is an important measurement. Daily weighing is a most valuable assessment of hydration and growth.

Serum osmolality may be affected by hyponatraemia, hyperglycaemia or uraemia, and may be unreliable under these circumstances. Similarly, glycosuria or proteinuria may affect urinary SG. We have found measurement of SG with Multistix SG Reagent strips (Bayer Australia, Pymble, NSW) reliable as an approximation to urinary SG, and the result is not affected by glycosuria. In practice we aim to keep the urinary SG between 1005 and 1010, increasing the fluid volume if the urine becomes more concentrated, and consider fluid reduction in the presence of very dilute urine.

Inappropriate antidiuretic hormone (IADH) secretion is a relatively common condition in both premature and full-term infants with severe lung or cerebral disorders. It may also be seen following neonatal surgery. The hallmark is dilute serum (low serum sodium and osmolality) with concentrated urine. Peripheral oedema is often present. The treatment is fluid restriction until the serum osmolality returns to the normal range (270–285 mmol/L).

Table 6.2 Energy requirements for optimal growth (at end of first week of life)

	Energy kcal/kg/day	Energy kJ/kg/day
Premature infant	120	516
Small for gestational age	140+	602
Term infant	100	403

Energy and macronutrients

Energy requirements for optimal growth depend on the baby's birthweight, gestational age and state of health. Ill babies are likely to be more catabolic and will have greater energy requirements. In addition, the smaller the infant the greater are the requirements per kilogram, and this is particularly so in infants who have suffered intrauterine growth restriction. Table 6.2 gives the energy requirements of various groups of infants for optimal growth. Of the recommended 120 kcal/kg/day of energy for the preterm infant only 25 kcal/kg/day are for energy storage for growth allowance.

Carbohydrate

The carbohydrate of human milk is predominantly lactose (90–95%) with small amounts of oligosaccharides (5–10%). Lactose (a disaccharide comprising glucose and galactose) must be metabolized to glucose for energy utilization in the brain and other organs. Approximately 40% of the infant's total energy requirement comes from the carbohydrate in milk. Because of concerns about the ability of preterm infants to utilize lactose and in an attempt to reduce osmolality, preterm formulas predominantly contain corn syrup (glucose polymers) as a carbohydrate source.

Fat

Fat in milk provides approximately half of the infant's energy requirements. Human milk fat is better absorbed than cows' milk fat. The mature infant absorbs about 90% of the fat in human milk, but infants weighing less than 1300 g absorb only 75–80% of fat from human milk, and less from artificial milk. Unsaturated fatty acids are better absorbed than saturated fatty acids, and medium-chain triglyceride better than long-chain triglyceride. Infants require 4–6 g fat/kg/day.

Considerable interest has developed in the role of long-chain polyunsaturated fatty acids (LC-PUFAs) in milk and their role in brain development. LC-PUFAs are present in human but not bovine milk, and fish oils are a particularly rich source. As accumulation of fetal LC-PUFAs is increased up to five times in the last trimester, prematurely born infants are thought to be particularly at risk of deficiency. Supplementation of milk with fish oils has shown enhanced maturation of the visual system in prematurely born infants, but this does not seem to confer long-term benefit. Routine supplementation of infant formulas with LC-PUFAs is the subject of ongoing research and is not currently routinely recommended for term infants . All ready-to-feed preterm formulas are supplemented with LC-PUFAs. Supplementation in term formulas increases cost. The predominant polyunsaturated fats are omega-6 (linoleic acid) and omega-3 (alpha-linolenic acid [ALA]), which are required for production of arachidonic and docosahexanoic acids, respectively.

Protein

Approximately 10% of the infant's energy requirements is provided by protein. The recommended daily intake is 2.5–3.5 g/kg/day for full-term infants and 3.0–3.8 g/kg/day for very premature infants. Milk protein is divided into curd (mainly casein) and whey (predominantly lactalbumin). Human milk contains more whey, and cows' milk considerably more curd. There are also important differences in the amino acid profile of human and cows' milk. Some low birthweight infants fed with a formula high in protein and especially high in the casein component develop a feeding acidosis or late metabolic acidosis. This is due to the inability of the preterm kidney adequately to excrete the acid produced from protein metabolism.

Minerals

The recommended minimal mineral requirements for optimal nutrition are shown in Table 6.3. In sick infants, particularly those receiving intravenous nutrition, it is important to monitor serum levels of these minerals and adjust intakes accordingly. Extra sodium may be required by the very-low-birth-weight (VLBW) infant, as there may be a high urinary loss for the first weeks of life. Potassium should not be given until adequate renal function has been established.

Trace elements

Recommended enteral requirements of trace elements are shown in Table 6.4. Copper and zinc have been shown to be essential trace elements for newborn infants. Other trace elements thought to be essential are chromium, manganese, iodine, cobalt and selenium. Breast milk and modern formula feeds contain some of these elements.

Fluoride is important in tooth development. Supplementation for infants and children is recommended in areas where drinking water is not fluoridated. The dose should be 0.1 mg/kg/day. Excessive fluoride intake during infancy may result in dental enamel fluorosis.

Table 6.3 Recommended enteral intake of minerals for term and VLBW infants (Koo & Tsang 1993)

	Enteral mineral intake (mmol/kg/day)	
	Term infant	VLBW infant
Sodium	2.5–3.5	3.0–4.0
Potassium	2.5–3.5	2.0–3.0
Chloride	5.0	1.5–4.5
Phosphorus	1.0–1.5	1.9–4.5
Calcium	1.2–1.5	3–5.5
Magnesium	0.6	0.3–0.6

Table 6.4 Recommended daily enteral intake of some trace minerals (Ehrenkranz 1993)

	Daily requirement (mmol/kg)	Daily requirement (µg/kg)
Zinc	7.7–12.3	500–800
Copper	1.9	120
Manganese	0.01	0.75
Chromium	0.001	0.05

Iron

Both preterm and term infants born to healthy mothers have sufficient iron stores at birth to double their haemoglobin mass. Depletion of these stores occurs at 3 months in premature and 5 months in term infants. If the baby is not receiving adequate iron in the diet by this age, iron deficiency anaemia will develop. Although the iron content of breast milk declines from 0.6 mg/L at 2 weeks to 0.3 mg/L at 5 months, breast milk provides sufficient iron for a term infant up to 6 months of age. Preterm infants (irrespective of which milk they receive) should be supplemented with oral iron from 6 weeks until the age of 12 months. They require approximately 1–2 mg/kg of elemental iron (30–60 mg ferrous sulphate) to prevent iron deficiency (see also p. 194).

Vitamins

The daily vitamin requirements for the newborn and young infant are shown in Table 6.5. The fat-soluble vitamins A, D, E and K are stored in the body and large doses may result in toxicity. Excess doses of water-soluble vitamins are readily excreted. The preterm infant probably requires more vitamin D (1000 IU). This is discussed in the section on rickets of prematurity (see p. 165). Much has been written about the supplementation of premature infants with vitamin E. However, there is no good evidence that this prevents late anaemia, or bronchopulmonary dysplasia. Its role in the prevention of retinopathy of prematurity is discussed on p. 229. Vitamin K is the only vitamin in which the normal breastfed infant may become seriously deficient. Vitamin K deficiency may cause haemorrhagic disease of the newborn (see p. 203).

Breastfeeding

Breast milk is the ideal food for normal full-term babies, but unfortunately in many Western societies its advantages are not fully utilized. The advantages of breastfeeding can be considered as those for the baby and those for the mother, although these are of course interrelated.

Advantages to the baby

Breastfeeding brings many benefits to the baby:
1 Nutritional. It provides the baby with a source of nutrition that changes with the baby's changing metabolic needs.
2 It confers an advantage in intellectual attainment (see below).
3 Breastfeeding is anti-infective (see below).
4 Antiallergic. The avoidance of foreign proteins in formula feeds reduces the risk of asthma and eczema in infants predisposed to these conditions.
5 Protection against various illnesses (e.g. gastroenteritis), although apparent protection against SIDS (sudden infant death syndrome) probably relates to maternal education, socioeconomic status and birthweight, rather than to breastfeeding *per se*.
6 Reduced likelihood and severity of cows' milk protein allergy.
7 Decreased incidence of infant obesity and subsequently type II diabetes, hypertension and hyperlipidaemia.

Advantages to the mother

The mother also gains from breastfeeding, in several ways.
1 Successful breastfeeding brings a sense of personal pride and achievement.
2 Promotion of a close mother–baby relationship, which provides security, warmth and comfort to baby.

Table 6.5 Recommended daily dosage for vitamin supplementation

Vitamin A	500–1500 IU
Vitamin D	400 IU
Vitamin E	5 IU
Vitamin C (ascorbic acid)	35 mg
Folate	50 μg
Niacin	5 mg
Riboflavin	0.4 mg
Thiamine	0.2 mg
Vitamin B_6	0.2 mg
Vitamin B_{12}	1 μg
Vitamin K	15 μg

3 Lactation helps the mother lose weight acquired in pregnancy.

4 Convenience – there is no preparation of formula. It can also be simply expressed, stored and given to the baby by others.

5 Lactational amenorrhoea remains the world's most important contraceptive by delaying the return of ovulation.

6 Oxytocin release during breastfeeding contracts the uterus and helps its involution.

7 Financial benefit, as breastfeeding is free.

8 It is possible to continue breastfeeding if a mother needs to return to paid work.

9 Breastfeeding confers some health advantages on the mother, as there appears to be some protection against ovarian and premenopausal breast cancer and osteoporosis.

A National Health survey in Australia in 2001 revealed 83% breastfeeding at hospital discharge, with rates of 48%, 23% and 1% at 6 months, 1 year and 2 years, respectively. These figures are similar in the UK. National Health and Medical Research Council (NHMRC) targets for Australia are 90% at discharge, 60% at 3 months and 50% at 6 months. Women of higher socioeconomic groups are more likely to initiate breastfeeding and continue for longer. In 1991 UNICEF and the World Health Organization introduced the global baby-friendly hospital initiative to improve these figures. The '10 steps' to successful breastfeeding are intended as a standard of good practice (Table 6.6).

The physiology of lactation

During pregnancy there is a marked increase in the number of ducts and alveoli within the breast in response to oestrogens, progesterone and placental lactogen. In the third trimester prolactin secreted by the anterior pituitary sensitizes the glandular tissue with the secretion of small amounts of colostrum. The flow of milk after birth is under the control of the let-down reflex. The baby rooting at the nipple causes afferent impulses to pass to the posterior pituitary, which secretes oxytocin. This stimulates the smooth muscle fibres surrounding the alveoli to force the milk into the large ducts. After birth there is an increase in prolactin levels, which maintains milk production. The hormonal maintenance of lactation is summarized in Fig. 6.2.

Table 6.6 The '10 steps' to successful breastfeeding (WHO 1989)

Step 1	Have a written breastfeeding policy that is routinely communicated to all healthcare staff
Step 2	Train all healthcare staff in the skills necessary to implement this policy
Step 3	Inform all women (face to face and with leaflets) about the benefits and management of breastfeeding
Step 4	Help mothers initiate breastfeeding shortly after delivery
Step 5	Show mothers how to breastfeed and how to maintain lactation (by expressing milk) even if they should be separated from their infants
Step 6	Give newborn infants no food or drink unless 'medically' indicated. No promotion of formula milks
Step 7	Practise 'rooming-in'. All mothers should have their infant's cots next to them 24 h a day
Step 8	Encourage breastfeeding on demand
Step 9	Give no artificial teats or pacifiers to breastfeeding infants
Step 10	Foster the establishment of breastfeeding support groups and refer mothers to them

Stress inhibits oxytocin release and may reduce milk production. This may cause the baby to cry more, thereby heightening maternal stress and further inhibiting milk production. This may be an important factor in the failure of long-term lactation (see below).

Milk production is controlled by endogenous (maternal) and exogenous (baby) factors:

1 *Endogenous.* In the first weeks of lactation, prolactin secretion occurs in response to feeding and controls milk production.

2 *Exogenous.* After a few weeks of successful breastfeeding the baby exerts the major control on breast milk production. The amount of milk produced is related to effective and frequent removal of milk from the breast by the baby.

Nutritional aspects

Human milk is uniquely adapted to the requirement of babies, with low levels of protein and minerals compared with the milks of other species. The energy content of human milk (67 kcal/100 mL) is

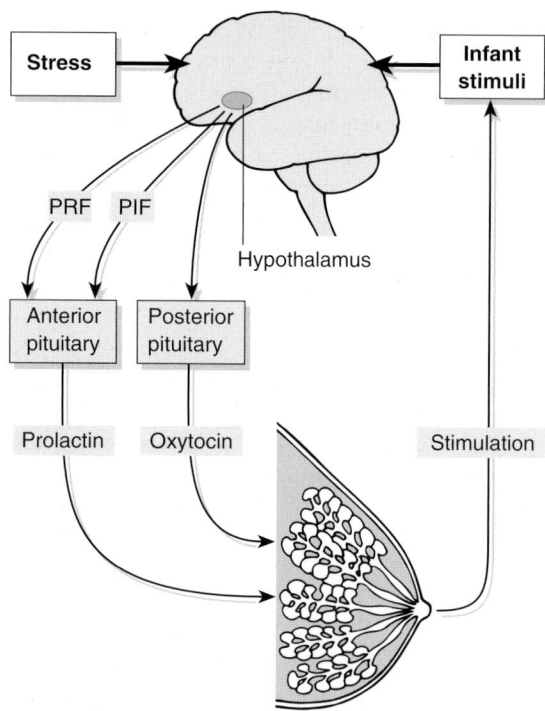

Figure 6.2 The hormonal maintenance of lactation. PIF, prolactin inhibiting factor; PRF, prolactin releasing factor.

Table 6.7 Proteins in human milk and cows' milk (g/100 mL) (Reproduced from Hambraeus *et al.* 1984.)

	Human milk	Cows' milk
Total protein	0.89	3.30
Caseins	0.25	2.60
Total whey protein	0.64	0.70
α-Lactalbumin	0.26	0.12
α-Lactoglobulin	–	0.30
Lactoferrin	0.17	Trace
Serum albumin	0.05	0.03
Lysozyme	0.05	Trace
IgA	0.10	0.003
IgG	0.003	0.06
IgM	0.002	0.003
Others	0.07	0.15

mineral level in human milk results in a low renal solute load for the immature kidney. Although calcium and phosphate levels in cows' milk are higher than in human milk, their absorption from cows' milk is much lower.

Variations in breast milk

Early breast milk contains a higher sodium and protein concentration than milk from mothers who have fed their infants for several months. The high sodium content in early milk reflects the young infant's inability fully to conserve sodium by the kidneys, a mechanism that matures in the weeks following birth. The amount of lactose in breast milk increases with postnatal age as the intestinal disaccharidase enzyme mechanism matures. Interestingly, up to 90% of milk is taken from the breast in the first 4 min of feeding; the rest of the 'feed' is largely non-nutritive. Bottle-fed infants have quite a different pattern of intake, less than 40% of the feed being taken in the first 5 min.

It is now known that the milk constituents of mothers who deliver prematurely are different from those of women who deliver at full term. Preterm milk contains a higher protein and sodium content than term milk, supporting the suggestion that preterm milk is better suited to premature infants than milk from established breastfeeding mothers. In addition, preterm milk contains considerably more immunoglobulin (IgA) and other

provided by fat (54%), carbohydrate (40%) and protein (6%). Human milk has a very low protein content of only 0.9 g/100 mL, with a whey:casein ratio of 0.7. A larger proportion of the nitrogen in human milk is derived from non-protein sources compared with cows' milk. Human milk contains twice the amount of lactalbumin as cows' milk (and is immunologically different), but no lactoglobulin, which is a significant component of the protein constitution of cows' milk. The levels of amino acids such as taurine, aspartic acid, glutamic acid and asparagine are especially high. Human milk fat is better absorbed than cows' milk fat because of the smaller size of the emulsified fat globules and the presence of lipase in human milk (see p. 245).

The main differences between human and cows' milk are shown in Table 6.7. There is a higher proportion of unsaturated fatty acids and a lower proportion of saturated fatty acids in human milk than in cows' milk. Human milk contains more vitamins A, C and E and nicotinic acid than does cows' milk, but less vitamin B_1, B_2, B_6, B_{12} and K. The low immune factors, and is more protective against necrotizing enterocolitis, than term milk. The composition of preterm human milk varies markedly but there is a progressive decline in energy, lactose and fat content over time. For mothers whose breast milk supply exceeds preterm requirements, feeding with energy and fat-rich 'hind milk' may increase weight gain.

Anti-infective properties of breast milk

Breastfeeding is an effective method of protection from infection while a baby's immunological system is developing. Breastfed infants are less likely to develop gastroenteritis, necrotizing enterocolitis (NEC) (see p. 254), otitis media and other serious infections, such as septicaemia and meningitis. This is due to numerous host resistance factors in human milk, which include:

- *Immunoglobulins*. IgA is the most important immunoglobulin secreted in breast milk, and is in very high concentrations in colostrum.
- *Cells*. Breast milk contains vast numbers of macrophages, polymorphs, and both T and B lymphocytes.
- *Lysozyme*. This acts to lyse the Escherichia coli cell membrane.
- *Lactoferrin*. This binds iron, which is necessary for some bacteria to multiply.
- *Antiviral properties* possibly due to secretory IgA or interferon production by lymphocytes.
- *Probiotics: bifidus factor and lactobacilli*. The stool of breastfed babies is more acid than that of artificially fed infants. This, together with the carbohydrate bifidus factor, encourages lactobacilli to flourish, which has the effect of inhibiting the growth of E. coli. Unfortunately, a single artificial feed is enough to upset this delicate balance and the gut flora changes as a result.

Contraindications to breastfeeding

These are uncommon and can be divided into maternal and infant contraindications.

In the mother
1 Acute illness – a relative contraindication, as illness is usually over quickly.

2 Chronic illness – neoplasms, mental illness (depending on medications and safety), tuberculosis (active treatment).
3 Breast infection/abscess – Management is either temporay expression of that breast or continue feeding depending on serverity
4 Human immunodeficiency virus (HIV) infection in the mother can be transmitted to the baby through the cells in breast milk. In developing countries the risk of gastroenteritis from contaminated feeds outweighs the risk of acquiring HIV infection from breast milk, but in developed countries, where clean water is taken for granted, breastfeeding by HIV-positive women is contraindicated (see also p. 66).
5 Illicit drugs – breastfeeding should occur before administration of planned illicit drugs and be delayed for at least 12 hours after the drug has been taken.

In the infant
1 Acute illness – this may be temporary and the expression of breast milk should be encouraged.
2 Mechanical problems – severe cleft lip and/or palate.
3 Metabolic problems – galactosaemia, phenylketonuria, lactose intolerance.
4 Breast milk jaundice (see Chapter 13) – interruption of breastfeeding may rarely be considered for a few days in order to make a diagnosis or until the jaundice falls to a safer level. Usually diagnosis is made by exclusion of other pathological causes.

Excretion of drugs in breast milk
The question of excretion of drugs (medically administered or illicit) as well as environmental toxins in breast milk has caused great concern and anguish to many mothers. Unfortunately, there is little scientific information on this subject. The factors that enhance the transfer of drugs in breast milk include
1 the lipid solubility of the drug;
2 pH – the pH of milk is 6.6–7.4, so that basic drugs such as antihistamines, aminophylline, opiates and antidepressants are more likely to be excreted in higher concentrations;
3 degree of ionization – unionized drugs are more likely to be excreted;
4 protein binding – drugs that are not protein bound show a greater tendency to be excreted;

5 molecular weight – drugs of low molecular weight are excreted to a greater extent.

Table 6.8 provides a guide to the safety of drugs given to breastfeeding mothers.

In addition, infants with glucose-6-phosphate dehydrogenase deficiency (see p. 198) may haemolyse if exposed to nitrofurantoin, sulfonamides or sulfasalazine via breast milk.

Techniques of breastfeeding

Establishment of lactation

Preparation for breastfeeding should begin in the antenatal period. Antenatal expression of colostrum may result in an increase in the duration of breastfeeding and a reduction in milk engorgement but may induce labour.

The infant should be put to the breast as soon as possible after delivery, and the timing and duration of feeds should be responsive to the needs of the baby. Breastfeeding at night should be encouraged. Supplementing breast milk with water or glucose reduces the duration of breastfeeding with no compensating benefit, and should be strongly discouraged.

The baby should never be pulled off the breast. The jaw should be released by depressing with the finger at the corner of the baby's mouth. Feeds should be started on alternate breasts. Nipple creams and sprays are unnecessary; application of breast milk to nipples post-feed accelerates healing.

Problems with breastfeeding

Ill or preterm baby
The mother should be encouraged to express by hand within a few hours of birth, as frequent breast expression up to 8–10 times a day increases lactation. A pump should only be used if it is comfortable and convenient and the nipples are not already traumatized. Current recommendation is to commence use of an electric pump on day 1.

Jaundiced baby
The sleepy, jaundiced baby should be encouraged to breast feed first but may need to take expressed breast milk from a bottle, so that an adequate intake of milk may be given and documented.

Table 6.8 A guide to the use of common drugs in breastfeeding mothers (Reproduced from Read *et al.* 1984.)

Unsuitable for breastfeeding mothers	Only use if mother and infant can be monitored	Safe to use in breastfeeding mothers
Gold salts	Aminoglycosides	Codeine
Indometacin	Cotrimoxazole	Non-steroidal anti-inflammatories
Phenylbutazone	Ethambutol	Paracetamol
Chloramphenicol	Isoniazid	Salicylates*
Tetracyclines	Clonidine	Cephalosporins
Phenindione	Diuretics	Erythromycin
Lithium	Antidepressants	Metronidazole*
Iodides	Carbamazepine	Penicillins
Oestrogens (high dose)	Phenytoin	Rifampicin
Antimetabolites	Primidone	Beta blockers
Atropine	Carbimazole	Digoxin
Ergotamine	Oral contraceptives	Heparin
Opiates (high dose)	Thiouracils	Hydralazine
Amiodarone	H_2 antagonists	Methyldopa
Dapsone	Antihistamines	Warfarin
Doxepin	Theophylline	Barbiturates*
Vitamin D (high dose)		Benzodiazepines*
		Sodium valproate
		Corticosteroids*
		Progestogens
		Bulk laxatives
		Kaolin
		Inhaled bronchodilators

* Only if low-dose regimens.

Test weighing
This is a technique performed to assess the volume of milk obtained while the baby is suckling at the breast. The weight of the infant (dressed or undressed) before a feed and after a feed is compared. If the baby is gaining weight satisfactorily and seems contented, test weighing is unnecessary. If there is genuine concern regarding the volume obtained at the breast, test weighs may be indicated. However, it must be emphasized that an isolated test weigh may be very misleading and provoke anxiety: it is unlikely to produce a realistic indication of the

amount or nature of milk a baby is receiving because of variations in intake from feed to feed and the changing composition of milk within the feed.

Insufficient breast milk

While in hospital the mother will require a great deal of support and reassurance and continued nipple stimulation to establish an adequate supply of milk. After discharge social and emotional problems may influence the milk supply.

Reasons for low supply include maternal anxiety, inadequate sucking stimulus due to inappropriate feeding routines and behaviours, and inadequate glandular response. The most common reason for early weaning is the mother's perception of inadequate milk production.

Milk engorgement

This can largely be prevented by demand feeding. Once breast engorgement has occurred, hot packs before feeding and cold packs after feeding are helpful. The mother should only express sufficient milk to soften the areola, to enable the baby to latch on to the breast.

Overfeeding

Posture feeding to reduce milk flow is no longer recommended when there is excessive milk production as it has been shown to be ineffective.

Cracked nipples

Cracks are caused by incorrect positioning of the baby on the breast. Nipple soreness may be due to positional soreness, nipple fissure, infection such as *Candida*, and dermatitis. Rarely is it necessary to take the baby off the breast, and there is little evidence that this practice accelerates healing. Nipple care with the application of lanolin or Masse cream and exposure to sunlight and fresh air may help heal the cracks. Hindmilk left on the nipples to dry after a feed may aid the healing process.

Inverted or retracted nipples

There is no evidence that inverted or retracted nipples inhibit the woman's ability to breastfeed her baby successfully, or that treatment prior to birth with nipple exercises or shields improves breastfeeding rates.

Sleepy babies

A baby may be sleepy in the first day or two after delivery, and this state may relate to analgesia and anaesthesia or mild birth asphyxia.

'Fighting the breast'

This is often associated with maternal anxiety and is aggravated if there are difficulties in getting the baby to the breast. Careful support and reassurance are necessary to establish successful lactation under these circumstances.

Twin feeding

If the twins are full term and vigorous, twin feeding should be possible even from day 1. Often the twins are small and do not readily suckle at the breast, so that expression may be necessary initially. It is an individual choice as to whether the babies are fed together or separately.

Weaning (changing from breast milk to another milk)

The decision on when to wean is an individual one between mother and baby. If breastfeeding has been established for more than 3–4 months, weaning should be a gradual process over at least 2–3 weeks. The last feed to be stopped should be the evening feed. If weaning takes place before 6 months, it is advisable to put the infant on a formula milk. Mutual weaning has many advantages, but often there are overwhelming reasons for maternal-led weaning.

Advice to breastfeeding mothers

If there are problems with breastfeeding after discharge from hospital, midwives and/or health visitors can provide help and support. Most countries have a wide range of community resources well equipped to deal with the mother under stress. Lactation consultants are readily available both in hospital and after discharge. Breast feeding support groups include the National Childbirth Trust (NCT), the Australian Breast Feeding Association and the Le Leche league in New Zealand.

Iron supplementation

Full-term infant

Babies receive sufficient supplemental iron in breast milk alone, at least until 6 months of age, and probably until 9 months. At about 6 months some iron-containing foods, such as cereal, egg yolk and meat broths, should be slowly introduced. Breast milk contains sufficient vitamins for the full-term infant until solids are introduced.

Preterm infant

The preterm infant needs supplemental iron whether breastfed or not. Ferrous sulphate is introduced on day 21 of life in a dose of 0.5 mL/day. Similarly, the premature infant requires extra vitamins, which can be commenced on day 14.

Breast milk bank

There are many advantages to feeding infants with breast milk, namely the nutritional balance of breast milk, its antimicrobial properties and the avoidance of foreign protein. For these reasons, milk banks have been established in order to provide breast milk for infants in whom artificial feeds may be disadvantageous. The practice of breast milk banking was placed in doubt with the worldwide epidemic of HIV/AIDS (p. 66), but by carefully screening donor mothers, milk banking is enjoying renewed enthusiasm. Donor mothers are invariably those who are well-established breastfeeders. Many are encouraged to collect the drip milk (that issuing from the non-feeding breast). This milk has a considerably lower fat content, which can be boosted by expressing any excess milk from the breasts after the infant has completed a feed. The milk is collected in sterile plastic bottles and stored in the mother's own domestic refrigerator at 4°C for not longer than 48 h. It is then delivered to the milk bank and frozen (–20°C) prior to heat treatment.

A major advantage of breast milk is its antimicrobial nature. Sterilization of the milk by boiling destroys all these properties. Pasteurization by the Holder method (62.5°C for 30 min) preserves IgA and lysozyme, but unfortunately cells are very sensitive and easily destroyed. A bacteriological sample is taken prior to pasteurization, and if any toxin-producing organisms are cultured the milk is discarded. A second sample is taken after pasteurization and, if free of pathogens and with a cell count below 100 000 organisms/mL, it is refrozen until required. Milk is not accepted from women who are HIV- or hepatitis B-positive.

Breast milk and intelligence

There has been considerable debate as to whether babies who have been breastfed subsequently have a higher intelligence quotient (IQ) than those given formula milk in the early months of life. This debate is beset with the difficulties of self-selection, as it is often women of higher socioeconomic class who elect to breastfeed, and intelligence has a major genetic influence.

Lucas *et al.* (1992, 1994) have conducted a number of intervention studies on premature babies. In one study mothers who elected not to breastfeed agreed to have their babies randomized to receive either banked donor milk or preterm formula. A second group of babies was studied where the mothers had elected to breastfeed, but if complements were required the baby would be randomly allocated to receive either banked donor milk or preterm formula. These studies show as clearly as is currently possible that at 7–8 years babies who had received human milk had a 10-point higher IQ than those who had never received breast milk.

Breast milk fortifiers

The preterm infant fed unfortified human milk receives inadequate energy, protein, calcium, phosphate and vitamins to equal fetal accretion rates. Human milk fortifiers are presented in sachets, and when added to expressed breast milk (EBM) improve weight gain and indices of protein nutritional status without adversely affecting protection against infections and NEC or rates of food intolerance.

Artificial feeding/formulas

If a mother fails in her attempts to breastfeed or does not wish to undertake breastfeeding, she must not be made to feel inadequate or guilty. Successful bottle feeding is much better than unsuccessful breastfeeding. Mothers make an informed decision not to breastfeed because of early return to work, adoption and previous lack of success.

Cows' milk

Unmodified cows' milk is not recommended during the first 12 months of life because:
- iron content is low and of poor bioavailability;
- higher levels of protein, sodium, potassium, phosphorus and calcium compared with human milk or formula;
- high renal solute load;
- lack of vitamin C and essential fatty acids;
- potential gastrointestinal tract blood loss, secondary to cow's milk colitis.

Cows' milk can be introduced into the infant's diet during the second 6 months of life as custard, yoghurt and cheese. Complementary feeding is not recommended until 6 months of age.

Cows' milk-based formulas

Commercially produced infant formulas that are reconstituted with water are sold as powders or 'ready-to-feed' liquids. The infant milk manufacturers produce milks that are similar to mature breast milk and are often marketed as 'breast milk substitutes'. The World Health Organization has set down very strict criteria in the International Code of Marketing of Breast-milk Substitutes. More recently, formula feeds have been developed that are better suited to the needs of premature infants.

The milk pharmaceutical industry has modified cow's milk in attempts to mimic human milk in nutritional content (Table 6.9). These modifications increase the cost of infant formulas. Casein-dominant formulas are usually cheaper than whey-dominant ones.

Modification of cows' milk-based formulas

Starter formulas are suitable from birth to 1 year. *Follow-on formulas* have slightly higher protein and electrolyte levels and are usually casein-dominant. They are often recommended from 6 months of age.

Soy formulas have higher levels of aluminium and phyto-oestrogens than cows' milk-based formulas but no adverse effects have been substantiated. There is no benefit over cow's milk formulas as a supplement for the breastfed infant and no proven

Table 6.9 Modifications to cows milk based formulas

Component	Usual form in cows' milk	Modification
Protein	Casein dominant	Whey dominant Protein Hydrolysates of whey, casein or amino acids Added nucleotides
Fat	Long-chain triglycerides	Medium-chain TGs Added LC-PUFAs
Carbohydrate	Lactose	Lactose-free Lactose, sucrose- and fructose-free Added thickening agents Added prebiotics
Minerals	High Na, K, calcium, phosphate	Demineralized

benefit in prevention of atopic disease. Soy-based formulas have low lactose content and are suitable for treatment of infants with galactosaemia. Some are sucrose free and suitable for sucrose intolerance.

There is no medical indication for selecting a *goats' milk-based* infant formula. Modified fresh goats' milk is not recommended because of low vitamin content.

Major nutrients

Protein modification

Whey/casein

Breast milk is 60–70% whey dominant whereas cows' milk is 60% casein dominant. Infant formula can be either whey or casein dominant. Whey-dominant formulas form an easier to digest curd in the stomach, are more similar to breast milk and are probably more suitable for young babies.

Hydrolysates

In hydrolysed formulas the protein molecules have been partly or completely broken down to smaller molecules, which may be less allergenic. In the absence of breast milk, partially hydrolysed formula is recommended for allergy prevention for infants with a first-degree family history of allergy such as asthma, atopic dermatitis, allergic rhinitis and food protein allergy to cows', goats' or soy protein. Formulas may be hydrolysed whey or casein or amino acids.

Nucleotides are present in breast milk and are progressively being introduced into formulas because of their potential to benefit the development of the gastrointestinal tract, immune system and intestinal microflora, and help iron absorption.

Fat modification

Long-chain polyunsaturated fatty acids (LC-PUFAs) are present in breast milk as omega-3 (alpha-linolenic acid → docosahexanoic acid [DHA]) and omega-6 (linoleic acid → arachidonic acid [AA]) and are major structural components of brain, retina and myelin for nerve sheaths. As preterm infants are deficient at birth in LC-PUFAs and cannot readily form DHA, LC-PUFAs are considered an essential supplement of preterm formulas. Although many formulas for term infants contain added LC-PUFAs, clinical trials are still underway to see whether they confer long-term benefits. Alteration of fat content in modified cows' milk formulas from long chain triglycerides (LCT) to medium chain triglycerides (MCT) occurs in some preterm formulas and semi- and complete elemental formulas to enhance absorption.

Carbohydrate modification

Lactose intolerance (LI) results from the deficiency of the enzyme lactase and may be primary (very rare) or secondary following damage to the gut lining from conditions such as gastroenteritis, malnutrition, protein allergy, celiac disease or inflammatory bowel disease. Lactose-free cow's milk-based formulas are usually the preferred choice for secondary LI, whereas more elemental formulas will be required for prolonged LI, especially with evidence of other malabsorption. Several of the soy formulas are both lactose- and sucrose-free and can be used for primary LI or lactose and sucrose intolerance.

Thickening agents

Thickening agents such as rice starch, carob bean flour or pre-gelatinized corn starch may be added to a standard formula or may come as an anti-reflux formula substituted for lactose. These formulas may stop regurgitation but do not affect gastrooesophageal reflux disease.

Prebiotics and probiotics

The industry is in a phase of research and development with respect to the benefits of prebiotics (carbohydrates) and probiotics ('good' anaerobic bacteria of bifidus, lactobacilli, etc).

Elemental or partially elemental formulas

These have modified protein (hydrolysates of whey or casein, or amino acids), carbohydrate (glucose polymers, lactose free) and fat (variable amounts of MCT). They are used in cases of allergy or intolerance to cows', goats' or soy protein, fat malabsorption, short gut syndrome, chylous effusions and sometimes severe infantile colic.

Other modified milks required in the management of specific malabsorption conditions are shown in Table 6.10. The management of these conditions requires the support of a metabolic physician or other specialist and the close support of an experienced nutritionist.

Techniques of artificial feeding

Volumes

The amounts suggested in the first section of this chapter should be given.

Table 6.10 Adapted formulas for various malabsorptive conditions

Condition	Recommended formula
Allergy/intolerance to cows'/goats' or soy milk	Hydrolysed formula or Partially elemental formula
Fat malabsorption (cystic fibrosis, biliary atresia, short gut syndrome)	Elemental or partially elemental formulas
Lactose intolerance	Lactose-free
Sucrose intolerance	Sucrose-free
Fructose intolerance	Special CHO-modified (cows' or soy)
Galactosaemia	Lactose-free milks (cows' or soy)
Phenylketonuria	Amino acid formula (low protein)
Other inborn errors of metabolism	Other specialized milks

Interval between feeds

In general, term infants weighing less than 3 kg are fed 3-hourly initially. Infants over 3 kg can be 'demand' fed or fed 4-hourly. It is reasonable to delete the night feed if the infant does not wake, once he or she is over 3 kg in weight.

Sterilization

A suitable technique for teats and bottles should be followed. One commonly used is the 'Milton method'. Water used in the preparation of feeds must be bacteriologically safe. This may be conveniently achieved by boiling the water for 10 min before it is used for feed preparation.

Preparation of feeds

Guidelines suggested by milk manufacturers for their products should be carefully followed. The preparation of overconcentrated feeds is an important cause of hypernatraemic dehydration.

Feeding the preterm infant

The nutritional reference standard for the term newborn is breastfeeding exclusively. A similar standard is not available for the preterm infant but the estimated nutrient intrauterine accretion rates for the fetus at corresponding gestational ages are surrogates. Data have been derived from fetal cadavers and non-invasive neutron activation techniques. Advisable intakes of nutrients have been calculated on the factorial approach of summation of intake and losses

Growth

In utero the fetus grows at about 15 g/kg/day and this is usually the goal for preterm infants of birthweight <2 kg. For infants of birthweight >2 kg weight gain expected is >20 g/day with growth in length of 0.7–1.0 cm/week and in head circumference 0.7–1.0 cm/week. The long-term goal of neonatal nutrition is to allow maximum attainment of potential growth and development.

Preterm infants have low body reserves of nutrients and high requirements compared with term infants (Tables 6.1–6.4) because most nutrient accretion occurs in the last 3 months of pregnancy. Early undernutrition may contribute to long-term problems such as poor bone mineralization and syndrome X (Barker hypothesis). The short-term nutritional goal is to mimic the growth and development that occurs *in utero*.

Feeding the very-low-birthweight (VLBW) infant

Few subjects in neonatal medicine generate as much controversy as the appropriate way to feed the very premature infant. Some ill VLBW infants will not tolerate milk feeds and require total parenteral nutrition (see p. 55). For those to whom milk may safely be given there is sometimes a choice between breast milk (expressed from the infant's own mother – EBM – or banked breast milk – BBM) or a formula feed. Unfortunately, there are now few human breast-milk banks in developed countries, but pasteurization and/or freezing EBM will reduce some of its unique immunological properties. Specially adapted formula milks have been developed for the needs of premature babies that meet their nutritional requirements better than standard formula feeds.

The following are the general principles on which feeding the VLBW baby is based:

Breast milk

Expressed breast milk from the biological mother is the preferred milk for preterm and low-birthweight infants. Breast milk expressed from the mother who delivers preterm has many important properties that make it the milk of choice for the preterm infant. These include
1 reduced risk of infection owing to the anti-infective properties described earlier (p. 254);
2 possible reduced risk of NEC in premature infants (p. 55);
3 the presence of growth factors in milk, which may be absorbed intact through the baby's gut;
4 advantageous for cognitive development (p. 282);
5 enhanced absorption, less steatorrhoea;
6 contains protein of high quality and bioavailability, plus unique fats and carbohydrates.

Breast or human milk fortifiers (HMFs)

Although the composition of preterm breast milk is more appropriate for the nutritional needs of the preterm infant than term breast milk, it does not meet the fetal accretion rate of nutrients. Human milk fortifiers can be added to EBM when a preterm infant (<32 weeks' gestation) is fully enterally fed, to boost the energy, protein, sodium, calcium, phosphorus and vitamin levels.

Low-birthweight formulas

Table 6.11 shows the typical contents of low-birthweight formulas compared with formulas for mature infants. The former often contain more sodium, potassium, protein and carbohydrate than breast milk or regular artificial feeds. We continue to feed the preterm infant on one of these formulas until the infant's postconceptual age is 35 weeks, and then change to a regular formula feed.

Preterm milks are available as ready-to-feed formulas, usually as 81 kcal/100 mL, have high levels of nutrients and low osmolality (<325 mosmol/L). They are supplemented with LC-PUFAs and nucleotides, and have a high Ca:phosphate ratio and variable proportions of MCTs.

Enteral vs. parenteral feeds

Early exposure of the baby's gut to enteral feeds has been shown to mature gut function. Low-volume hypocaloric feeds (20 mL/kg) significantly reduce the time for a baby to reach full feeding compared with babies who do not have early feeding. This effect is probably mediated through the stimulation of gut hormones.

Practical management

In developing a policy for feeding the VLBW infant, the following principles should be considered:

1 Early introduction of breast milk is beneficial even if the milk is given in small volumes (trophic feeding for bowel adaptation).
2 Avoid milk feeding in the first 5–7 days in babies at very high risk of NEC (critically ill, severe intrauterine growth restriction, particularly if absent diastolic flow on antenatal Doppler studies).
3 Once feeding with breast milk is established, supplement the milk with either breast milk fortifiers or low-birthweight formula.
4 The nasogastric route is preferred. Nasojejunal feeding is associated with a significantly higher risk of death and should not be used unless there is a particular indication.
5 There appears to be no advantage of continuous feeding over bolus feeding, which is more physiological. In babies with gastro-oesophageal reflux continuous feeding may be more appropriate to reduce reflux.
6 Total parenteral nutrition (TPN) (p. 55) should be used only when milk feeding is contraindicated, or as a supplement to milk feeding where a low volume of milk is indicated. Use TPN for the shortest acceptable period of time.

A slow stepwise daily incremental increase in enteral feeding of EBM is best tolerated in infants <30 weeks' gestation. During this period of gut adaptation nutritional requirements are delivered as supplemental parenteral nutrition via a long, peripheral or central intravenous (i.v.) line.

Additional nutritional supplements

The volume of milk tolerated by preterm infants is usually about 160 mL/kg/day, but for infants with chronic

Table 6.11 Typical contents of various milks fed to mature and immature infants (contents per 100 mL of milk)

	Mature human milk	Modified milk formula	Demineralized whey formula	Preterm formula
Energy (kcal)	70	65	68	80
Protein (g)	1.34	1.7	1.45	2.0
Sodium (mg)	15	25	19	35
Calcium (mg)	35	61	35	90
Phosphorus (mg)	15	49	29	50
Carbohydrate (g)	7.0	2.8	7.0	6.6–8.6
Fat (g)	4.2	2.6	3.82	4.8

neonatal lung disease it is often only 120–140 mL/kg/day, and with high metabolic rates growth may be sub-optimal even when EBM is fully fortified with HMF. Under these circumstances growth may be assisted by additional nutritional supplements, including

- carbohydrate – glucose polymers (4 kcal/g);
- fat – MCT oil (9 kcal/g);
- carbohydrate and fat – Duocal (Scientific Hospital Supplies, Baulkham Hills, NSW);
- protein – Promod (Abbott Australia Kumell, NSW) (4 kcal/g).

Iron

The preterm infant has sufficient iron stores at birth to double haemoglobin mass by 3 months, at which time, without iron supplementation, iron deficiency anaemia may develop. Preterm infants <32 weeks' gestation should be supplemented with 1–2 mg/kg of elemental iron as ferrous sulphate daily from 6 weeks of age.

Total parenteral nutrition (TPN)

TPN is not the preferred method for feeding infants and should be used only when appropriate enteral feeding is not possible. Supplemental parenteral nutrition is frequently practised whilst the preterm infant (<30 weeks' gestation) slowly adapts to increasing enteral feeds.

Indications

The main indications for TPN are as follows:

- Preterm infants <30 weeks' gestation and/or <1000 g.
- Preterm infants >30 weeks but unlikely to receive full feeds by day 7.
- Severe intrauterine growth restriction (IUGR) with abnormal Doppler flow studies.
- NEC.
- Gastrointestinal tract anomalies.

Methods of delivery of TPN

The solutions used in TPN are highly irritant and may cause severe tissue damage if subcutaneous extravasation occurs. For this reason, administration of TPN through a long peripheral or central venous line (see pp. 56, 309) is advisable.

The TPN regimen aims to provide carbohydrate, fat, protein, electrolytes, minerals, vitamins and trace elements. TPN can be conveniently ordered and administered through standardized bags with modifications as necessary to dextrose, sodium, calcium and phosphate. Generally amino acid bags will be left connected for 48 hours with a long-life bacterial filter. Lipid emulsion syringes need to be changed daily.

Carbohydrate

This is usually in the form of 5%, 7.5% or 10% dextrose, and it is to this that the electrolyte and mineral mixture is added. Dextrose is mixed with the amino acid solution in the ratio of 3:1. This combined solution is both acidic and hypertonic.

Protein

This is provided as a mixture of crystalline L-amino acids. The provision of amino acids in these solutions does not closely match the amino acid requirements of ill infants, and regular serum and urinary amino acid profiles should be measured. The rate of infusion for protein is 2.5–4.0 g/kg/day, and the protein is mixed with the dextrose- electrolyte solution prior to infusion. Newer protein solutions have an amino acid profile similar to cord blood including all the essential amino acids.

Fat

Fat emulsions are made from soya bean oil, egg yolk lecithin and glycerol or olive oil, and contain a high proportion of essential long-chain fatty acids. Fats are protein bound in the plasma and may displace bilirubin from albumin, hence caution with infusion is necessary in jaundiced infants. Many 20% fat emulsions have appropriate phospholipid:trigly-ceride ratios and are rapidly cleared from plasma. Commencement at 1 g/kg/day as early as day 2 of life, increasing in 1 g/kg/day increments every day or up to 3 g/kg/day is recommended. Some infants, particularly those who are very ill with respiratory disease, appear to fail to clear the fat emulsion from the circulation and it accumulates in the lungs. The serum should be regularly examined for opa-lescence or the triglyceride (TG) concentration measured. The infusion is stopped if the TG level is high or if the serum is cloudy. Intravenous fat emulsions should be infused simultaneously with carbohydrate and protein solutions through a 'Y' connector distal to a bacterial filter.

Minerals

Sodium and potassium requirements are estimated daily and added to the dextrose as required. A mineral mix (e.g. Peditrace, [Pharmatel Fresenius Kabi N2, Auckland]) provides the necessary trace minerals.

Vitamins

Water-soluble vitamins (e.g. Solvito 0.5 mL/kg/day) and fat-soluble vitamins (e.g. Vitialipid 1 mL/kg/day) are added to the solutions. Vitialipid is mixed with fat emulsion, but is photosensitive and the syringe to which it is added should be protected from light.

Trace elements

Trace elements such as copper and zinc are present in a number of commercial TPN products. Other trace elements (Peditrace) should be added to the TPN solution when TPN is used for more than 7 days.

Clinical management

Individual neonatal units need to develop their own clinical and laboratory monitoring of TPN. However, the following procedures play a crucial part:
- Before infusion commences take a mandatory X-ray, with radio-opaque contrast if necessary, after insertion of a long/central line.
- Observe the infusion site closely, especially when a peripheral line used.
- Measure blood glucose 4–6 hourly for the first 3 days, twice a day when stable.
- Weigh every second day, and length and head circumference weekly.
- Observe serum for lipaemia or measure TG levels.

Laboratory tests

Laboratory investigations for monitoring of safety of TPN should include the following:
- Full blood count (FBC), electrolytes and creatinine – every second day for 1 week and then twice weekly.
- Plasma calcium, phosphate and magnesium twice weekly.
- Liver function tests if TPN >2 weeks.

Complications

Complications from TPN have been reduced with use of newer commercial products. However, the major areas of concern are as follows:

1 Infection. There is a constant risk of septicaemia when giving TPN. *Staphylococcus epidermidis* is the commonest cause of systemic infection. Regular monitoring for sepsis is required, including FBC, C-reactive protein (CRP) and blood cultures.

2 Hyperglycaemia. Premature babies do not tolerate glucose well. Four-hourly stick tests for glucose should be carried out. Insulin (0.1 U/kg) may be necessary. Minimal enteric feeds have a glucose-lowering effect.

3 Metabolic disturbances. Careful biochemical surveillance is essential in all infants receiving TPN (see above).

4 Cholestatic jaundice results from prolonged TPN, especially due to lack of hepatic stimulation in the absence of enteral feeding.

5 Hyperammonaemia.

6 Lipaemia and fat accumulation in the lungs. Lipid peroxidation when exposed to light is prevented with a silver foil covering lipid infusate or addition of vitamin C. Liberated free fatty acids from lipid infusate can displace bilirubin from albumin.

7 Metabolic acidosis.

8 Venous thrombosis (long-line).

9 Tissue injury due to extravasation (peripheral line).

Common feeding disorders

The most frequent problems are possetting, vomiting, colic, constipation, diarrhoea and failure to thrive, and these will be discussed below.

Vomiting

Possetting. Many babies have small spills of feed (posset), and this is considered normal.

Vomiting. This is a common symptom in the newborn and its causes may be non-organic or organic:

1 *Non-organic*: overfeeding; incorrect preparation of feeds; overstimulation or excessive handling of baby; crying; air swallowing.

2 *Organic*: infection (urinary tract infection, gastro-enteritis, meningitis, otitis media); gastro-oesophageal reflux, gastritis (meconium, blood), hiatus hernia; organic bowel obstruction, pyloric stenosis, small bowel obstruction, large bowel obstruction; transient gastrointestinal intolerance (e.g. prematurity, metabolic disorders); food allergy (cows' milk). Bile-stained vomiting must always be urgently investigated to exclude malrotation of the bowel (p. 249).

Investigation

The cause of infant vomiting can usually be determined if a careful history of feeding technique, description of the vomiting, preparation of the infant formula and other symptoms are assessed. The physical examination must be complete. A test feed is often necessary. If there is a possibility of underlying pathology but the history and physical examination are inconclusive, then appropriate investigations are necessary, for example:

1 abdominal X-ray (erect, supine): bowel obstruction;
2 ultrasound examination is very useful in the investigation of malrotation;
3 barium swallow: hiatus hernia, gastro-oesophageal reflux;
4 urine microscopy: urinary tract infection;
5 septic screen including urine for micro and culture: infection;
6 stool cultures and microscopy: infection;
7 24-hour oesophageal pH probe monitoring: gastro-oesophageal reflux.

Management of the vomiting baby

1 Identify and treat the cause wherever possible.
2 Maintain fluid balance: parenteral therapy may be indicated.

Organic causes of vomiting

It is appropriate to discuss some organic causes of vomiting:

Gastritis

This may be due to meconium or blood swallowed before or during birth. Characteristically it is associated with mucous vomiting.

Treatment. The routine aspiration of the stomach after birth, followed by lavage with normal saline where blood or mucus is present, may prevent the occurrence of vomiting. Where established mucus vomiting exists, gastric lavage with normal saline is usually all that is necessary.

Gastro-oesophageal reflux/hiatus hernia

Gastro-oesophageal reflux is a common cause of vomiting in the newborn infant. It results from an incompetent lower gastro-oesophageal sphincter and is particularly prevalent in preterm infants, as well as neurologically abnormal infants with severe hypo- or hypertonia. It frequently occurs following repair of diaphragmatic hernia and oesophageal atresia. The vomiting usually occurs at the end of a feed, and particularly when 'winding' the baby. Preterm infants are particularly prone to vomiting due to lax lower oesophageal sphincter tone, delayed gastric emptying and poor oesophageal contractility, all of which improve with maturity.

The character of the vomiting varies from small spills occurring just after feeds to large, sometimes projectile, occasionally blood-specked vomits. The natural history is for gradual improvement with growth of the infant, and cessation usually by the end of the first year of life in normal children.

Complications. These include
1 persistent vomiting leading to failure to thrive;
2 oesophagitis, hiatus hernia, oesophageal stricture;
3 obstructive apnoea, SIDS and 'near miss' SIDS;
4 recurrent aspiration of milk, with the development of a brassy cough, wheeze and stridor;
5 Sandifer's syndrome: this occurs in older, children with learning difficulties who show head-cocking trait associated with iron-deficient anaemia and reflux oesophagitis.

Investigations. Infants with mild symptoms do not require investigation. Many tests have been used to evaluate reflux. One commonly used test is a barium swallow with inversion of the infant during the procedure to show the degree of reflux present. A pH probe inserted into the middle third of the oesophagus may be useful, but does not detect non-acid reflux. Oesophagoscopy may be useful in a few infants.

General Measures. Certain general measures can help infants with reflux.

1 Studies have demonstrated the prone position with a 30–40° head-up tilt to be the position of choice. However, the increased risk of SIDS with this sleep position makes it untenable. Mild cases usually improve when the infant is nursed in a more upright position. Special chairs have been used, but are often inappropriate.

2 Thickening the feeds with an agent such as rice starch, carob bean flour or corn starch is usually effective, in combination with upright feeding. Sometimes the feed needs to be so thick that it must be spooned into the baby.

3 Antireflux milks use similar thickeners.

4 Acid suppression. H_2 receptor antagonists such as ranitidine have proven the most effective in a dose of 2 mg/kg three times a day. Antacids are not recommenced in the newborn period but may reduce stomach acidity in later infancy. Proton pump inhibitors are the most potent acid suppressors used after other therapies have failed, or they may be used as first line agents for selected infants with respiratory or neurological symptoms. Omeprazole in a dose of 0.7–3.3 mg/g/day is most extensively used.

5 Continuous feeding via nasogastric tube or gastrostomy or even transpyloric tube is sometimes required.

6 Surgery. Rarely fundoplication will be necessary when medical treatment fails or when respiratory complications occur.

Pyloric stenosis

This condition usually presents after the first month of life: rarely it may occur in the first week. It is characterized by projectile vomiting, more commonly in boys, and is associated with visible peristalsis and a palpable 'tumour'. There is often a family history.

Treatment is surgical and consists of a muscle-splitting operation of the pylorus (Ramstedt's operation).

Infant colic

Some apparently healthy infants, who are feeding well and gaining weight, cry at certain times during the day, but especially in the evening around 6 pm. The infant has attacks of screaming, draws up his or her legs and is unable to be comforted. The condition tends to disappear spontaneously at about 3 months. There is often no obvious cause, although many explanations have been given including: overfeeding, underfeeding, milk allergy, spoiling and boredom.

Treatment includes attention to feeding techniques, posture feeding and warmth to the abdomen (e.g. baths). The removal of dairy products from the maternal diet when breastfeeding occasionally helps. Dicycloverine (dicyclomine) hydrochloride (Merbentyl) 2–5 mL given 15 min before feeds may be useful. The daily maximum dose should not exceed 20 mL. Recently the manufacturers of Merbentyl have recommended not using this agent in infants under 6 months of age because of several case reports of apnoea.

Constipation

This term means hard, dry stool without regard to the frequency. Often when mothers talk of constipation they mean an absence of stools for 2–3 days, which may be normal. Breastfed babies are unlikely to be constipated and yet may not have a stool for several days.

Aetiological factors

There are several possible causes of constipation.

1 Inadequate or improper feeding, e.g. a milk formula that is too concentrated.

2 Anatomical abnormalities, e.g. anal stenosis, Hirschsprung's disease, fissure *in ano*.

Treatment

The management will depend on the underlying cause. Local anaesthetic cream (e.g. Xylocaine) is used for fissure *in ano*. Alteration of the feeds may be indicated, for example giving prune juice, orange juice or extra water. The addition of a stool-wetting agent such as dioctyl sodium increases the fluid in the stools. Milk of magnesia may be used as a mild laxative. Glycerine suppositories and/or small enemas may occasionally be indicated.

Diarrhoea

This term is used to mean loose frequent stools with stool volume >10 mL/kg/day. Acute diarrhoea lasts <10 days whilst chronic diarrhoea persists beyond 2–3 weeks. The pathological mechanisms include osmotic, secretory and inflammatory processes. Stools initially change colour from a dark green-black (meconium), through a greenish-yellow transitional stage, and attain the typical yellow colour by 4–5 days. Stools may normally be very frequent initially, especially in breast-fed babies, and this situation should not be confused with diarrhoea. Infants undergoing photo-therapy commonly have greenish loose stools, and these must be distinguished from diarrhoeal stools.

When an infant is having loose frequent stools, the following causes of diarrhoea should be considered:

1 maternal diet in a breastfed infant, e.g. excessive chocolate, Coca Cola, etc.;
2 incorrect formula preparation, overfeeding;
3 infective (viral, bacterial, protozoan);
4 sugar intolerance: transient or permanent;
5 steatorrhoea, e.g. cystic fibrosis.

Management will involve treatment of the specific cause whenever possible, and attention to fluid balance as necessary. Antidiarrhoeal drugs are not used in the newborn period.

Failure to thrive

This is a term used to describe infants whose weight gain is inadequate. Weight gain in the first year of life is not linear, but frequently occurs in spurts. Generally babies at least double their birthweight by 5 months, and treble it by 1 year. The infant who fails to thrive shows a characteristic fall-off in weight gain and linear growth. These measurements cross centile lines in a downward direction, and this is more significant than an infant whose measurements are on or below the third centile but who grows along a line parallel to the centile line. A fall in the incremental growth curve when gluten is introduced into the diet rouses suspicion of coeliac disease. Normal head growth may continue despite poor weight gain, as brain growth is the last to fail. A broad approach to management of an infant with failure to thrive can commence with classification into non-organic and organic causes.

PRINCIPLES OF MANAGEMENT

- Breast milk is the ideal food for normal babies both term and preterm.
- The preterm infant fed unfortified human milk receives inadequate energy and nutrients to equal fetal accretion rates.
- Unmodified cow's milk is not recommended during the first 12 months of life.
- Survival reflexes of suck, swallow, cough and gag are usually not developed until 34 weeks.
- The nutritional reference standard for the term newborn is the exclusively breastfed infant.
- Total parenteral nutrition should only be used when enteral feeding is not possible.

- Non-organic – inadequate parenting and poor nutrition.
- Organic – failure of intake, abnormal losses or failure of utilization.

References

Dear PRF. Nutritional problems in the newborn. *Hospital Update*, November 1984, 915–917.

Ehrenkranz, RA. Iron, folic acid and vitamin B$_{12}$. In: Tsang RC, Lucas A, Uauy RD, Zloken S (eds) *Nutritional Needs of the Preterm Infant*. Baltimore: Williams and Wilkins, 1993.

Hambraeus L, Fransson GB, Lönnerdal B. Human milk composition. *Nutrition and Abstracts and Reviews* 1984;**54**:4.

Koo W, Tsang RC. Calcium, magnesium, phosphorus, and vitamin D. In: Tsang RC, Lucas A, Uauy RD, Zloken S (eds) *Nutritional Needs of the Preterm Infant*. Baltimore: Williams and Wilkins, 1993.

Lucas A, Morley R, Cole TJ *et al*. Breast milk and subsequent intelligence quotient in children born preterm. *Lancet* 1992;**339**:261–264.

Lucas A, Morley R, Cole TJ, Gore SM. A randomised multicentre study of human milk versus formula and later development in preterm infants. *Arch Dis Child* 1994;**70**:F141–F146.

Read MD, Golightly PW, Grant E. *A Guide to Drugs in Breast Milk*. Boehringer Ingleheim, 1984.

WHO (World Health Organization) Protecting, Promoting and Supporting Breast Feeding: The special role of mateinity services, Geneva: WHO, 1989.

Further reading

Arenz S, Ruckerl R, Koletzko B, van Dires R. Breastfeeding and childhood obesity – a systematic review. *Int J Obesity Related Metab Dis: J Int Assoc Study Obesity* 2004;**28**:1247–1256.

Cooke RJ (ed.) Neonatal nutrition. *Semin Neonatology* 2001;**6**:363–449.

Hale T. *Medications and Mothers' Milk*, 11th edn. Texas: Pharmasoft Publishing, 2004.

Kuschel CA, Harding JE. Multicomponent fortified human milk for promoting growth in pretern infants. *Cochrane Database of Systematic Reviews* 2004.

NHMRC. *Dietary Guidelines for Children and Adolescents in Australia*. Ausralian Government Publishing Service, 2003.

Ronald E, Kleinman MD. *Pediatric Nutrition Handbook*, 5th edn. American Academy of Pediatrics Committee on Nutrition. Illinois: American Academy of Pediatrics 2003

Sear MA, Greene JM, William AR *et al*. Long term relation between breastfeeding and development of atopy and asthma in children and young adults: a longitudinal study. *Lancet* 2002;**360**:901–907.

Tsang RC, Lucas A, Uauy RD, Zloken S (eds.). *Nutritional Needs of the Preterm Infant*. Baltimore: Williams and Wilkins, 1993.

Tsang RC (ed.) *Nutrition of the Preterm Infant. Scientific Basis and Practical Guidelines*. Ashland, OH: AtlasBooks, 2002.

Internet resources

Unicef. International Code of Marketing of Breast-milk Substitutes (www.unicef.org/nutrition/index_24805.html). www.unicef.org/programmes

New Zealand Breastfeeding Authority. Baby Friendly Aotearoa New Zealand (www.babyfriendly.org.nz).

CHAPTER 7

7 Infection

Infection is an ever-present problem in the newborn. Infection is not only common, but also presents in many different ways involving almost any system in the body, and must therefore be considered in the differential diagnosis or as a possible complication of almost every condition affecting the newborn. The incidence of infection is approximately 5 per 1000 live births, and is more common in premature infants.

Historical aspects

Sepsis has always been one of the prime causes of neonatal mortality, and the history of neonatology runs hand in hand with the history of neonatal sepsis. The major nursery pathogens have been

1 1930s and 1940s – group A β-haemolytic streptococcus.

2 1940s and 1950s – coliform organisms.

3 Late 1950s and early 1960s –*Staphylococcus aureus* emerged as the major nursery pathogen, but towards the end of this era was largely eradicated by the routine use of hexachloraphene (Phisohex).

4 1960s – coliform organisms: these will always present a problem because there is no passive maternal immunization.

5 1970s – group B β-haemolytic streptococci became the major pathogenic organism in the neonatal nursery.

6 1980s – coagulase-negative staphylococci were recognized to be serious nosocomial pathogens, especially in extremely preterm, sick infants. Other 'new' pathogens included *Acinetobacter, Citrobacter, Serratia* and *Enterobacter* species.

7 1990s – emergence of multiresistant organisms such as methicillin-resistant *Staphylococcus aureus* (MRSA), expanded spectrum of β-lactamase Gram-negative bacteria (ESBL) and vancomycin-resistant enterococci (VRE).

The immature immune system

The immune system develops from early in fetal life, but is not functionally fully integrated until about 1 year of age. Immunity can be considered to be specific and non-specific.

Specific immunity

Specific immunity is mediated through lymphocytes, of which there are two types – B and T cells – and activation results in immunological memory. Neonatal lymphocytes do not function as efficiently as mature lymphocytes owing to a reduced production of cytokines.

B cells

When stimulated, B lymphocytes transform to plasma cells and produce immunoglobulin (Ig). IgM is the first type to be produced at 15 weeks' gestation, and IgG is first produced at 20 weeks. Initially fetal levels of the three major Ig types are minimal and remain very low at birth. Adult levels of IgM are attained by 1 year and of IgG at 5 years. IgG is the only Ig that crosses the placenta, and consequently at birth the baby has high levels of maternally derived IgG. This gives the neonate effective passive immunity, but the levels fall in the months after birth. IgG leads to bacterial cell lysis by opsonization and complement fixation and also neutralizes viruses and toxins. IgA is produced by secretory cells.

T cells

T cells are produced in the fetal bone marrow and migrate to the thymus; hence the term thymus (or T)-related lymphocytes. When stimulated by an infective agent they transform to perform one of three functions:

1 Produce cytokines such as interleukins, tumour necrosis factor and interferon gamma; performed by CD4+ helper cells, which are the primary effector cells.
2 Suppress the immune response of other cells.
3 Kill target cells.

Non-specific immunity

There are two main types of non-specific immunity:
- *Cellular*. Phagocytic white cells (neutrophils and monocytes) ingest bacteria (a process enhanced by complement and IgG) and are attracted to sites of inflammation by chemotactic chemicals such as complement and leukotrienes.
- *Humoral*. This includes complement, interferons (produced by virally activated cells), lactoferrin (binds iron and reduces growth of *E. coli*) and lysozymes.

Susceptibility of the neonate to infection

The neonatal immune system is much less efficient than the mature system, in a number of fundamental ways, predisposing the infant to infection. Exogenous factors may also predispose the infant to infection.

Endogenous factors

1 Low levels of Igs, particularly IgM and IgA.
2 Premature infants fail to receive normal passive IgG transfer during the last trimester of pregnancy.
3 Phagocytic action is less effective in the newborn.
4 Humoral activity is impaired and, in particular, complement levels are low.
5 As well as the premature infants being more prone to infection, intrauterine growth-restricted infants also appear to be more susceptible.

Exogenous factors

1 The baby is born bacteriologically sterile, with little competition from existing bacterial flora when exposed to potential pathogens. Babies exposed to very early antibiotic use, either as newborns or as fetuses, may be predisposed to colonization with potentially pathogenic organisms.
2 Breaches of the skin barrier such as long lines and cannulas allow entry of bacteria to the baby.
3 Drugs may further impair immune function, with corticosteroids being the main offenders.
4 Fat emulsions. Agents such as Intralipid appear to impair the phagocytic function of the white cells.
5 Hyperbilirubinaemia reduces immune function in several different ways.

Origins of infections

Infections may be acquired *in utero* (congenital), intrapartum or postnatally. Box 7.1 gives key guidelines for managing infections.

Congenital (intrauterine)

Transplacental

First trimester: TORCH infections: this is an acronym derived from the first letter of the following conditions:

Toxoplasmosis

Other, e.g. Coxsackie B virus, varicella, human immunodeficiency virus (HIV)

BOX 7.1 General Management Infection

- *Prevention.* Every effort should be made to prevent pregnant women from becoming infected. Infected infants should be isolated from pregnant nurses. Non-immunized women should be immunized against rubella before pregnancy.
- *Specific.* There is no specific treatment for congenital rubella, CMV and Coxsackie B infections.
- *General supportive measures.* These include maintenance of normal temperature and intravenous fluids.
- *Barrier nursing.* This is essential to prevent the spread of certain infectious agents.
- *Treatment of complications* such as convulsions, respiratory distress, congestive heart failure and hyperbilirubinaemia may be required.

Rubella
Cytomegalovirus (CMV)
Herpes simplex type 2

Second trimester: Treponema pallidum (syphilis).

Third trimester and labour:
1 Viral – varicella zoster, hepatitis B, Coxsackie B, echovirus, HIV.
2 Bacterial – group B β-haemolytic streptococcus, *Listeria monocytogenes*, *Haemophilus influenzae*, pneumococcus.
3 Protozoan – malaria.

Ascending infections

These occur after rupture of the membranes and represent the most common form of ante- and intra-partum infection. The most frequent pathogens are: bowel organisms (e.g. *Escherichia coli*, *Klebsiella*, *Pseudomonas*, *Proteus*, *Enterococcus fecalis*), group B β-haemolytic streptococcus, group A streptococcus and rarely *Staphylococcus aureus*.

Intrapartum

Organisms causing intrapartum infections colonize the infant during passage through the birth canal, although infection occurs in a relatively small proportion of births. Prolonged rupture of the membranes predisposes to intrapartum infection. Pathogens include: herpes simplex, *Neisseria gonorrhoeae*, hepatitis B, group B β-haemolytic streptococcus, *Chlamydia trachomatis*, *Candida albicans* and HIV.

Acquired infections

In the nursery (nosocomial):
1 bacteria – coagulase-negative staphylococci, *Staphylococcus aureus*, group B β-haemolytic streptococcus, coliforms, *Salmonella* spp., *Shigella* spp., anaerobic bacteria, *Pseudomonas* spp.;
2 viruses – coxsackie, rotavirus, respiratory syncytial virus, adenovirus, echovirus;
3 fungal – *Candida albicans*, *Candida parapsilosis*.

Congenital (TORCH) infections

Devastating effects on the fetus may result from intrauterine infections. Fortunately, such occurrences are rare, but constant vigilance is necessary to keep the incidence low. Several congenital infections

Table 7.1 Principles of Management of Congenital infection

Organism	Maternal treatment	Infant treatment
CMV		Ganciclovir for 3 months
Toxoplasmosis	Spiramyicin and sulfadiazine or pyrimethamine + sulfadiazine	Spiramycin alternating with pyrimethamine + sulfadiazine for 1 year
Syphilis	Penicillin	Penicillin for 10 days
Hepatitis B		Vaccination at birth, 1 and 6 months
HIV	Antiretroviral treatment from 28 weeks	Oral zidovudine for 4-6 weeks Deliver by elective caesarean section Avoid breastfeeding
Varicella		ZIG and, if vesicles, start aciclovir

have a similar clinical picture, and it is convenient to think about, and investigate, the TORCH group as a whole. Table 7.1 outlines the general principles of management of congenital infections.

Clinical features

Infection at the embryonic stage (first 12 weeks) may lead to multiple abnormalities (Fig. 7.1). With infection occurring later, the baby may be born with a viraemia and may have neonatal illness associated with jaundice, enlarged liver and spleen, anaemia and thrombocytopenia. The predominant features of the three most common prenatal infections are shown in Table 7.2. The investigation of infants with suspected congenital infections should include
1 review of maternal history for immunization and exposure to infectious agents;
2 serological tests, including quantitative IgM and specific antibody serology for TORCH infections, and polymerase chain reaction (PCR) to amplify DNA particles;
3 urine for CMV inclusions and viral culture;

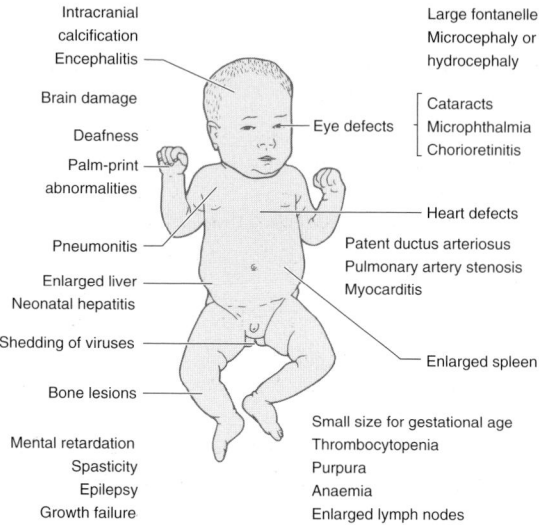

Intracranial calcification
Encephalitis

Brain damage

Deafness

Palm-print abnormalities

Pneumonitis

Enlarged liver
Neonatal hepatitis

Shedding of viruses

Bone lesions

Mental retardation
Spasticity
Epilepsy
Growth failure

Large fontanelle
Microcephaly or hydrocephaly

Eye defects [Cataracts / Microphthalmia / Chorioretinitis]

Heart defects

Patent ductus arteriosus
Pulmonary artery stenosis
Myocarditis

Enlarged spleen

Small size for gestational age
Thrombocytopenia
Purpura
Anaemia
Enlarged lymph nodes

Figure 7.1 Schematic representation of the clinical features of prenatal TORCH infections.

4 throat and nose swabs, cerebrospinal fluid (CSF) and faeces for viral culture;
5 computed tomography (CT)/ultrasound to detect intracranial calcification in toxoplasmosis, CMV and rubella, and X-rays of long bones to show periostitis in syphilis and viral osteopathy in rubella and CMV;
6 ophthalmological examination to detect chorioretinitis in toxoplasmosis and cataracts, retinitis and microphthalmia in rubella.

Rubella

Because of high immunization rates, congenital rubella syndrome currently affects less than 50 children each year in the UK. When maternal infection occurs before 8 weeks of pregnancy, 85% of infants will have symptoms; this rate falls to 52% if infection occurs at 9–12 weeks and 16% at 13–20 weeks. Congenital infection does not occur after 20 weeks' gestation. The risk of a fetus being damaged as a result of inadvertent rubella vaccination given to a pregnant woman is very small.

Cytomegalovirus (CMV)

This is the commonest congenital infection in the UK and occurs in 3–4 per 1000 live births, but only

Table 7.2 Relative clinical features of prenatal rubella, cytomegalovirus and toxoplasmosis

	Rubella	Cytomegalovirus	Toxoplasmosis
Eye involvement	++	++	+++
Microphthalmia	+	+	+
Chorioretinitis	+	++	++
Cataracts	++	–	–
Intrauterine growth retardation	+++	+	+
Brain	++	++	+++
Hydrocephaly	–	–	++
Microcephaly	+	++	+
Calcification	++	++	++
Deafness	+++	+++	++
Hepatosplenomegaly	++	++	++
Cardiac	++	–	+ –
Purpura	++	++	–
Pneumonitis	+	++	+
Bony involvement	++	+	–

15–20% of congenitally infected infants develop symptoms. Serious symptomatic infection may occur with exposure after 28 weeks' gestation. Diagnosis is made by identifying the virus in urinary squames or from a throat swab in the first week of life. Viral embryopathy predominantly occurs with primary maternal CMV infection, with maternal reinfection or reactivation occasionally resulting in neonatal CMV viruria.

CMV acquired postnatally is an important source of this condition and may be contracted from caregivers, infected blood (all blood products should be screened for CMV) and possibly breast milk.

In infants with symptomatic congenital CMV there is preliminary evidence that ganciclovir improves outcome if given for 3 months after birth.

Toxoplasmosis

Toxoplasmas are protozoal organisms that rarely cause congenital infection in the UK and Australia; such infection is considerably more common in France. Fetal infection after maternal seroconversion may be diagnosed by PCR or serological testing on fetal blood obtained by cordocentesis.

Maternal treatment is with either spiramycin alone or pyrimethamine together with sulfadiazine (not before 16 weeks' gestational age (GA)). Only 25% of infected babies show neonatal symptoms or signs, and symptoms may not appear for several years. The classical features are the triad of chorioretinitis, hydrocephalus and periventricular calcification.

The congenitally infected baby (even if asymptomatic) should be treated with spiramycin (100 mg/kg/day) for 4–6 weeks, alternating with pyrimethamine (1 mg/kg/day) and sulfadiazine (50 mg/kg/day) for 3 weeks, over one year (Kieffer *et al.* 2002). Folinic acid 5–10 mg intramuscularly (i.m.) every 2–4 days prevents the side effects of pyrimethamine.

Syphilis

The incidence of this condition has recently increased in developed countries. Congenital infection is seen if maternal infection occurs after the fourth month of gestation. Penicillin is an effective treatment for mother and fetus. Classically the infant at birth is found to have persistent snuffles, skin eruptions and widespread metaphyseal bony lesions. However, many infants show no symptoms at birth.

Interstitial keratitis is the commonest feature of congenital infection, and hepatomegaly is present in almost all cases. Treatment of maternal syphilis in pregnancy usually eradicates infection in the infant. The mother will have positive VDRL (venereal disease research laboratory) and TPHA (*Treponema pallidum* haemagglutination assay) tests, and the infant will also be positive as a result of passive transfer of IgG to the fetus. More specific investigations are necessary.

The fluorescent *Treponema* antibody absorption (FTA-ABS) test should be performed for both IgG and IgM. The IgG response will remain positive for several weeks but should be negative by 6 months. The IgM response should be negative at birth. If positive, the infant should be treated for congenital syphilis with parenteral benzylpenicillin (50 000 U/kg) twice daily for 10 days (Zenker & Berman 1991). Prior to treatment the CSF should be examined. It is recommended that all neonates born with a positive VDRL test should be treated at birth.

Hepatitis B

This is largely a disease of developing countries, but with worldwide travel it is now relatively common in the UK and Australia. Mothers who develop acute hepatitis B infection in the third trimester of pregnancy have a 70% risk of the infant developing the disease, but the neonatal disease is rarely severe or fatal. More commonly, mothers who are chronically hepatitis B 'surface antigen' positive pass the infection vertically to their baby via the placenta. Forty percent of children with persistent hep B infection will die in adult life of hepatocellular carcinoma or chronic liver disease.

All women should be screened for hepatitis B at booking, with serological tests for surface antigen (HBsAg). But they are at greatest risk of infecting their babies if they are also HBe antigen (HBeAg) positive. If a woman has antibody to HBe (antiHBe), then the risk of serious disease to her infants is very small. Therefore, women who are HBsAg positive and negative for HBeAg and have antiHBe are at low risk of their infants developing severe disease, but the infants may become chronic carriers of HBsAg and at risk of developing carcinoma of the liver. Symptoms of liver disease in the neonatal period are rare in affected babies.

Prevention of transmission is possible by immunizing infants born to women who have acute hepatitis B in the last trimester of pregnancy, or where the mother is HBsAg positive.

Treatment of the baby is with vaccination and hepatitis B immunoglobulin (HBIG). The first dose of vaccine is given within 12 h of birth, with further immunization at 1, 2 and 12 months after birth. Follow-up should ensure that seroconversion occurs. HBIG (200 IU i.m.) should be given within 12 hours of birth. Women positive for hepatitis B should be encouraged to breastfeed.

Hepatitis C

Perinatal transmission of hepatitis C virus (HCV) occurs in pregnant women with anti-HCV-positive tests. Pregnant women who are anti-HCV positive should have the appropriate antibody and antigen testing. Infants born to pregnant women who are HCV RNA positive have a 6–8% risk of acquiring the infection, which is usually chronic. There is no evidence that breastfeeding increases the risk of perinatal transmission. Currently women in high-risk groups, such as women with substance dependency, sex industry workers, and those with hepatitis B or who are HIV positive, are tested for HCV antibodies.

Human immunodeficiency virus (HIV/AIDS)

The HIV retrovirus causes AIDS and damages the immune system, with consequent frequent severe infections that eventually lead to death on average 2 years after AIDS is first diagnosed. HIV is an important perinatal pathogen, but with effective treatment the risk of transmission from mother to infant can now be virtually eliminated. In worldwide terms HIV/AIDs is common, with over 40 million people infected, 90% of whom live in the developing world. In the UK HIV/AIDS is relatively rare (6 per 10 000 women), but the incidence in London is six times higher. The UK has a rapidly increasing population of asylum seekers from sub-Saharan Africa, and consequently the prevalence of women who are HIV-positive is increasing throughout the country.

Women are infected with HIV in the following ways:
• heterosexual intercourse with infected partners (33%);
• needle sharing amongst intravenous drug abusers (25%);
• no known risk factors (36%);
• miscellaneous (6%).

It is clear that a significant proportion of infected women will be missed by identifying risk groups and for that reason all women should be offered routine screening for HIV in early pregnancy after appropriate counselling. Most women of childbearing age with HIV are asymptomatic, and symptomatic AIDS (advanced HIV) is rare in pregnancy. Women at particularly high risk of transmitting HIV to their babies are those with symptomatic HIV/AIDS, a falling or low CD4 T-lymphocyte count or high viral load (>10 000 copies/mL). It is estimated that in 80% of cases mother to infant transmission of HIV occurs from 36 weeks of gestation, during labour and at delivery; <2% occurs in the first and second trimesters of pregnancy.

Management

In developed countries, the risk of vertical transmission from mother to child for a non-breastfeeding woman is 15–20%, and with appropriate management and advice in pregnancy and early infancy this can be reduced to <2%. Management can be considered under the following headings.

Antenatal. Antiretroviral therapy from 28 weeks of gestation until delivery. Zidovudine monotherapy reduces the risk of vertical transmission by 50%. Highly active antiretroviral therapy (HAART) with multiple drugs such as zidovudine together with nevirapine or lamivudine may be recommended depending on local circumstances, the presence of high maternal viral load and the health of the mother. The local specialist in HIV should be consulted in each case.

Avoid chorionic villus sampling or second trimester amniocentesis wherever possible. If these are considered necessary HAART may be indicated.

Intrapartum. Avoid allowing spontaneous membrane rupture by performing a planned caesarean section at 38 weeks. This has been shown significantly to reduce the risk of mother–infant transmission in addition to prenatal drug treatment.

Neonatal. At delivery the baby should be considered to be potentially infective. Gloves, mask and goggles should be worn. In developed countries, discourage breastfeeding as HIV may be transmitted to the infant through breast milk. It is estimated that breastfeeding doubles the risk of the infant being infected with HIV.

All babies born to HIV-positive women should be treated with oral zidovudine for 4–6 weeks after birth.

There is a high risk of HIV infection for babies born to mothers who
• follow incomplete course of antiretroviral therapy in pregnancy;
• have maternal high viral load (>50 copies/mL); or
• have maternal CD4 count <200/mL.
These babies should be treated with HAART (e.g. zidovudine, lamivudine and nevirapine). The precise regimen will depend on local expert advice.

The baby should have HIV-PCR assessment on day 1 (do not send cord blood, which may be contaminated by maternal blood), and this should be repeated at 4–6 weeks, 3–4 months and again at 4–6 months (the latter only in infants born very preterm).

Parvovirus B19

This virus most commonly causes a mild illness known as erythema infectiosum (fifth disease). It is characterized by mild systemic symptoms, including fever and a distinctive facial rash with a 'slapped cheek' appearance. Parvovirus B19 infection in pregnancy, which is often asymptomatic in the mother, can cause severe anaemia with resultant hydrops and fetal death, but the risk of death is less than 10% after proven maternal infection.

Varicella

Maternal chickenpox developing in the period of a week before or 5 days after birth predisposes the infant to a very high risk of potentially fatal varicella. Zoster immunoglobulin (ZIG) 2 mL should be given immediately to infants at high risk of congenital chickenpox. The infant is then carefully watched and, at the first sign of a vesicle, the antiviral agent aciclovir is given intravenously for 10 days. This treatment should prevent serious infections. Varicella in the first and second trimesters rarely causes congenital defects. If the pregnant woman is not immune to varicella zoster, and the infection occurs before 20 weeks' gestation, then she should receive ZIG as soon as possible after contact.

Intrapartum infection

At birth it may be difficult to decide whether a baby is infected or not. The following factors should be considered:

1 maternal features of sepsis, e.g. fever, high white cell count, tender uterus, offensive or purulent liquor;
2 duration of rupture of membranes: if the membranes have been ruptured for more than 18 h, chorioamnionitis is expected;
3 duration of labour: a prolonged labour beyond 12 h carries an increased risk of systemic infection;
4 frequent vaginal examinations and instrumental delivery further increase the risk of infection;
5 the presence of fetal distress or birth asphyxia increases the likelihood of infection.

Critically ill infants with infection may exhibit respiratory distress, shock and renal failure. They may develop disseminated intravascular coagulation with internal and external bleeding.

Often congenital bacterial infections have a less dramatic clinical presentation, with lethargy, vomiting, diarrhoea, jaundice, apnoea or mild respiratory difficulty. The organisms detailed below may cause intrapartum infection. Box 7.2 summarizes the evaluation and management of intrapartum infection.

BOX 7.2 Evaluation and management of intrapartum infection

● Recognize risk factors for early infection	Maternal infection (chorioamnionitis)
	Prolonged rupture of membranes
	Premature delivery
	Fetal distress
	Serious infection in a previous child
● Undertake appropriate investigations	Surface swabs
	Gastric aspirate
	Blood cultures ($\pm$ lumbar puncture)
	Full blood count, CRP
● Start antibiotics if significant risk of neonatal infection	Penicillin (or ampicillin), gemtamicin $\pm$ metronidizole
	Continue for 48 hours if culture negative
● Clinical course	The early signs of infection are variable and may be subtle
	Maintain a low tolerance for starting antibiotics

Investigations

Swabs are taken from the throat, nose, umbilicus, rectum and auditory canal. A gastric aspirate specimen is examined for pus cells and organisms on Gram staining. The superficial swabs merely reflect contamination, but gastric aspirate and ear swabs probably reflect intrapartum exposure to organisms. The gastric aspirate is useful because it provides early information about the infecting organisms and may therefore influence the initial choice of antibiotics. Blood cultures are essential, and a lumbar puncture should be considered.

Ancillary investigations include a full blood count with differential white cell count. Neutropenia, thrombocytopenia and a toxic white cell reaction suggests infection. An elevated C-reactive protein (CRP) estimate (>20 mg/L) suggests infection.

Group B β-haemolytic streptococcus (GBS)

This is the commonest cause of serious intrapartum infection, and although the prognosis has improved it is fatal in 10–20% of cases depending on gestational age and age of onset. Vaginal or rectal colonization with GBS is found in 15–30% of pregnant women, and 10–20% of infants born to colonized women will themselves be colonized, but far fewer than this are infected. In the UK and Australia the incidence of early-onset GBS infection in the neonate is approximately 0.4–1.0 in 1000 liveborn infants. The possibility of early-onset GBS infection should be considered in any infant presenting with respiratory distress in the first 12 h of life.

Two forms of neonatal GBS sepsis are recognized: *early-onset* disease presents with septicaemia, respiratory distress and septic shock, which if not suspected and treated early is rapidly fatal. The second form is *late onset*, characterized by meningitis, which usually develops some time after 5–7 days. Various serotypes of GBS are described, and all are implicated in early-onset disease, although type III has been more frequently associated with late-onset disease. Late-onset disease may be acquired from infected breast milk or from a caregiver other than the mother. Recurrent neonatal GBS infection is reported in 1% of neonates.

Some neonates appear to be particularly susceptible to this infection if their mother has low circulating anti-GBS IgG, and if the baby is born prematurely his or her white cells are particularly poor at killing this organism.

Eighty percent of babies who develop early-onset disease show at least one of the following risk factors:

- chorioamnionitis;
- low birthweight;
- prolonged rupture of the membranes (>18 hours);
- birth following prolonged labour;
- frequent vaginal examinations in labour;
- a sibling previously infected with GBS.

Presentation and diagnosis

Most babies presenting with early-onset disease develop symptoms in the first 4–6 hours of life. The baby may initially develop signs of respiratory distress, which clinically and radiologically may be indistinguishable from respiratory distress syndrome (RDS). Shock, renal failure and convulsions may also occur within the first 12 hours of life in affected infants. GBS infection must be considered as a possible cause of any baby presenting with early-onset illness.

All at-risk babies should have surface swabs taken at birth as well as a gastric aspirate for culture. Symptomatic babies should have blood cultures taken immediately after birth, and lumbar puncture should be considered even in suspected early-onset presentation. Latex particle agglutination tests are unreliable as early predictors of infected babies. A full blood count may show a neutropenia and/or thrombocytopenia.

Management

Early administration of intravenous antibiotic is essential, as is supportive treatment to maintain the baby in good condition and early recognition of complications of the infection. Where the diagnosis is unconfirmed penicillin (or amoxicillin) together with gentamicin is the best choice, and these two drugs act synergistically against GBS. When the diagnosis is confirmed, benzylpenicillin should be administered for 7–10 days.

Prevention

As early-onset GBS infection in the neonate occurs in only 1% of colonized women, two strategies to reduce the risk have been described. In the USA all women are screened at 35–37 weeks for GBS colonization, and those found to be positive are treated with intrapartum penicillin; this approach has resulted in a significant reduction in early-onset GBS disease. Others have shown that this approach increases the risk of other forms of neonatal infection particularly from Gram-negative organisms. In the UK there is no national policy, but the Royal College of Obstetricians and Gynaecologists (RCOG, 2003) recommends an at-risk strategy. Penicillin G is given 4-hourly to woman in labour with two or more of the following risk factors (some centres will treat women with only one risk factor):

- Preterm labour <37 weeks' gestation
- Prolonged membrane rupture >18 hours
- Maternal fever (>38°C) in labour

Escherichia coli

The K1 strain of *E. coli* is particularly associated with perinatal infection and may cause septicaemia or meningitis. The sensitivity of *E. coli* to antibiotics is variable.

Listeria monocytogenes

This is a not uncommon perinatal pathogen and may invade the fetus through intact membranes. Characteristically, infected infants pass meconium *in utero*, and if this is seen in premature infants *Listeria* should be strongly suspected. The organism has a predilection for the lungs and brain. Hydrocephalus is a common sequel to *Listeria* meningitis. The organism is usually sensitive to ampicillin.

Herpes simplex

Neonatal herpes simplex infection is a rare but devastating condition. The herpes simplex virus (HSV) can be classified as either type 1 or 2. Type 1 infection is generally limited to the lips and mouth (cold sores), but recently has become more common as a cause of genital infection probably as the result of increased oral sex. Infection with type 2 virus is usually due to sexual contact and involves the genitalia. Up to a third of sexually active women have

antibodies to herpes simplex type 2 virus. Neonatal infection now occurs as a result of HSV type 1 and 2 in equal proportion. The neonate is most commonly infected as a result of vaginal delivery, and if the mother has an active genital lesion there is a particularly high risk of neonatal infection. In most babies there is no history of genital herpes and the women are asymptomatic. The virus enters the baby through skin, eye or mouth and may disseminate to the brain or other organs.

The risk of an infant being infected from a parent, nurse or midwife with cold sores is small, but not negligible. Careful hand-washing is all that is necessary to avoid this risk. Rarely, paronychia may be due to herpesvirus, and staff with this type of active infection must not handle infants.

Presentation and diagnosis

Neonatal HSV presents in one of three ways:

- Neurological symptoms. Approximately one-third of babies present with encephalopathic signs of meningoencephalitis, most commonly at 10–14 days.
- Systemic symptoms. These babies present in the first few days of life with signs of major overwhelming illness including shock, respiratory failure and often severe hepatitis and coagulation disorders. Meningoencephalitis may also develop.
- Cutaneous symptoms, including rash and keratoconjunctivitis, in the second week of life. These babies rarely become seriously ill.

HSV infection must be considered in the differential diagnosis of any ill baby. Viral cultures should be taken from blood, CSF and skin lesions. Always consider HSV infection when lumbar puncture reveals an excess of white cells that is bacterial culture negative. Rapid diagnosis is made by immuno-fluorescence or PCR amplification from blood and CSF. In babies with encephalopathy the electro-encephalogram (EEG) may show a characteristic appearance. Brain imaging may also show specific abnormalities.

Management

Rapid administration of the antiviral aciclovir (30 mg/kg 8-hourly) for at least 14 days improves the outcome, but the prognosis remains poor. In babies with systemic disease 35–60% die, and of those with neurological disease 10–15% die. HSV-2 has a worse prognosis than HSV-1. The outcome for surviving infants is poor, with over 50% being left severely disabled. The prognosis is good for cutaneous disease, but late neurodevelopmental sequelae have been reported in up to 30%.

Chlamydia trachomatis

Chlamydia is found in the vagina of 4% of pregnant women. Up to 70% of infants born through an infected cervix will acquire chlamydia, but most show no symptoms. Chlamydia conjunctivitis and, less commonly, pneumonia occur in a relatively small proportion of infants. The conjunctivitis is purulent and is clinically indistinguishable from that of gonococcal ophthalmia. Specific culture media are necessary for this organism. Infants should be treated with tetracycline eye ointment and oral erythromycin.

Others

Pneumococcus, *Haemophilus influenzae* and anaerobic organisms may cause significant perinatal infection. Anaerobes are contracted from the birth canal and require special culture media for their identification. The first two organisms are probably haematogenously spread from maternal septicaemia. They may cause profound shock in the infant, indistinguishable clinically from group B β-haemolytic streptococci.

Antibiotic policy

Many of these organisms cause severe and rapidly developing symptoms. Successful treatment depends on a high index of clinical suspicion, because in the most severe cases positive cultures may not be available until after the infant has died. Broad-spectrum antibiotic cover is required. Ampicillin will usually cover GBS, *Listeria*, pneumococcus and *Haemophilus*. Gentamicin is usually effective against coliforms. If anaerobes are suspected then metronidazole is the appropriate antibiotic. Ampicillin (100–200 mg/kg/day i.v.) and gentamicin (5 mg/kg/day i.v.) are recommended for

cases of suspected intrapartum infection, and should be started as early as possible.

Late-onset (acquired or nosocomial) infection

Late-onset refers to signs of infection that develop more than 48 hours after birth. The implication of this is that the infection has been acquired from the baby's environment or caregivers rather than vertically from the mother. It may, however, be very difficult to differentiate infections acquired during delivery from those acquired postnatally. Almost every bacterium and virus known to infect humans may cause clinical infection in the newborn. *Staphylococcus* species are probably the most important group of infections infants acquire in the neonatal unit.

When a nosocomial infection is suspected, the following risk factors should be reviewed:
1 direct contamination by the hands of medical staff or parents due to faulty hand-washing techniques;
2 frequently performed procedures, such as intubation, insertion of catheters, humidification of oxygen, parenteral nutrition and exchange transfusions, all predispose sick babies to infection; and
3 cross-infection: the routes of neonatal cross-infection are illustrated in Fig. 7.2.

Clinical features

There are no pathognomonic signs of infection or any totally reliable way to make an early diagnosis in the laboratory. The doctor must have a high level of suspicion for infection and not be too reliant on

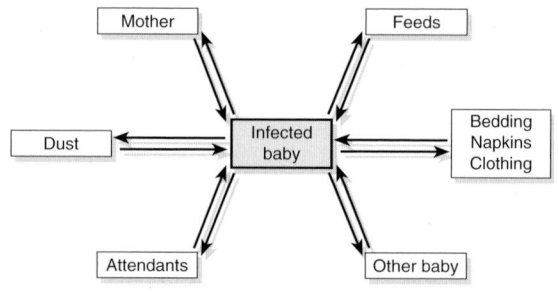

Figure 7.2 Routes of neonatal cross-infection.

blood tests to make the diagnosis. If in doubt treat the baby.

Symptoms of acquired infection are generally non-specific and include pyrexia, hypothermia, lethargy, hypotonia, irritability, poor feeding, weak cry, respiratory distress, apnoea, cyanosis, jaundice, hepatomegaly, abdominal distension, vomiting, diarrhoea, failure to thrive, rashes, purpura and a bulging fontanelle.

Investigations

If infection is suspected, the following investigations may be useful in finding the causative organism.

Deep cultures

Blood, urine, CSF and tracheal aspirate are sent to the microbiology laboratory for culture and antibiotic sensitivity testing.

Full blood count and film

Leukocytosis, leukopenia and thrombocytopenia may occur. Changes suggestive of infection may be seen in the cell morphology of the blood film, and include toxic granulations, vacuolations of neutrophils and Döhle bodies. There is frequently a left shift towards the more primitive cells in the neutrophil series.

Others

Because infection is often insidious in its presentation, attempts have been made to use screening tests to predict whether infection is likely to be the cause of illness or not. The best evaluated of these are

1 C-reactive protein. This is an acute-phase protein released at times of stress, including infection. The test is weakly positive if the level is 10–20 mg/L, and strongly positive if >20 mg/L. It has been shown to be 62% sensitive for infection (Kite *et al*. 1988).

2 Nitroblue tetrazolium (NBT) test. This examines neutrophils for uptake of the nitroblue dye, which indicates bacterial activation. If more than 13 of 100 neutrophils take up the dye the test is considered to be positive. This test has a 77% sensitivity.

3 Plasma elastase α1-proteinase inhibition. Testing provides a sensitive but non-specific index of infection

in the first 24 h after birth. Sequential testing serves as a guide to the cessation of antibiotic treatment (Rodwell *et al*. 1992).

Common acute acquired infections

Septicaemia

Apart from perinatally acquired GBS and *E. coli*, the most common organisms to cause septicaemia in the newborn unit are coagulase-negative staphylococci. This should not be dismissed as a contaminant if it is both cultured from blood culture bottles and the infant is unwell; it must be treated as a pathogen. It is particularly likely to occur when total parenteral nutrition is administered, especially if a silastic catheter 'long-line' is *in situ*. The 'long-line' should be removed when antibiotics are started if the infant is ill. Preservation of the long-line with successful antibiotic therapy is possible in less ill patients.

Other organisms include *Staphylococcus aureus*, *Pseudomonas* spp., *Proteus* spp., *Klebsiella*, *Serratia* and *Candida albicans*. Disseminated intravascular coagulation (DIC) syndrome may occur and meningitis may also be associated with septicaemia.

Methicillin-resistant staphylococcal aureus (MRSA) is an emerging problem in most intensive care units and requires rigorous treatment as well as preventative measures to stop its spread to other patients.

If *Candida* septicaemia is suspected the urine should be examined for budding hyphae. This is the most sensitive investigation for systemic candidiasis as blood culture may take some time to prove the diagnosis. If the infant has thrush in the groin this may contaminate the urine sample, and in such cases a suprapubic aspiration should be performed or a catheter sample obtained. *Candida* antigen may help in confirming the diagnosis. An ultrasound scan of kidneys may also be helpful as it shows increased echogenicity due to the presence of hyphae balls.

Treatment of septicaemia

General supportive measures. Intravenous fluids, incubator care, heart rate/respiratory/blood pressure monitoring of vital signs.

Specific therapy. The clinical dilemma is whether to treat blindly without knowing which organism is causing the infection. A best-guess policy is required, but review of all cultures taken over the previous few weeks is helpful to establish whether the infant has been colonized by potentially pathogenic organisms. Knowledge of the sensitivities of 'local' pathogens is also important in order to choose the best antibiotics.

It is usual to commence with two or three antibiotics until bacteriological culture and sensitivity results are obtained. Flucloxacillin or vancomycin and gentamicin are a good combination, but for severe infection a combination of ampicillin, cefotaxime and gentamicin is valuable. Once the organism and sensitivity have been identified, the appropriate antibiotic should be administered for 2–3 weeks.

Meningitis

Meningitis is more common, and mortality and morbidity rates higher, in the first month of life than at any other age. The organisms most usually encountered are *E. coli* and group B β-haemolytic streptococci. In addition to the other organisms seen with septicaemia, epidemics of *Listeria monocytogenes* occur. Table 7.3 shows the most common causes of pathogens in developed countries.

Many of the early clinical manifestations are nonspecific. Coma, convulsions, opisthotonus, increasing head size and a bulging fontanelle are late signs of meningitis.

Investigations
1 A lumbar puncture must be done in all infants with suspected meningitis. The CSF is often turbid

Table 7.3 Common causes of neonatal meningitis and outcome

Organism	Proportion (%)	Mortality (%)	Severe/moderate disability (%)
GBS	50	12	25
E. coli	20	15	25
Other Gram-positive	18	Low	30
Other Gram-negative	7	Low	25
Listeria	5	15	25

and cloudy, with an elevated white cell count, low sugar and high protein. Positive cultures on CSF are obtained in about 50% of cases of suspected bacterial meningitis. A premature neonate may normally have up to 12 white cells/mm³ in the CSF and a term baby up to 5 white cells/mm³, but if all these cells are granulocytes meningitis cannot be excluded.
2 Blood cultures are positive in about 50% of neonates with bacterial meningitis.
3 A full blood count may reveal variable pictures of neutropenia, neutrophilia and toxic changes.
4 Counterimmune electrophoresis: this technique can provide a rapid diagnosis of some bacterial pathogens.

Management
● *Initial therapy for suspected meningitis in the first week of life.* Combination of ampicillin, gentamicin and cefotaxime together.
● *Initial therapy for suspected meningitis after first week of life.* Combination of ampicillin, cefotaxime and an aminoglycoside together.

Always consider herpes simplex as a cause of meningitis and add aciclovir (see p. 69).

Once the organism has been identified then microbiological advice as to the most appropriate antibiotic should be sought. Meningitis due to group B streptococcus should be treated with both gentamicin and penicillin for at least 2 weeks. Listeria is best treated with ampicillin and gentamicin. Be aware of local patterns of antibiotic resistance. Meropenem may be indicated where a multiply resistant Gram-negative organisms is known to be prevalent.

Rapid sterilization of the CSF is essential and it is recommended that a second lumbar puncture be performed after 48 hours of therapy to ensure that the CSF is sterile.

Continue intravenous antibiotics for at least 2 weeks in GBS infection and for at least 3 weeks in Gram-negative infections. There is no evidence that intrathecal antibiotics improve outcome.

Ultrasound brain imaging should be performed in all infants with meningitis to detect progressive hydrocephalus, which may need treatment.

Outcome
Post-meningitis hydrocephalus is a well-recognized complication particularly in *Listeria* meningitis.

Brain abscess may occur particularly with *Citrobacter* and *Enterobacter* meningitis. Deafness is a recognized complication, and a screening test for hearing should be performed on discharge from hospital.

Approximately 50% of all babies with neonatal meningitis will show some neurodevelopmental problems at 5 years of age. The risk of severe or moderately adverse outcome is shown in Table 7.3. Box 7.3 outlines the principles of managing neonatal meningitis.

Systemic candidiasis

Diagnosis of this condition depends on a high clinical suspicion for the organism. It may rarely be congenital, associated with maternal vaginitis, or acquired in a baby receiving neonatal intensive care. *Candida albicans* accounts for over 90% of infections although *C. parapsilosis* is also seen rarely. Preterm infants undergoing intensive care are particularly vulnerable to *Candida* sepsis. Risk factors include:

- parenteral nutrition;
- central vascular catheter;
- mechanical ventilation;
- course of antibiotics.

BOX 7.3 Principles of management of neonatal meningitis

- Perform lumbar puncture if baby is at risk of meningitis or if baby is ill
- Perform full infection screen (50% of babies will also have septicaemia)
- If baby <1 week old start ampicillin, gentamicin and cefotaxime together
- If baby >1 week old start ampicillin, cefotaxime and aminoglycoside together
- Always consider herpes simplex and add aciclovir if in doubt
- Repeat lumbar puncture after 48 hours to establish CSF is sterile
- Once sensitivities are known stop inappropriate antibiotics
- Continue treatment for at least 2 weeks if GBS and >3 weeks if other organism
- Ultrasound imaging weekly to assess ventricular size
- If persistence of symptoms consider cerebral abscess (MRI or CT brain scan)
- Perform hearing test on recovery

The best method of diagnosis is to identify budding hyphae in urine from a suprapubic stab. The organism may also be isolated from arterial and/or venous blood cultures. Diagnosis may also be strongly suspected by observing 'fungal balls' on renal ultrasound scan or a pathognomonic appearance on ophthalmoscopy.

Treatment is with amphotericin B, usually in a liposomal formation (AmBisone) as it is less toxic. 5-Flucytosine acts synergistically with amphotericin and may be added in severe infection. Fluconazole may be used in amphotericin resistance or increasingly as a first-line antifungal agent. Central vein lines should be removed on starting treatment.

Death has been reported to occur in 40% of babies who are infected at <37 weeks' gestation.

Prophylaxis
Fluconazole (6 mg/kg every 72 h) prophylaxis in the first 4 weeks of life in extremely low birthweight (ELBW) infants has been shown to reduce significantly the incidence of colonization and systemic infection by *Candida*.

Lower respiratory tract infections

In the newborn, pneumonia is relatively common and is usually bacterial. Particular organisms involved are Gram-negative bacilli (e.g. *E. coli, Klebsiella, Pseudomonas*), group B streptococcus and *Staphylococcus* species. Rarer bacterial pathogens include *Listeria monocytogenes* and anaerobic bacilli. Non-bacterial pathogens include *Chlamydia trachomatis, Mycoplasma pneumoniae, Ureaplasma urealyticum, Candida albicans*, CMV and *Pneumocystis carinii*. Pneumonia may be contracted *in utero* and be present at birth (congenital), or acquired after birth (nosocomial). Congenital pneumonia may be due to ascending infection associated with prolonged rupture of the membranes, or less frequently to a transplacental infection. Viral pneumonitis is rare but may occur with CMV, Coxsackie virus, respiratory syncytial virus and rubella infection. The clinical picture may mimic that of the respiratory distress syndrome (RDS). Staphylococcal infections may be associated with pneumatocoeles, empyema, abscesses and pneumothoraces. Treatment consists of antibiotics and respiratory support (see Chapter 11).

Urinary tract infection

The incidence of urinary tract infection is approximately 3 per 1000 live births. Symptoms and signs are non-specific, and therefore this condition must be constantly borne in mind. The main problem is that it is difficult to obtain uncontaminated urine. Ideally one should strive to obtain a clean-catch midstream specimen after cleansing the external genitalia with sterile water. Suprapubic aspiration of the bladder may be used to obtain uncontaminated urine, but care is necessary with this method to avoid complications. Often urethral catheterization is necessary to obtain a satisfactory collection.

Treatment should be with an appropriate antibacterial agent for 10–14 days. With all proven urinary tract infections in the newborn it is mandatory to follow the child for the first year of life, carrying out monthly cultures of urine. In addition, creatinine estimations at regular intervals, ultrasound examination of the kidneys and micturating cystourethrography to detect underlying anatomical abnormalities of the urinary tract should be performed. For details see Chapter 22.

Conjunctivitis ('sticky eyes')

Mild eye infections are very common and are referred to as 'sticky eyes'. Purulent conjunctivitis may be either a congenital or an acquired infection. Conjunctivitis is sometimes secondary to a blocked nasolacrimal duct. Usually the organisms involved are *Staphylococcus aureus*, *E. coli*, *Pseudomonas* spp., *Chlamydia trachomatis* and *Neisseria gonorrhoeae*. Reddened swelling in the region of the lacrimal sac (dacrocystitis) may occur following infection of a blocked nasolacrimal duct. The term ophthalmia neonatorum is reserved for infection with *N. gonorrhoeae*.

Management

Conjunctival swabs should be taken and sent promptly to the laboratory. If ophthalmia neonatorum or *C. trachomatis* are suspected, swabs need to be taken by laboratory staff and applied to culture plates in the ward. Conjunctival scrapings need to be taken for Giemsa staining and cell culture. If maternal gonorrhoea is suspected, prophylactic treatment of the newborn's eyes with 1% silver nitrate eyedrops may prevent purulent conjunctivitis.

With mild conjunctivitis, or 'sticky eyes', frequent eye toilet with normal saline may be all that is required. More florid infections will need the frequent instillation of antibiotic drops (e.g. chloramphenicol or sulfacetamide) after cultures have been taken and eye toilet carried out. After the conjunctivitis has settled somewhat, antibiotic ointment may be used.

Treatment of gonococcal ophthalmia involves local irrigation with crystalline penicillin in normal saline solution and systemic penicillin for 10 days. In severe ophthalmia the drops must initially be instilled every 10 min for an hour, then hourly for 4–6 h depending on the response. For the treatment of chlamydia, (see p. 70).

Omphalitis and funisitis

Infections of the umbilical cord (funisitis) and umbilical stump (omphalitis) are usually due to *E. coli*, other Gram-negative bacteria or *Staphylococcus aureus*. Infection may arise as the result of chorioamnionitis. Because of the potential seriousness of the spread of infection to the portal vein and subsequent portal hypertension, infection in this area must be treated promptly. If there are signs of spread with surrounding cellulitis, parenteral antibiotics such as flucloxacillin and gentamicin are necessary after appropriate swabs and cultures have been taken. Topical treatment with an antibiotic is also necessary. Routine cord care has evolved over recent years from cleansing with methylated spirits to the use of normal saline and, currently, tapwater.

Infection of the skin and subcutaneous tissues
Paronychia

Reddening of the skin in the nailfold is common and may proceed to pus formation when staphylococcal infection is present. Topical treatment consists of applications of 1% aqueous gentian violet and is usually all that is necessary to eradicate *Candida albicans* or minor bacterial infections. Parenteral and topical antibiotics are indicated if systemic spread is suspected with bacterial infection.

Pustules

These may be single or in crops and must be distinguished from toxic erythema (see p. 261). Treatment consists of 1% chlorhexidine washes and sometimes systemic antibiotics. *Staphylococcus aureus* is the most frequently found pathogen.

Thrush

Infection with this yeast is common, particularly if there has been *Candida albicans* colonization of the maternal genital tract. It is also likely to occur in association with the use of broad-spectrum antibiotics and in debilitated neonates receiving total parenteral nutrition. It commonly occurs in the mouth and looks like milk curds that cannot be removed with a swab stick. The infection usually occurs towards the end of the first week of life. In the napkin area it appears as a spreading centrifugal rash. It sometimes occurs as a secondary infection following ammoniacal dermatitis. Napkin psoriasis is a rare condition that starts in the napkin area and may become widespread, usually secondary to thrush. The treatment of oral candidiasis consists of the use of nystatin mouth drops or gel instilled every 6 h for 1 week. For the napkin area, nystatin cream applied four times daily is usually sufficient. One per cent aqueous gentian violet may be used in both of these sites, but tends to cause staining of clothes. Treatment of systemic candidiasis is discussed on p. 73.

Gastroenteritis

Gastroenteritis usually occurs in epidemic form in neonatal nurseries. Outbreaks have in the past been associated with enteropathogenic *E. coli*, occasionally with *Salmonella* spp. and *Shigella* spp., but currently the most frequent nursery pathogen is human rotavirus.

Because the neonate withstands salt and water loss poorly, dehydration may rapidly occur. The infant shows signs such as loss of skin turgor, sunken eyes and fontanelle, dry mouth and oliguria.

Treatment consists of isolation from non-infected infants and replacement of electrolytes and water. Antibiotics are of no value unless there is evidence of systemic bacterial infection.

Prevention of acquired infections

The procedures detailed below will help to reduce and control infections.

Labour ward

1 Fastidious care in hand-washing.
2 The use of gloves for vaginal examinations, insertion of scalp electrodes and instrumental deliveries.

Nursery

1 Careful hand-washing is the key to reducing nosocomial infection. All staff and visitors should on entry into a neonatal unit wash their hands carefully with an antiseptic such as iodine or chlorhexidine. An alcohol hand rub should then be used before and after handling each infant.
2 Cleansing of incubators and equipment.
3 Routine baths for babies using hygienic soap solutions.
4 Aseptic surgical techniques for procedures such as intubation, umbilical catheterization, intravenous cannulation and lumbar punctures.
5 Isolation techniques for infectious babies.
6 Avoidance of overcrowding and restriction of nursery 'traffic' to a minimum.

Adjunctive therapy

Intravenous immunoglobulin therapy

A number of studies have evaluated the role of intravenous immunoglobulin (IVIG) infusion in infants with suspected or proven sepsis. Although most of these showed a modest reduction in mortality compared with controls, a recent Cochrane review (Ohlsson & Lacy 2006) concluded that there is insufficient evidence to support the routine use of IVIG in infants with suspected or proven infection.

Granulocyte transfusion

Septic premature infants often develop neutropenia, and attempts have been made to bolster the immune response in these babies by giving transfusions of granulocytes. Very few babies have been subjected to randomized controls, and to date there is no evidence that granulocyte transfusion reduces mortality.

G-CSF treatment

Haemopoietic colony stimulating factors (CSFs) for granulocytes (G-CSF) or granulocyte-macrophages (GM-CSF) have been evaluated either for prophylaxis or in the management of septic infants in a number of studies, but the number of enrolled infants remains small and no clear benefit has been shown.

References

Hughes RG, Brocklehurst P, Heath P. *Prevention of Early Onset Neonatal Group B StreptococcalD disease.* Recommendations from Green-top Guideline No 36. Royal College of Obstetricians and Gynaecologists, 2003, London.

Kieffer F, Thulliez P, Brezin A *et al.* Treatment of subclinical congenital toxoplasmosis by sulfadiazine and pyrimethamine continuously during 1 year. *Archives de Pediatrie* 2002;**9**:7–13.

Kite P, Millar MR, Gorham P, Congdon P. Comparison of five tests used in diagnosis of neonatal bacteraemia. *Arch Dis Child* 1988;**63**:639–643.

Ohlsson A, Lacy JB. Intravenous immunoglobulin for suspected or subsequently proven infection in neonates (Cochrane review). The Cochrane Library, Issue 3. Chichester, John Wiley & Sons, 2006.

RCOG. Green-top guideline No 36. 2003, London.

Rodwell RL, Leslie AL, Tudehope DI. Early diagnosis of neonatal sepsis using a haematological scoring system. *J Pediatr* 1988;**112**:761–767.

Rodwell RL, Taylor KM, Tudehope DI, Gray PH. Capillary plasma elastase L1-proteinase inhibitor in infected and non infected neonates. *Arch Dis Child* 1992;**67**:436–439.

Zenker PN, Berman SM. Congenital syphilis: trends and recommendations for evaluation and management. *Pediatr Infect Dis J* 1991;**10**:516–522.

Further reading

Heath PT, Nik Yusoff NK, Baker CJ. Neonatal meningitis. *Arch Dis Child Fetal Neonatal Ed* 2002;**88**:F173–F178.

Isaacs D, Moxon RE. *Handbook of Neonatal Infections. A Practical Guide.* London: W.B. Saunders, 1999.

Remington JS, Klein JO (eds). *Infectious Diseases of the Fetus and Newborn Infant*, 5th edn. Philadelphia: W.B. Saunders, 2001.

Royal College of Obstetricians and Gynaecologists. *Management of HIV in Pregnancy*. Guideline No 39.

CHAPTER 8

8 | # The low birthweight infant

Newborn infants may be classified according to birthweight, gestational age or size (large or small) for gestational age (Table 8.1). A low birthweight infant may be either preterm or small for gestational age, or both (Table 8.1). The problems these infants develop depend on whether the infants have been born too early or are born too small for the duration of gestation. The paediatrician therefore needs an objective test for the assessment of gestational age; the Dubowitz examination (Dubowitz *et al.* 1970), or its abbreviated version, the new Ballard examination (Ballard *et al.* 1991), is recommended. The Ballard examination quantifies six neurological and six physical parameters and should be performed with the baby fully exposed under a radiant heat warmer (Fig. 8.1).

The expanded New Ballard Score includes extremely premature infants and has been refined to improve accuracy in more mature infants.

The preterm infant (prematurity)

Clinical management of preterm labour

Premature birth has become the foremost problem of obstetric practice today. Although the high mortality and morbidity associated with preterm delivery have prompted a great deal of research into ways of predicting preterm birth with the hope of prevention, only limited benefits have resulted. Where possible, the woman in preterm labour <32 weeks' gestation should be transferred to a perinatal

Table 8.1 Classification of newborn infants according to birthweight, gestational age or size for gestational age

Factor	Terminology	Incidence (%)
Birthweight		
< 2500 g	= Low birthweight (LBW)	6.5
< 1500 g	= Very low birthweight (VLBW)	1.3
< 1000 g	= Extremely low birthweight (ELBW)	0.6
Gestational age (completed weeks after last normal menstrual period)		
< 37 weeks	= Preterm	8.4
> 41 weeks	= Post-term	0.6
Size for gestational age		
Weight between 90th and 10th centiles for gestation + 2 SD to − 2 SD from mean	= Appropriate for gestational age (AGA)	95
Weight < 10th centile for gestation	= Small for gestational age (SGA)	≈10
Weight > + 90th centile for gestation	= Large for gestational age (LGA)	≈10

SD, standard deviation.

(a)

Skin	Sticky friable transparent	Gelatinous red, translucent	Smooth pink, visible veins	Superficial peeling &/or rash, few veins	Cracking pale areas, rare veins	Parching deep cracking no vessels	Leathery cracked
Lanugo	None	Sparse	Abundant	Thinning	Bald areas	Mostly bald	
Plantar surface	Heel–toe 40–50 mm:−1 <40 mm: −2	>50 mm no crease	Faint red marks	Anterior transverse crease only	Creases ant. 2/3	Creases over entire sole	
Breast	Imperceptible	Barely perceptible	Flat areola no bud	Stippled areola 1–2 mm bud	Raised areola 3–4 mm bud	Full areola 5–10 mm bud	
Eye/ear	Lids fused loosely: −1 tightly:−2	Lids open pinna flat stays folded	Slightly curved pinna; soft; slow recoil	Well-curved pinna; soft but ready recoil	Formed & firm instant recoil	Thick cartilage ear stiff	
Genitals male	Scrotum flat, smooth	Scrotum empty Faint rugae	Testes in upper canal Rare rugae	Testes descending Few rugae	Testes down Good rugae	Testes pendulous Deep rugae	
Genitals female	Clitoris prominent Labia flat	Prominent clitoris Small labia minora	Prominent clitoris Enlarging minora	Majora & minora equally prominent	Majora large Minora small	Majora cover clitoris & minora	

Maturity rating	
Score	Weeks
−10	20
−5	22
0	24
5	26
10	28
15	30
20	32
25	34
30	36
35	38
40	40
45	42
50	44

(b)

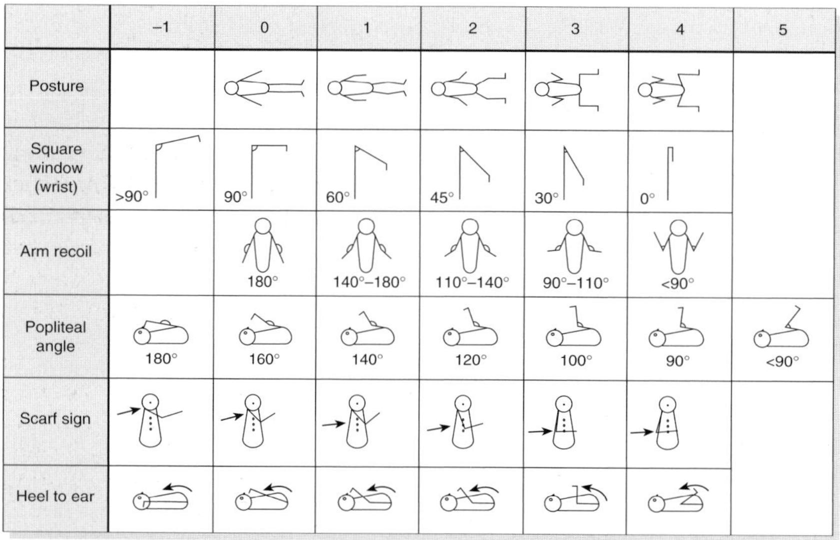

	−1	0	1	2	3	4	5
Posture							
Square window (wrist)	>90°	90°	60°	45°	30°	0°	
Arm recoil		180°	140°–180°	110°–140°	90°–110°	<90°	
Popliteal angle	180°	160°	140°	120°	100°	90°	<90°
Scarf sign							
Heel to ear							

Maturity rating	
Score	Weeks
−10	20
−5	22
0	24
5	26
10	28
15	30
20	32
25	34
30	36
35	38
40	40
45	42
50	44

Figure 8.1 The expanded New Ballard Score (see also p. 77). (Reproduced with permission from Ballard *et al.* 1991.)

intensive care unit where optimal delivery, resuscitation and subsequent management of her infant can be carried out. *In utero* transfer should only be attempted when the preterm labour is not advanced or can be safely and effectively suppressed with tocolytic agents. Obstetric management of preterm labour is rarely clearcut and is a balanced decision between the relative risks to mother and fetus of continuing the pregnancy versus those of a preterm birth.

When a patient is admitted with a diagnosis of possible 'preterm labour', the management plan depends on the following criteria:

1 Is the patient in active preterm labour?
2 Is there an underlying cause for the onset of labour?
3 Should steroids be given to the mother to enhance fetal lung maturity?
4 Should drugs be used to reduce uterine activity?

5 Are the mother and fetus at risk of infection?

6 Where is the baby to be delivered?

7 How is the baby to be delivered?

In general, there are few clearcut answers to these questions.

Suppression of preterm labour is sometimes possible and desirable with tocolytic agents such as beta-mimetics (e.g. terbutaline), calcium channel blockers (e.g. nifedipine), magnesium sulphate, oxytocin receptor antagonists (e.g. atosiban) or prostaglandin synthetase inhibitors (e.g. indometacin). Temporary suppression may enable *in utero* transport to a tertiary perinatal centre or the acceleration of fetal lung maturity with glucocorticoids. Suppression of labour is contraindicated in the presence of intrauterine infection, congenital anomaly, signs of fetal compromise or significant antepartum haemorrhage.

The inhibition of preterm labour by these drugs may allow for two doses of antenatal corticosteroids to accelerate fetal lung maturity. Betamethasone has been shown to be associated with fewer adverse effects than dexamethasone. Meta-analyses have consistently shown that corticosteroids given for 48 hours before delivery significantly reduce the incidence and severity of respiratory distress syndrome and the incidence of intraventricular haemorrhage, and possibly improve neurodevelopmental outcome.

Causes or risk factors for preterm delivery

Preterm breech presentation

The preferred mode of delivery for the preterm breech fetus has been the subject of considerable controversy. The hazards to the fetus of vaginal breech delivery include difficulty with delivery of the head and, rarely, entrapment of the aftercoming head. Although caesarean section in the preterm breech may be associated with some difficulties, it is probably the preferred method of delivery beyond 25 weeks' gestation.

Outcome for the preterm infant

Decision-making in the management of the extremely preterm delivery is influenced by the improved short- and long-term outcomes observed with the advances in perinatal care. Aggressive obstetric management and intervention for fetal reasons in late second-trimester deliveries is

practised in many tertiary perinatal centres, and these attitudes are partly responsible for the improved outcomes obtained. Practitioners in perinatal units should develop their own guidelines for the management of extremely preterm labour.

Published survival rates vary markedly from centre to centre, but also depend on the inclusion or exclusion of the following infants:

1 those with lethal congenital abnormalities;

2 birthweight <500 g or gestation <24 weeks;

3 born alive but not resuscitated or not resuscitatable;

4 considered previable and not admitted to intensive care;

5 those dying after the neonatal period (day 28).

Representative figures for survival rates are presented by birthweight and gestational age in Table 8.2. Figure 8.2 shows the risk of adverse outcome (death and severe neurodisability) for geographically identified populations of very immature babies born in Europe and Australia.

Transportation

The transportation of preterm infants to regional intensive care units presents special problems and it is recommended that high-risk preterm infants be transferred *in utero* where possible. Women in preterm labour <32 weeks' gestation should be delivered in a tertiary perinatal centre. When this is not

Table 8.2 Typical survival rates analysed by gestational age and birthweight for groups for Australian and New Zealand intensive care nurseries when baby is resuscitated and admitted for intensive care (Abeywardana 2006)

Gestation at birth (weeks)	Survival (%)	Birth weight (g)	Survival (%)
22 or less	<10	400–499	25
23	20	500–749	65
24	60	750–999	85
25	75	1000–1249	95
26	85	1250–1500	98
27	90	<1500	98
28–29	95		
30–32	99		

Source: Abeywardana S. Reports of the Australian and New Zealand Neonatal Network Sydney 2004, ANZNN 2006.

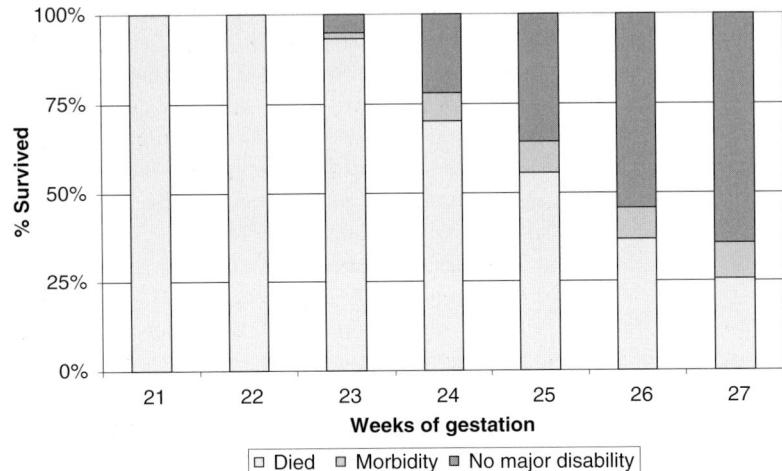

Figure 8.2 Incidence of mortality and severe morbidity from five geographically based studies. (Reproduced with permission from *Acta Paediatrica*.)

feasible, consideration should be given to transportation of infants of less than 1500 g birthweight. This decision will be influenced by the expertise and facilities of the referring hospital, as well as the safety and availability of transportation.

If an infant is to be transferred to an intensive care unit, then the unit with the best transport facilities should undertake the transfer. This usually means a team from the referral unit going out with a specially equipped transport incubator to retrieve the baby. It is essential that the infant be carefully assessed and completely stabilized before transportation. Procedures such as the insertion of an intravenous line, intubation and the initiation of mechanical ventilation are performed prior to transport if indicated. Trying to intubate in an ambulance is an uncomfortable experience! Neonatal transport is fully discussed in Chapter 26.

Specific problems of the preterm infant

During the final 3 months of intrauterine life most organ systems are undergoing important structural and functional development. Premature birth requires rapid adaptation to extrauterine life before these organ systems are adequately developed. The incidence and severity of all complications of prematurity are normally related to gestational age and birthweight. The main problems are:

1 perinatal asphyxia;

2 thermal instability;

3 lack of primitive survival reflexes – suck, swallow and gag – which may predispose the infant to milk aspiration;

4 jaundice;

5 pulmonary diseases – apnoea, respiratory distress syndrome, transient tachypnoea of the newborn, pneumothorax, pneumonia and bronchopulmonary dysplasia;

6 metabolic disturbances – hypoglycaemia, hypocalcaemia, hypomagnesaemia, hyponatraemia, hypernatraemia, hyperkalaemia;

7 patent ductus arteriosus – congestive heart failure;

8 neurological problems – intracranial haemorrhage (especially intraventricular haemorrhage), periventricular leukomalacia, ventricular dilatation;

9 susceptibility to infection, both perinatal acquisition and nosocomial;

10 gastrointestinal intolerance and necrotizing enterocolitis (NEC);

11 ophthalmic problems – retinopathy of prematurity, myopia, strabismus;

12 surgical lesions – undescended testes, inguinal and umbilical hernias;

13 haematological problems – haemorrhagic disease of prematurity, disseminated intravascular coagulation, iron deficiency anaemia;

14 renal immaturity – inability to concentrate urine, and inability to excrete an acid load with a low renal bicarbonate threshold, resulting in late metabolic acidosis. Late metabolic acidosis may be associated

with failure to gain weight satisfactorily. Treatment with sodium bicarbonate and a more appropriate formula or expressed breast milk should result in a satisfactory response.

The specific problems of prematurity are discussed in the appropriate chapters.

Supportive care of the preterm infant

Resuscitation

Perinatal consultation should occur between all clinical staff to optimize care of mother and preterm infant. Perinatal asphyxia is a major risk of preterm delivery, and personnel competent in neonatal resuscitation should always be present. Airway stabilization with continuous positive airway pressure or mechanical ventilation has been widely practised in infants <32 weeks' gestation. The use of pulse oximetry in the delivery room is used to assess the response to resuscitation. If intubation is required, the prophylactic use of exogenous surfactant is recommended.

Monitoring

Heart rate, respiratory rate, blood pressure and temperature must be monitored continuously, with appropriate alarm signals, if cardiopulmonary disease is present.

Oxygen therapy

Many sick preterm infants require oxygen therapy to relieve hypoxia. Oxygen is a toxic substance in the preterm infant, and may cause retinopathy of prematurity. It must therefore be administered with the utmost care and the response continuously monitored with a pulse oximeter and/or transcutaneous Po_2 monitoring. Regular measurements of P_aO_2 are made in premature infants requiring extra oxygen to minimize complications such as retinopathy of prematurity and chronic lung disease. It is dangerous to treat ill premature infants where adequate blood-gas oxygen monitoring is not available. Research studies are currently underway to determine target O_2 saturation levels but in the interim the arterial oxygen tension should probably be maintained between 50 and 80 mmHg (6.2–10 kPa) and O_2 saturation at 85–95%. Whether oxygen is administered directly into the incubator, via a headbox, nasal prongs, continuous positive airway pressure tube or endotracheal tube, its use must be monitored very carefully. Oxygen should be warmed to 35–37°C, humidified to 28–38 mg H_2O/L, and the inspired concentration continuously recorded with high and low alarms set.

Continuous oxygen monitoring

1. Transcutaneous oxygen monitors (± transcutaneous carbon dioxide monitor). These devices utilize a small heating element to heat the skin to 43–44°C and induce hyperaemia to arterialize the capillary blood and oxygen (±CO_2) diffusing through the skin, which is monitored continuously.
2. Pulse oximetry utilizes analysis of light transmitted through tissues to measure haemoglobin oxygen saturation in arterial blood.
3. An oxygen-sensitive probe attached to the tip of an umbilical arterial catheter provides a continuous readout of arterial oxygen tension.

Intermittent oxygen monitoring

Arterial catheterization of an umbilical (p. 304) or peripheral artery (p. 307) provides a readily available site for sampling arterial blood for blood gases, electrolytes and blood glucose, and continuous blood pressure monitoring. Intermittent arterial stabs are less reliable for monitoring P_aO_2, and capillary sampling is not reliable.

Blood pressure

Arterial blood pressure is an important variable to measure. If an indwelling arterial catheter is *in situ*, it can be attached to an electronic pressure transducer to measure blood pressure. Alternatively, a mechanical oscillometric device can be used, attached to a blood pressure cuff. Normal blood pressure ranges are shown on p. 177. Blood pressure varies with gestational age and birthweight and normally increases over the first 24 h of life. Maintenance of an adequate and stable cerebral blood flow is important to avoid cerebral ischaemic and haemorrhagic damage. Mean blood pressure should probably be kept above the infant's gestational age in weeks and postnatal age in days for the first 4 days of life, with the aid of crystalloid infusion and inotropic agents.

Thermoregulation

Body temperature must be maintained in the normal range (36.5–37.0°C per axilla) by nursing the preterm infant under an open radiant heat source or in a closed incubator (see Chapter 9).

Feeding

Infants of less than 34 weeks' postmenstrual age do not have a good suck or swallow reflex and should usually be fed via an orogastric or nasogastric tube. Premature infants with small gastric capacity require frequent feeding (sometimes every 1–2 h) and should be started on 1–2 mL/kg per feed, increasing in increments of 1–2 mL/kg, as tolerated. The frequency of feeds is dependent on gestational age but generally those <34 weeks commence on 2-hourly feeds and those >34 weeks are fed 3-hourly. Gastric aspirate must be checked before the next feed. Occasionally, this regimen is not tolerated, and a continuous infusion of milk via an orogastric or nasojejunal tube will be necessary. This feeding technique is particularly applicable to infants of birthweight <1000 g or <29 weeks' gestational age (see Chapter 6).

Parenteral fluids

Sick babies and infants of less than 1500 g or 32 weeks' gestation may need parenteral fluids with 10% dextrose infusion into the umbilical or a peripheral vein. Sometimes intravenous alimentation with dextrose, crystalline L-amino acid solution and fat emulsion will be necessary (see Chapter 6) as enteral feeding is slowly introduced.

The fluid requirements of ill preterm infants depend on a variety of factors, including postnatal age, renal function and transepidermal water loss. Consequently, the fluid intake is estimated on the basis of urine output, weight, serum electrolytes and urinary concentration. Water requirements will be increased for phototherapy (approximately an extra 20 mL/kg/day) and open radiant incubators (approximately an extra 20 mL/kg/day). Sick preterm infants, especially those with respiratory distress syndrome (RDS) and patent ductus arteriosus, should receive restricted fluid volumes until renal output is well established. The use of servocontrol humidity and temperature incubators decreases insensible water loss in preterm infants.

In addition, the electrolyte requirement for premature infants is increased owing to the poor conservation by the immature kidneys. Close monitoring of serum electrolytes, including calcium, is necessary in order to replace losses adequately. Infants with severe late metabolic acidosis should have their maintenance sodium as sodium bicarbonate.

Jaundice

This is extremely common in the preterm infant and must be followed with frequent bilirubin estimations. Jaundice of prematurity is a diagnosis of exclusion after other causes have been eliminated. Preterm infants are more prone to bilirubin encephalopathy than term infants, and factors that affect the entry of free bilirubin into the brain include low albumin levels, acidosis, hypoxia, hypoglycaemia, hypothermia, certain drugs and starvation. Guidelines for the management of hyperbilirubinaemia are shown on p. 136.

Respiratory distress syndrome (RDS)

(see Chapter 10)

Even with the advent of tocolytic suppression of preterm labour and use of antenatal corticosteroids, RDS remains the major problem of prematurity today. Most preterm infants who die have hyaline membranes demonstrated at autopsy, but may also have evidence of intraventricular haemorrhage, patent ductus arteriosus, pneumothorax, NEC and bronchopulmonary dysplasia.

For infants of birthweight <800 g or <26 weeks' gestation it may be desirable to intubate and ventilate from birth to provide initial airway stabilization. For other infants <32 weeks' gestation, airway stabilization at birth with continous positive airway pressure (CPAP) is widely practised. Exogenous surfactant should be administered via the endotracheal tube prior to 2 h of age. Babies of birthweight <2000 g with RDS are best managed in an intensive care nursery.

Vitamins

A single intramuscular dose of 0.5–1.0 mg of vitamin K is adequate unless the baby is receiving broad-spectrum antibiotics, when twice-weekly injections are necessary to compensate for loss of the endogenous vitamin K normally produced by bowel flora. Sick preterm infants requiring intravenous alimentation should receive additional multivitamins.

Preterm infants who require total parenteral nutrition (TPN) receive supplemental water and fat-soluble vitamins. Preterm formulas are supplemented with vitamins. Preterm infants <32 weeks' gestation should have human milk fortifier added to expressed breast milk (EBM). Once a preterm infant <34 weeks' gestation is tolerating full feeds a multivitamin preparation such as Pentavite 0.5 mL or Abidec drops 0.6 mL is given.

Anaemia

Some sick preterm infants will be anaemic at birth or develop anaemia in the first week of life as a result of frequent blood sampling, and will require a transfusion with packed red blood cells cross-matched against mother and baby. The venous haematocrit should be maintained at more than 0.35% (haemoglobin 12 g/dL) in all sick babies with RDS. However, during the physiological trough of anaemia preterm infants may tolerate a haemoglobin concentration of 7 g/dL (haematocrit 0.25%), especially if there is an adequate reticulocyte response (>5%). To prevent iron deficiency anaemia, so prevalent after 3 months of age, all preterm infants less than 1800 g birthweight or 34 weeks' gestation should receive supplemental iron (ferrous sulphate 0.5 mL/day) from the age of 3 weeks.

Preparation for discharge

The transition from hospital to home is a crucial step in the future wellbeing of the family. Once the requirements for intensive care are over, the baby will still need monitoring, incubator care and gavage feedings. This can be a very frustrating time for the parents, who have already experienced so much. Early discharge for low birthweight infants can be safely practised and may promote attachment. The baby may be discharged at 1900–2300 g, provided feeding is progressing well, weight gain is steady, the mother is handling her baby competently and the home situation is good.

Small for gestational age infant

Although several synonyms have been used to describe the growth-restricted infant, including Clifford syndrome, dysmaturity, light for dates, small for dates and intrauterine growth restriction, the preferred term, based on common usage, is now 'small for gestational age' (SGA). There has been no such uniformity in the definition of SGA. From a statistical viewpoint, infants born at any gestational age and weighing more than two standard deviations below the mean can be defined as SGA. However, because they share common clinical problems, infants of birthweight at or below the 10th centile for gestational age are often regarded as SGA. Furthermore, many neonates with birthweights above the 10th centile will demonstrate evidence of acute or chronic weight loss, and should therefore fall into the spectrum of the growth-restricted infant. Variables such as sex, race and altitude should be considered when determining growth curves, because a birthweight below the 10th centile in one population may not fall below the 10th centile growth curve in another, even though growth restriction may be present in both instances. Table 8.3 lists important factors that

Table 8.3 Determinants of birthweight

Maternal factors before conception:
Stature
Weight
Genotype
Race
Age
Parity
Socioeconomic status (occupation, education, income)

Factors at or around conception:
Fetal genotype
Singleton or multiple conception
Fetal sex
Genetic anomaly (chromosomal or major gene locus)

Factors between conception and birth:
Altitude
Fetal or maternal infection (rubella, malaria)
Maternal work
Maternal cigarette smoking
Maternal diet
Maternal alcohol, drugs, medications

predict birthweight of an individual fetus or neonate (customized fetal growth curves) or for a given population.

Classification of SGA infants

Subdividing the heterogeneous SGA population into more homogeneous groups offers the potential to establish a better understanding of the underlying cause of the problem, and therefore more accurate prognoses and more appropriate plans for postnatal management.

It is important to attempt to define the neonate 'starved' as a result of intrauterine growth restriction (IUGR). These babies show growth failure greatest for weight, then length; head circumference is the least affected. There is little subcutaneous fat, the skin may be loose and thin, muscle mass is decreased, especially buttocks and thighs, and the infant often exhibits wide-eyed, anxious facies. This type can be distinguished from the uniformly growth-retarded type, which implies either a fetal cause (e.g. chromosomal) or a very early insult.

Subcutaneous fat can be objectively assessed by measuring the circumference of the mid-upper arm or by measuring skinfold thickness with special calipers. A simpler measurement is the Ponderal index. This is derived from accurate measurements of the infant's length and weight and calculated from the formula:

$$\text{Ponderal Index (PI)} = \frac{\text{Birthweight in (g)}}{\text{Length}^3 \text{(cm)}} \times 100 \qquad (8.1)$$

A normal PI is ≥2.41 and a low PI is <2.41. Table 8.4 shows the major differences between the proportionate and the disproportionate SGA infant.

Causes of IUGR

The causes of IUGR can be classified according to whether they are fetal, placental or maternal (Table 8.5). The growth failure can be classified as 'intrinsic', which implies an abnormality at the time of conception or within the first trimester (fetal and some maternal causes), or 'extrinsic', implying a later onset of growth restriction (placental and some maternal causes).

Table 8.4 Classification of the growth-restricted fetus and the SGA infant

Proportionate (type I IUGR)		Disproportionate (type II IUGR)
Symmetrical	vs	Asymmetrical
Normal Ponderal Index	vs	Low Ponderal Index
Intrinsic cause	vs	Extrinsic cause
Hypoplastic	vs	Hypotrophic

Many growth-restricted infants exhibit a mixture of classifications.

Table 8.5 Cause of intrauterine growth restriction

Fetal	Placental	Maternal
Chromosomal abnormalities	Toxaemia of pregnancy	Maternal disease
Prenatal viral infection	Multiple pregnancy	Alcohol
Dysmorphic syndromes	Small placental size	Smoking
X-rays	Site of implantation	Malnutrition
	Vascular transfusion in monochorial twin placentas	Altitude

Intrinsic fetal growth restriction

Early-onset growth restriction, which tends to give rise to an SGA infant who is proportionate, symmetrical and hypoplastic and has a normal PI, is more likely to have an intrinsic cause of growth failure. During the first trimester, global insults include chromosomal anomalies (e.g. trisomy syndromes), perinatal infections (e.g. TORCH: toxoplasmosis, other, rubella, cytomegalovirus, herpes simplex type II), dwarfing syndromes (e.g. achondroplasia, chondrodystrophic dwarfism, Russell–Silver syndrome), maternal recreational drug abuse (e.g. alcohol, narcotics, cocaine) and exposure to teratogenic drugs and ionizing radiation.

Constitutional growth restriction relates to parental stature and racial and ethnic factors. These infants, often referred to as having type I growth restriction, show symmetrical growth restriction, with similar growth reductions in weight, length and head circumference. They do not exhibit a head-sparing effect and, because of a decreased number of cells, as well as decreased cell size, do not have the potential for normal growth. Fortunately, this group comprises only about 10–30% of all SGA babies in modern Western societies, but if they are evaluated after the first trimester by ultrasound assessment of biparietal diameter, an inappropriately low assessment of gestational age may result.

Extrinsic fetal growth restriction

Later onset of fetal growth restriction results from disorders of the placenta or from maternal problems. Extrinsic mechanisms operate during the latter half of pregnancy and are associated with impaired delivery of oxygen and nutrients from the placenta. These factors may become operative at different times during pregnancy, resulting in less predictable effects on fetal growth. Maternal factors include hypertension (e.g. essential, pregnancy-induced, renal), diabetes mellitus with vascular complications, renal disease, cardiac disease, sickle-cell disease and collagen disorders. Maternal smoking, alcohol and narcotic abuse and maternal hypoxia (e.g. cardiac disease, pulmonary disease, residence at high altitude) may also cause IUGR.

Placental factors

These all have the common feature of diminished placental blood flow, which may become more severe later in pregnancy. Twins will show a normal rate of intrauterine growth until the demands of the two fetuses outstrip the placental blood supply. This usually occurs at about 32 weeks' gestation, and fetal growth rates fall off from this time. SGA infants occur in 24–40% of twin pregnancies. Placental disorders associated with IUGR include chronic villitis, haemorrhagic endovasculitis, chorioangioma, chronic abruptio placentae, hydatidiform degeneration, single umbilical artery and twin–twin transfusion syndrome.

Specific problems of the growth-restricted fetus and sga infant

When considering the problems of SGA babies, it seems more appropriate to compare them with their gestational age peers rather than with babies of similar birthweight.

When IUGR results from restricted nutrient supply, the fetus adapts to maximize the prospect of good outcome by sparing brain growth, accelerating pulmonary maturity and increasing the red cell mass (polycythaemia). These features may initially represent important adaptational strategies, but they later become pathological when deprivation is more extreme and fetal distress supervenes. Table 8.6 summarizes the problems that these fetuses and babies may face.

Neonatal period

Perinatal asphyxia. Fetuses with chronic distress do not tolerate the additional hypoxic stress of delivery well, and they readily develop hypoxia and acidosis.

Congenital malformations. There is a 20-fold increased incidence of congenital malformation in SGA babies compared with their normal birthweight peers.

Infection. There is a ninefold increased incidence of infection. This is partly explained by the greater incidence of TORCH infections, but also relates to a greater incidence of acquired infection.

Table 8.6 Anticipated problems in the fetus/neonate who is small for gestational age (SGA)

Fetus	Newborn	Subsequent outcome
Stillbirth	Asphyxia	Impaired growth
Fetal distress	Hypoglycaemia	Intellectual deficit
Meconium aspiration	Meconium aspiration syndrome	Cerebral palsy (due to asphyxia)
Oligohydramnios	Polycythaemia	
Congenital malformation	Hyperviscosity	
Deformations	Hypothermia	
Cord compression	Hypocalcaemia	
Premature rupture of membranes	Infection (impaired immune system)	
Preterm delivery	Pulmonary haemorrhage	
	Transient neonatal hyperglycaemia	

Hypoglycaemia. SGA infants have deficient hepatic and cardiac muscle glycogen stores and a limited capacity for gluconeogenesis. Hypoglycaemia is usually asymptomatic, but minor or major symptoms may develop if appropriate treatment is not instituted.

Hypocalcaemia. The increased incidence of hypocalcaemia relates to the birth asphyxia and not to SGA infants *per se.*

Polycythaemia. This is a common problem, especially when there has been prolonged intrauterine hypoxia resulting in elevated levels of erythropoietin.

Thermal instability. Maintenance of body temperature is a problem to the SGA infant, but less so than for the preterm infant. This probably relates to the large surface area to body weight ratio.

Respiratory distress. Respiratory distress in the SGA infant may be due to meconium aspiration, polycythaemia, massive pulmonary haemorrhage or pneumonia, but is not usually due to RDS. Growth restriction in extremely preterm infants does not protect them against RDS or subsequent chronic neonatal lung disease.

Infancy and childhood

Growth

In the neonatal period the infant loses little weight and begins to gain weight rapidly after birth. However, this growth spurt is often not maintained and a permanent deficit in somatic growth may persist into childhood.

Full-term growth-restricted infants stand a good chance of catching up, particularly if growth restriction is due to maternal factors. Infants who are both severely preterm and growth restricted are much less likely to reach average size than infants of the same degree of prematurity but who are normally grown. If catch-up growth is going to occur, it usually does so by 6 months. Infants with intrinsic causes of fetal growth restriction exhibit minimal or no catchup growth and remain lighter, shorter and with smaller head circumference at 3 years of age.

Development

The ultimate outcome relates to the cause of aberrant growth, the timing and duration of intrauterine insult, the severity of growth restriction, the degree of asphyxia, the postnatal course and the socioecomonic status of the infant's family.

A number of follow-up studies have shown that SGA infants born at term are prone to more developmental, behavioural and learning problems than infants born mildly preterm, and males are more vulnerable than females. A baby who is both SGA and premature is predisposed to a greater risk of serious neurological abnormalities than if he or she were only premature or only SGA. If catch-up in head growth occurs, then the eventual IQ score is higher than in those infants whose head remains small.

The Barker hypothesis

A large number of epidemiology studies have shown a relationship between small birth size and the subsequent risk of type 2 diabetes, insulin resistance, hypertension, cardiovascular disease and stroke. This is thought to be mediated through insulin-like growth factor 2 (IGF-2) and is referred to as the Barker hypothesis after David Barker, who first made these observations. This programming is thought to be due to an evolutionary adaptation whereby the growth-restricted fetus alters its physiology in expectation of a particular postnatal environment in that longer term growth is restricted, which is an advantage in a hostile environment where food is not plentiful. This has been referred to as the 'thrifty phenotype'. In a modern society where food is plentiful this phenotype is predisposed to atherogenesis and cardiovascular disease in later life.

Management

The appreciation that a fetus is growth restricted or that a baby is SGA will greatly influence management.

If IUGR is suspected, careful monitoring of fetal and uteroplacental function will be necessary, with tests such as serial ultrasound scans, Doppler assessment of umbilical flow, cardiotocography and Lecithin/Sphinomyelin (L/S) ratio on amniotic fluid prior to early delivery.

A considered decision regarding the best method and timing of delivery will need to be made. If it is elected to deliver vaginally, then continuous intrapartum fetal heart rate monitoring should be undertaken. A paediatrician or other skilled resuscitationist should attend the delivery and suction the trachea under direct vision, if necessary, to prevent meconium aspiration.

If severely growth restricted, the baby should be transferred to a special care nursery for observation for signs of respiratory distress, hypoglycaemia and temperature instability. Usually incubator care will be necessary.

If catch-up growth is to occur and the child is to reach his or her full growth and intellectual potential, adequate and early feeding is essential. The SGA infant should commence feeds at 2 h of age, if possible, and initially feeding should be every 2 h with dextrose. Estimates of blood glucose should be made before alternate feeds. The first feed should be full-strength breast milk or formula. Feeding regimens are discussed in Chapter 6. The expected weight of the SGA infant should be calculated by estimating the 50th percentile weight for the infant's gestation and then feeding the infant to a weight halfway between that weight and the actual weight. The infant should receive at least 60 mL/kg on day 1, and increase up to 200 mL/kg of expected weight.

If the infant develops hypoglycaemia (heel-prick estimate <2.6 mmol/L despite early feeding), 10% dextrose is given by uninterrupted intravenous infusion, in addition to the oral feed.

A capillary haematocrit should be performed at 4–6 h of age. If this is greater than 70%, a venous haematocrit is indicated. If the venous haematocrit is greater than 70%, or if the baby has symptoms of polycythaemia, an isovolaemic, dilutional exchange transfusion with plasma (30 mL/kg) is indicated.

A careful examination for congenital malformations should always be made. The most common anomaly is a single umbilical artery. The baby should be examined for features suggestive of intrauterine infection, such as hepatosplenomegaly, petechiae, cataracts and microcephaly. If an intrauterine infection is likely, or even if there is no obvious cause for growth retardation, a cord blood immunoglobulin M (IgM) level and appropriate

TORCH serology should be performed. In case the infant is infected, he or she should be isolated and barrier nursed.

When two or more dysmorphic features are present, chromosome analysis should be undertaken.

PRINCIPLES OF MANAGEMENT

- Perinatal consultation between clinical staff optimizes management of mother and preterm or growth-restricted infant.
- Infants <33 weeks' gestation require specialized neonatal care.
- The decision whether to actively resuscitate a marginally viable preterm infant (22–25 weeks) depends on individual policy of the neonatal intensive care unit and parental choice.
- Extremely preterm infants requiring intubation at birth should receive prophylactic surfactant.

References

Abeywardana S. *Report of the Australian and New Zealand Neonatal Network 2004*. Sydney: ANZNN, 2006.

Ballard JL, Khoury JC, Wedig K et al. New Ballard Score, expanded to include extremely premature infants. *J Pediatr* 1991;**119**:417–423.

Dubowitz LMS, Dubowitz V, Goldberg C. Clinical assessment of gestational age in the newborn infant. *J Pediatr* 1970;**77**:1.

Levene MI, Dubowitz LMS. Low birth weight babies: long-term follow-up. *Brit J Hosp Med* 1982;Nov:487–493.

Further reading

MacDonald MG, Mullett MD, Seshia MK (eds). *Avery's Neonatology: Pathophysiology and Management of the Newborn*, 5th edn. Philadelphia: Lippincott-Raven, 2005.

Peebles D (ed.) Fetal growth restriction. *Semin Fetal Neonat Med* 2004;**9**.

Rennie JM, Roberton NRC (ed.) *Textbook of Neonatology*, 3rd edn. Edinburgh: Churchill Livingstone, 1999.

Spitzer AR. *Intensive Care of the Fetus and Neonate*, 3rd edn. St Louis: Mosby, 1996.

CHAPTER 9

9 Thermoregulation

The full-term infant is a homeotherm but his or her ability to regulate body temperature is not as effective as that of older children or adults. The small for gestational age (SGA) infant, and particularly the preterm infant, have greater problems than the normally grown full-term baby in maintaining body temperature. After birth, deep body and skin temperature of the term newborn can drop at a rate of approximately 0.1°C and 0.3°C per minute, respectively, unless immediate action is taken

An infant's temperature depends on the site at which the measurement is made. Normal central (or core) temperature ranges between 36.7°C and 37.3°C, and can be measured by a rectal thermometer; however, this is not routine practice and should be avoided. Axillary temperature approximates to core temperature, and the thermometer needs to be left for at least 2 min. It is the preferred route for recording temperature in newborn babies. Skin temperature is lower than core temperature and is recorded by taping a thermistor to the abdomen. Normal abdominal temperature is 35.5–36.5°C in a term infant and 36.2–37.2°C in small premature infants. If the difference between abdominal and peripheral (e.g. toe) temperature is large, then the infant is vasoconstricted to conserve heat (or because he or she is infected or shocked). If the difference is small, the infant is vasodilated and attempting to lose heat.

The World Health Organization classifies a core body temperature for newborns of 36–36.4°C as mild hypothermia, 32–35.9°C as moderate and <32°C as severe hypothermia.

Mechanisms of heat loss

Heat is lost from the body to the environment via the following four standard physical mechanisms:

- *Evaporation*. When a moist baby is exposed to room temperature there is conversion of water to vapour, with subsequent loss of heat.
- *Radiation*. Heat is dissipated down a concentration gradient via the surrounding air.
- *Conduction*. There is direct heat loss from the skin to cooler objects, such as a cold wrap, cold towel or wet nappy.
- *Convection*. Heat loss occurs via a current of moving air.

Mechanisms to conserve heat

When exposed to cold the normal baby tries to conserve heat by a variety of means:
1 Peripheral vasoconstriction.
2 Increased heat production through
   (a) increased basal metabolism with increased oxygen consumption;
   (b) increased voluntary muscular activity;
   (c) involuntary muscular activity – shivering. Shivering is virtually non-existent in preterm infants and their ability to increase muscular activity is limited;
3 Non-shivering thermogenesis. Full-term infants are born with a layer of brown fat, mainly around the neck, between the scapulae and along the aorta. Brown fat can be rapidly metabolized to generate heat, and this is under the control of the sympathetic nervous system.

Why is the newborn prone to heat loss?

There are several reasons why the newborn is particularly susceptible to heat loss:
1 Large surface area to body weight ratio. A preterm infant's limited ability to flex limbs and trunk increases the exposed surface area for heat loss.

2 Limited ability to shiver.

3 Deficiency of subcutaneous fat tissue.

4 Relative deficiency of brown fat and glycogen.

5 The baby is often born covered in liquor, vernix, meconium or blood. Moist skin predisposes to loss of heat and fluid by evaporation.

Prevention of excessive heat loss

Labour ward

The provision of warmth and prevention of heat loss is the first essential step in resuscitation of the newborn. The baby must be dried completely with a prewarmed, sterile wrap. Additional measures to reduce heat loss in the immediate postnatal period fall into two groups: (i) barriers to heat loss and (ii) external heat sources.

Interventions in the first group focus mainly on reducing evaporative heat losses and include wraps and/or head coverings made from a variety of materials. Transparent plastic coverings such as bubble wrap and single layer gowns are effective in the delivery suite for full-term healthy newborn infants and those with birth weights >2000 g, respectively, and the intervention with polyethylene wrap is preferable for infants of <33 weeks' gestation. In some centres very immature babies are placed into a prewarmed plastic bag with a drawstring around the baby's neck to allow access to mouth and nose. This is a very effective way of reducing heat and insensible water losses.

Interventions in the second group include heated mattresses and radiant warmers. For a healthy term newborn skin-to-skin contact, (where the infant is thoroughly dried and placed on the mother's chest and abdomen with a light blanket around them), can reduce radiant and conductive heat loss, promote temperature stabilization and improve bonding.

Nursery

1 Very low birthweight (VLBW) infants do not have a superficial layer of keratin, and consequently water and heat are lost through the permeable skin. Adequate ambient humidity in the incubator will prevent this.

2 Reduce radiant and convective heat loss by dressing the infant whenever possible.

3 Prevent radiant heat loss from the infant by avoiding positioning him or her near a cold window. A warm incubator (particularly if double walled) will also reduce radiant loss, and heat loss is further limited by a perspex heat shield over the infant.

4 Avoid placing the infant in draughts. A perspex shield over the infant with the foot end blocked off will prevent draughts in the incubator.

5 Never place an infant on a cold surface or in a cold cot.

6 Whenever possible the infant should be clothed, especially with a bonnet, bootees and jacket, to reduce thermal gradients.

Thermoneutral environment

The thermoneutral environment is the ambient temperature at which oxygen consumption and energy expenditure are at a minimum to maintain vital activities.

If an infant is cold, he or she will attempt to keep warm via the mechanisms listed above, including shivering, vasoconstriction and increased activity. These are energy-requiring processes. Similarly, an infant who is too hot will vasodilate and sweat (also using extra energy) to stay cool. The ambient temperature at which the infant uses the least energy to maintain body temperature is referred to as the thermoneutral environmental temperature (Fig. 9.1).

The thermoneutral temperature in an individual infant depends on birthweight and gestational age. Hey (1971) has devised charts to predict the appropriate incubator temperature for various groups of infants (Fig. 9.1). The thermoneutral temperature also varies depending on whether the infant is nursed dressed or undressed. These charts were devised by measuring the oxygen consumption of normal infants and may not be reliable for critically ill babies (Table 9.1).

Incubator care

Ill or small infants are nursed in incubators, which are of two types, closed and open.

Closed incubator

These are designed to reduce heat loss. The baby is enclosed in a perspex box with various ports and doors for access. A heater keeps the air warm, which

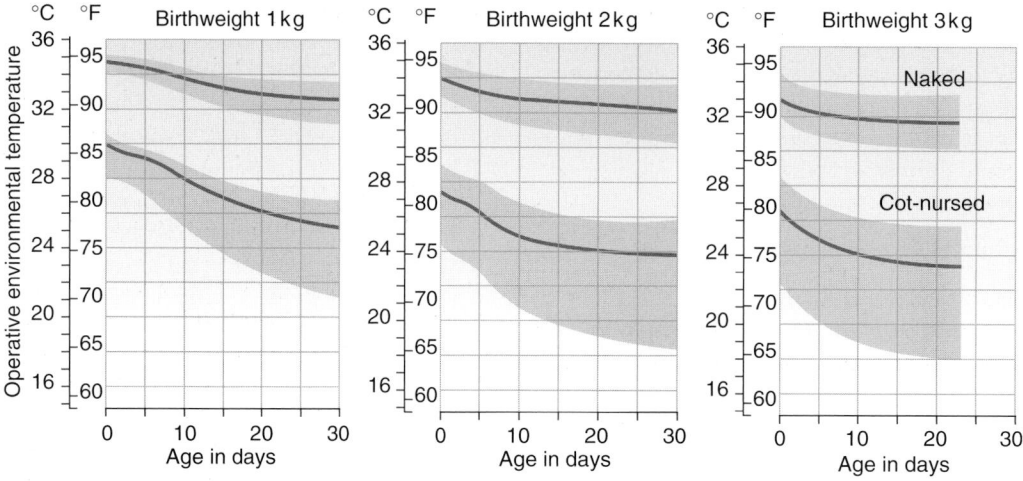

Figure 9.1 The thermoneutral temperature range for three birthweight groups of healthy babies. The upper graph represents infants nursed naked and the lower is for clothed babies. (Reproduced with permission from Hey 1971.)

Table 9.1 The mean temperature needed to provide thermal neutrality for a healthy baby nursed naked in draught-free surroundings of uniform temperature and moderate humidity. (Reproduced with permission from Hey 1975)

Birthweight (kg)	Operative environmental temperature*			
	35°C	34°C	33°C	32°C
1.0	For 10 days →	After 10 days →	After 3 weeks →	After 5 weeks
1.5	—	For 10 days →	After 10 days →	After 4 weeks
2.0	—	For 2 days →	After 2 days →	After 3 weeks
>2.5	—	—	For 2 days →	After 2 days

*To estimate operative temperature in a single-walled incubator, subtract 1°C from incubator air temperature for every 7°C by which this temperature exceeds room temperature. Clothed babies require lower incubator temperatures.

is circulated by a fan. With modern incubators the infant can be nursed in either air mode or baby mode. In the former a thermistor within the incubator detects the environmental temperature and regulates the heater to maintain air at a constant preset temperature. The baby's temperature must be checked regularly. Baby mode (sensor-controlled) incubators rely on a thermistor attached to the baby, so the heater is regulated to keep the infant's temperature constant. Overheating can occur if the thermistor becomes detached from the baby.

Incubators usually have the facility to humidify the ambient air. This is valuable in infants of 1500 g and below to prevent excessive evaporative water and heat loss from the immature skin. All VLBW or cold infants (temperature <35°C) should be nursed in humidified incubators. However, such incubators carry the risk of bacterial contamination with *Pseudomonas aeruginosa* or, less commonly, *Serratia* spp., which colonize the water reservoir and may lead to neonatal infection. The water should be changed every 24 h and cultured to detect these organisms. Normally humidification is only necessary during the first week of life in VLBW infants, because after this time the formation of a keratin layer waterproofs the skin.

Open incubator (radiant warmer)

The infant lies on a mattress under a heating element which delivers radiant heat energy. A thin, clear plastic blanket (bubblewrap or clingfilm) reduces insensible water loss. It works on a servo-controlled mechanism by means of a thermistor on the baby's abdominal wall, and the radiant heater is automatically switched on and off to maintain body temperature at a preset level (usually 36.5°C).

The great advantage of this device is that it gives easy access to the infant for surgical or nursing procedures. It is also useful for rapidly warming cold babies (see below). Its disadvantages are obvious in that heat loss is large and transepidermal water loss considerable, particularly in the most immature babies. Careful fluid and electrolyte balance is essential (see p. 45). In some units a perspex heat shield with one end closed is placed between the infant and the radiant heater to reduce water loss and prevent draughts. In general closed incubators are associated with fewer complications than open radiant incubators.

Skin covering

The use of semipermeable non-adhesive dressings lowers the transepidermal water loss without any increased risk of colonization with bacteria. Emolients are also considered to be effective in preventing water loss and protecting skin from cracking and fissuring. Their effect lasts only for about 3 hours necessitating repeated application.

Ventilator humidity

It is important to use adequate humidification in all ventilator circuits as there can be high fluid and heat loss in babies being ventilated.

Phototherapy

Excessive transepidermal water loss can still occur in babies receiving phototherapy despite stable temperature and humidity. Such babies require careful monitoring of their fluid balance

Transport

This presents a major challenge as temperature control can be particularly difficult in very low birthweight babies. Despite adequate incubator temperature, there is often a high radiant heat loss, epecially in cold weather. This can be reduced by covering the incubator and wrapping the baby in blankets. Evaporative heat loss can be reduced by placing the baby in plastic bags. Heated mattresses can also be used during transport, with the baby getting heat by conduction.

Neonatal cold injury

Prolonged exposure to a cold environment increases oxygen consumption and glucose utilization, and consequently the baby readily becomes hypoxic and hypoglycaemic. There is peripheral cyanosis with redness of the face, refusal to feed and lethargy, followed by oedema and sclerema (localized hardening of the subcutaneous tissue). Cold-stressed babies may develop apnoeic spells, worsening of their respiratory distress syndrome, severe metabolic acidosis, hypoglycaemia, pulmonary haemorrhage and intracranial haemorrhage.

Hypoglycaemia and metabolic acidosis are most likely to occur when the infant is being warmed. Restoration of metabolic processes creates a demand for glucose and this should be anticipated. Regular stick tests for glucose must be performed. As blood pressure and perfusion improve the products of anaerobic metabolism are washed out into the circulation, causing a severe metabolic acidosis.

Therapeutic hypothermia

Controlled mild-to-moderate hypothermia (33–34°C) has been proposed as treatment for potentially brain-injured- and near-term babies. This technique has shown beneficial effects in experimental animal models, and now there is increasing evidence of its beneficial neuroprotective effect in babies born with moderate asphyxia. The therapeutic value of mild hypothermia is discussed in more detail on p. 22.

References

Hey EN. The care of babies in incubators. In: *Recent Advances in Paediatrics* (eds D. Gairdner & D. Hull). London: Churchill Livingstone, 1971, pp. 171–216.

Hey EN. Thermal neutrality. *Brit Med Bulle* 1975; **31**:69–74.

Further reading

Leone TA, Finer NN. Fetal adaptation at birth. *Curr Paediatr* 2006;**16**:373–378.

Lyon A. Temperature control in the newborn infant. *Curr Paediatr* 2006;**16**:386–392.

CHAPTER 10

10 Respiratory disorders

At birth major cardiopulmonary changes take place in order to prepare the baby for extrauterine existence. The fluid in the fetal lung is rapidly replaced by air. Associated with lung inflation and increased oxygenation there is a marked decrease in the pulmonary vascular resistance, with consequent increased pulmonary blood flow and closure of the ductus arteriosus, foramen ovale and ductus venosus. As a result the lungs take over the respiratory function previously carried out by the placenta. Many pathological processes can interfere with this normal sequence of events. Respiratory disorders in the newborn present in three different ways:
1 respiratory distress;
2 apnoea and bradycardia (see Chapter 12); and
3 upper airway obstruction (see Chapter 12).

Respiratory distress

Respiratory distress is a general term used to describe respiratory symptoms and is not synonymous with respiratory distress syndrome (RDS) or hyaline membrane disease. It is assessed clinically by the following signs:
1 Tachypnoea – a respiratory rate greater than 60/min.
2 Expiratory grunt – the infant expires against a closed glottis, which maintains a higher residual lung volume, thus preventing alveoli from collapsing and thereby improving gaseous exchange. It occurs particularly in preterm infants with RDS.
3 Chest retraction or recession – this may be intercostal, lower costal, sternal or substernal.
4 Flaring of the ala nasae – this represents the infant's use of accessory respiratory muscles.
5 Cyanosis in air – the cyanosis is central and should be differentiated from peripheral cyanosis

associated with poor circulation due to cooling, polycythaemia or shock.

Diagnosis

The presence of two or more of the above signs persisting for 4 h or more suggests respiratory distress. There are many causes of respiratory distress in the newborn (Table 10.1). A critical evaluation of the cause of respiratory distress should always be undertaken. Diagnosis will be made by a full clinical history, physical examination and appropriate investigation, including a chest X-ray. Perinatal history should include gestational age, the presence of polyhydramnios or oligohydramnios, anomalies on ultrasound, risk factors for sepsis, the passage of meconium, depression at birth and duration of membrane rupture. Physical examination includes observation, vital signs, palpation of dextrocardia and hepatomegaly, and auscultation of the lungs for air entry, symmetry and adventitial breath sounds.

Investigations for respiratory distress

1 Bacteriological cultures on blood, urine, cerebrospinal fluid (CSF) and gastric aspirate.
2 Viral cultures and rapid-yield immunodiagnostic tests.
3 Haematocrit and full blood count.
4 Lecithin/sphingomyelin (L/S) ratio or 'shake test' on gastric or tracheal aspirates (or on amniotic fluid when available; see p. 95).
5 Chest transillumination with a cold light source if pneumothorax suspected.
6 Passage of nasogastric catheters for choanal and oesophageal atresias.

Table 10.1 Common causes of acute respiratory distress

Primary respiratory
Transient tachypnoea of the newborn (or retained fetal
  lung fluid)
RDS (hyaline membrane disease)
Pneumonia
Pneumothorax; pneumomediastinum; pulmonary
  interstitial emphysema
Aspiration syndromes, e.g. meconium, milk, blood
Pulmonary hypoplasia, e.g. Potter's syndrome,
  oligohydramnios
Surgical conditions, e.g. choanal atresia, Pierre Robin
  sequence, diaphragmatic hernia, lobar emphysema,
  oesophageal atresia with tracheo-oesophageal fistula
Massive pulmonary haemorrhage
Chronic neonatal lung disease, e.g. bronchopulmonary
  dysplasia, Wilson–Mikity syndrome, chronic pulmonary
  insufficiency of prematurity
Secondary to extrapulmonary pathology
Following birth asphyxia
Persistence of fetal circulation (or persistent pulmonary
  hypertension)
Congenital heart disease
Anaemia
Polycythaemia
Cerebral damage
Infection
Metabolic disease

7 The nitrogen washout test to differentiate from
cyanotic congenital heart disease (see p. 181).

Treatment of respiratory distress

Supportive care

The supportive care of the infant with respiratory
distress is similar regardless of aetiology. Infants
with mild respiratory distress require frequent
observations of respiratory and heart rates, temperature, blood pressure and signs of respiratory distress, whereas infants with more severe respiratory
distress require continuous monitoring of these
parameters with appropriate alarm signals.
Accurate fluid balance charts are essential. Adequate
thermoregulation may be obtained in a closed incubator or in an open, radiant heat source incubator.

Oxygen

Oxygen is a useful and life-saving therapeutic
agent, but is potentially dangerous, particularly in

the preterm baby, when it may damage the eyes
(retinopathy of prematurity) and the lungs (bronchopulmonary dysplasia). When administered, it
should be warmed to 34–37°C and 90–100% humidified. Oxygen therapy is discussed in Chapter 8.

Fluids

Infants with acute moderate to severe respiratory
distress should not be breastfed or bottle fed. With
mild respiratory distress gavage feeding may be
adequate, but with severe respiratory distress fluids
via intravenous and/or arterial routes will be
required. Usually a 10% dextrose solution is used
and other electrolytes added after 24 h, depending
on serum levels.

Acid–base studies

With moderate or severe respiratory distress assessment of the arterial acid–base status, with samples
from an intra-arterial catheter, or capillary blood
gases may be necessary. Continuous transcutaneous monitoring of Po_2 and Pco_2 decreases the
requirement for blood sampling and enables rapid
detection of fluctuations in clinical status. If respiratory acidosis is severe (pH <7.20 with Pco_2
>60 mmHg, 8 kPa), assisted ventilation may be nec-
essary. For a severe metabolic acidosis an infusion of
sodium bicarbonate may be indicated. Arterial catheterization is indicated when there is a need for frequent sampling for gas analysis, and is used for
direct aortic blood pressure monitoring (see p. 177).

Assisted ventilation

In more severe cases respiratory support may be necessary, but the further management depends on the
size of the infant and degree of respiratory distress.

Mild respiratory distress

1 Colour – presence of central cyanosis.
2 Chest recession.
3 Grunt and flaring of the alae nasae.
4 Heart rate – hourly recordings.
5 Respiratory rate – hourly recordings.
6 Temperature – 4-hourly measurements.
7 Blood pressure – 4-hourly.

  If there is deterioration with an increasing respiratory rate, onset of cyanosis or falling blood pressure, then more intensive monitoring is necessary.

Moderate to severe respiratory distress

1 Heart rate monitoring with alarm system for bradycardia.
2 Respiratory monitoring with alarm system for apnoea.
3 Transcutaneous Po_2 and Pco_2 or pulse oximetry.
4 Regular arterial blood-gas monitoring (4-hourly).
5 Hourly blood pressure monitoring.
6 Twenty-four-hour fluid balance chart.

Umbilical artery catheterization

This is a useful technique in infants who require regular blood-gas estimations and it can also be used for direct aortic blood pressure monitoring. Indications for the insertion of an umbilical artery catheter (UAC) include
1 infants requiring intensive care or ventilatory support;
2 infants with increasing respiratory distress;
3 infants with severe recurrent apnoea.

The technique for insertion of a UAC is described on p. 304.

Incubator therapy

See Chapter 9.

Fluid balance and feeding

See Chapter 6.

Blood pressure monitoring

See Chapter 17.

Transient tachypnoea of the newborn (retained fetal lung fluid)

This occurs in approximately 1–2% of all newborn infants. Tachypnoea is generally the outstanding feature. Transient tachypnoea of the newborn (TTN) is usually benign and self-limiting, with symptoms rarely persisting beyond 48 h.

Pathogenesis

Most of the fetal lung fluid is squeezed out during descent through the birth canal or within the first few breaths after birth, but some is reabsorbed into the pulmonary capillaries and lymphatics. Occasionally, there is an excess of fluid or the clearance mechanisms are inefficient. In these cases retained fluid causes respiratory distress.

Predisposing factors for TTN are prematurity (34–36 weeks), heavy maternal analgesia, birth asphyxia, prelabour caesarean section, breech presentation, male sex, hypoproteinaemia and excessive fluid administration to the mother in labour. Polycythaemia may produce a similar clinical picture resulting from hyperviscosity with resultant pulmonary plethora.

Diagnosis

The diagnosis of TTN is confirmed by chest X-ray and the clinical course. Resolution of the respiratory distress within 48 h confirms the clinical diagnosis retrospectively. Chest X-ray shows streakiness caused by interstitial fluid, fluid in the lung fissures and perihilar cuffing. Pleural effusions and cardiomegaly may also sometimes be seen.

Treatment

TTN does not usually require respiratory support, other than extra inspired oxygen. Regular blood-gas measurements should be performed in the first hours of the illness. In more severe cases continuous positive airway pressure may aid resolution. If the blood gases deteriorate, the diagnosis should be reconsidered or complications such as pulmonary hypertension or pneumothorax may have developed. Sometimes the typical picture of TTN evolves over several days into one of RDS.

Respiratory distress syndrome (hyaline membrane disease)

Respiratory distress syndrome (RDS) is a specific clinical entity occurring predominantly but not exclusively in preterm infants owing to a lack of surfactant (a surface tension-lowering agent) in the alveoli. It has a characteristic clinical course and specific X-ray changes.

Incidence

Although there have been a number of recent advances in the management of premature delivery,

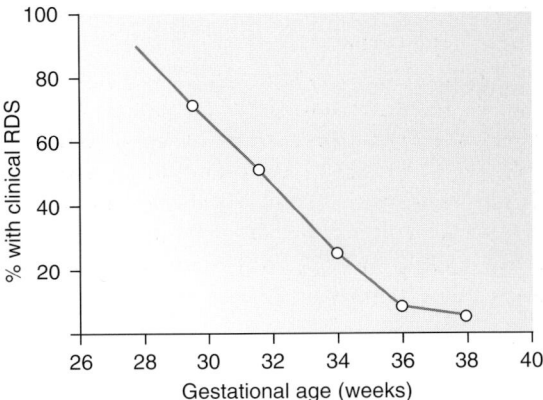

Figure 10.1 Incidence of RDS related to gestational age.

including suppression of labour, estimation of L/S ratios and the use of steroids and exogenous surfactant, the incidence of this condition has remained remarkably static. It is related to the degree of prematurity and is unusual in full-term infants (Fig. 10.1).

Predisposing factors

1 Prematurity.
2 Infant of a diabetic mother.
3 Antepartum haemorrhage.
4 Second twin.
5 Hypoxia, acidosis, shock.
6 Male sex.
7 Prelabour caesarean section (many factors involved).

Historical background

This important condition was first described in 1903 when hyaline membranes were demonstrated in the lungs of dead premature infants (Comroe 1977). Further important landmarks in the understanding of the disease have included the demonstration in the 1950s that this condition was associated with the deficiency of a substance, called surfactant, that prevented alveolar collapse. In the 1970s a method for detecting a deficiency of surfactant became available, and corticosteroids were used to accelerate lung maturity. In the 1980s exogenous surfactant became available for administration into the lung in affected infants.

Aetiology and pathogenesis

The lack of surfactant results in alveoli remaining unexpanded (atelectatic) and gaseous exchange is impaired. Surfactant is a phospholipid secreted by the type II alveolar cells of the lung and is stored in lamellar bodies. The major active component is lecithin, but other phospholipids and protein must be present for full activity. These surface-active agents are released into alveoli, reducing the surface tension and helping to keep the alveoli open.

Lung maturity can be assessed by measuring the L/S ratio either on amniotic fluid obtained by amniocentesis or on gastric aspirate, which reflects the L/S ratio of the swallowed liquor. An L/S ratio <1.5 predicts a high risk of RDS (70% incidence); a ratio of 1.5–2.0 predicts a 40% risk of developing RDS; and a mature ratio >2 indicates a very small risk unless the mother is diabetic (Roberton 1981). In diabetic pregnancies the presence of phosphatidylglycerol (PG) in the liquor suggests that the infant will not develop RDS.

Surfactant is secreted into the fetal lung at 30–32 weeks' gestation. It forms a surface film over the alveoli and because of its molecular structure is poorly compressible, thereby preventing the alveoli from collapsing down to their unexpanded state. The action of surfactant can be understood by the LaPlace equation:

$$P = \frac{2\sigma}{r} \qquad (10.1)$$

where P is the pressure required to inflate a sphere, σ the surface tension and r the radius (Fig. 10.2).

The equation explains why, in the presence of high surface tension, large alveoli tend to become larger and small ones remain collapsed. Assuming that both small and large alveoli receive equal perfusion with blood, there will be a ventilation/perfusion (V/Q) imbalance. This results in severe biochemical disturbances, with hypoxia and acidosis, which give rise to a deterioration in pulmonary perfusion, thus causing further deterioration in V/Q. This may become progressively more severe and lead to persistent pulmonary hypertension (see p. 189).

When the lungs of an infant who has survived for several hours after birth are examined at autopsy, hyaline membranes may be demonstrated lining

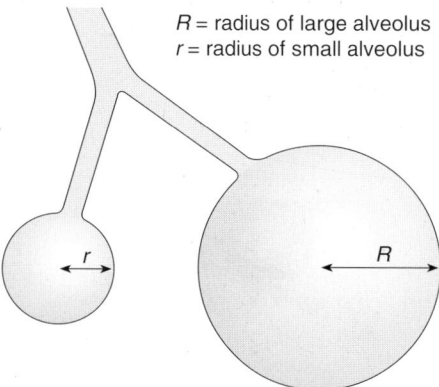

R = radius of large alveolus
r = radius of small alveolus

Figure 10.2 Schematic representation of two alveoli demonstrating LaPlace's law (see text for details).

the respiratory bronchioles and alveolar ducts. The term hyaline membrane disease is derived from the examination of pathological material.

Clinical features

The signs of RDS start immediately after birth or become obvious in the first 6 h of life. In the absence of surfactant each breath the infant takes is like the first breath in an effort to expand the alveoli. Fatigue contributes to the respiratory failure. The clinical course is usually associated with worsening of the symptoms, with a peak severity at 48–72 h, although occasionally maximum severity may occur in infants less than 12 h old. In the early stages the infant lies in a 'frog-like' position due to poor muscle tone, and may have difficulty with copious pharyngeal secretions, which require suctioning for clearance. As the disease progresses the infant shows a need for increasing oxygen to abolish cyanosis, the expiratory grunt may diminish and prolonged apnoea may occur. Apnoea is a late sign of respiratory failure and, if it occurs in the first 6 h of life, infection (particularly due to group B β-haemolytic streptococcus) is a likely cause. The breath sounds are decreased and there may be a fall in blood pressure. The infant is oliguric initially and has evidence of increasing peripheral oedema. At about 48 h a diuresis often occurs, with a concomitant clinical improvement in less severely affected infants.

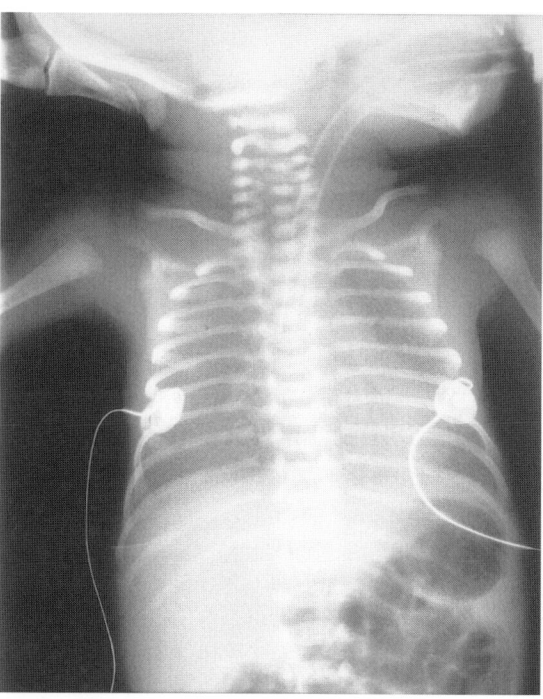

Figure 10.3 Chest radiograph showing the characteristic 'ground glass' appearance of RDS.

Radiology

The X-ray is usually characteristic, showing under-aeration and a fine reticular or granuloreticular pattern, often referred to as 'ground glass'. In addition, air bronchograms are seen in the lung fields (Fig. 10.3). Severe cases with near-total atelectasis may show complete opacification of the lung fields ('white out'). The appearance of the chest X-ray may not correlate well with the clinical severity of RDS. Extremely preterm infants, in whom lungs are not fully developed, may actually have clear lung fields.

Laboratory abnormalities

Arterial oxygen tension is usually decreased. Arterial carbon dioxide tension initially may be normal (when breathing faster to compensate for respiratory difficulty), but is usually increased. Blood pH may reflect respiratory acidosis (from hypercarbia), metabolic acidosis (from tissue hypoxia) or mixed acidosis.

Treatment

Surfactant replacement therapy

Pulmonary surfactant, a multicomponent complex of several phospholipids, neutrolipids and specific proteins, is synthesized and secreted into alveolar spaces by type II epithelial cells. Pulmonary surfactant reduces the collapsing forces in the alveoli, conserves mechanical stability to the alveoli, and maintains the alveolar surface relatively free of liquid. Preterm infants are deficient in endogenous surfactant and administration of exogenous surfactant in such cases reduces the pressure required to open the lung, increases the maximum lung volume, and prevents lung collapse (atelectasis) at low pressure. Surfactant is primarily composed of phospholipids (85%) and proteins (10%). Dipalmitoylphosphatidylcholine (DPPC) is the predominant phospholipid in surfactants. The structure of DPPC is suited to form a stable monolayer generating the low surface tension required to prevent alveolar collapse at end expiration.

However, phospholipids alone do not make up for all the biophysical properties of pulmonary surfactant. The contribution of surfactant proteins, especially the low molecular weight SP-B and SP-C, is essential for structural organization and functional durability of surfactants. They both promote the rapid dispersion of phospholipids at the air–liquid interface and account for the sustained low surface tension activity after dynamic compression. However, in several laboratory investigations, SP-B has been found to reduce surface tension to a greater extent than SP-C. SP-B also participates in intracellular and extracellular regulation of surfactant structure and function, and without SP-B, SP-C is not expressed properly. Congenital absence of SP-B is lethal, with respiratory failure occurring soon after birth. In contrast, SP-C deficiency is not associated with respiratory failure at birth, but may lead to interstitial lung disease in later childhood. The structure and function of the SP-B and SP-C proteins, including the effect of their mutations on lung function, have been the subject of recent reviews, which show a clear difference between the structures of SP-B and SP-C, and thus predicting differing functions. There are two other surfactant proteins, SP-A and SP-D, which are only marginally involved in the surface tension-lowering ability of pulmonary surfactant but play an important role in the innate lung defence barrier against pathogenic organisms (Sinha *et al.* 2007).

The development and use of surfactant replacement therapy has revolutionized the treatment of RDS. Numerous preparations including animal-derived surfactants and equally effective newer synthetic surfactants are now available. Surfactants can be used either prophylactically in 'at risk' infants (born less than 27 weeks' gestation) or as a rescue treatment in bigger babies only if they develop respiratory distress.

Establish adequate gas exchange

Oxygen

The aim of treatment is to maintain the $P_a o_2$ within the normal range. This is done in mild cases by increasing the inspired oxygen concentration ($F_I o_2$). In more severe cases respiratory support may be necessary, but the further management depends on the size of the infant and degree of gaseous exchange abnormality.

Infants <1500 g. Although continuous positive airway pressure (CPAP) may be administered shortly after birth, smaller infants are more likely to require mechanical ventilation. The goal of mechanical ventilation is to achieve adequate pulmonary gas exchange while decreasing the patient's work of breathing. Indications for mechanical ventilation are as follows:

1 apnoea;

2 $F_I o_2$ exceeding 60% to maintain $P_a o_2 > 60$ mmHg (8 kPa);

3 rising $P_a co_2$ that exceeds 60 mmHg (8 kPa), particularly if there is a falling pH (<7.25).

Infants >1500 g. CPAP should be considered early if $F_I o_2$ exceeds 30–40% to maintain $P_a o_2 > 60$ mmHg (8 kPa). Mechanical ventilation is recommended if

1 there is severe or recurrent apnoea;

2 there is worsening respiratory distress, increased work of breathing or respiratory fatigue;

3 $F_I o_2$ exceeds 60% to maintain $P_a o_2 > 60$ mmHg (8 kPa) while on CPAP;

4 a rising $P_a co_2$ exceeds 60 mmHg (8 kPa), particularly if there is a falling pH (<7.25).

Details of CPAP and mechanical ventilation are described in Chapter 11.

Supportive treatment

Chest physiotherapy

Infants receive regular position changes and airway suctioning to reduce the risk of mucus retention, airway plugging and pulmonary collapse. Routine chest physiotherapy is of no proven value in management of RDS. Active chest percussion and cupping is only practised for problematic secretions and collapse/consolidation demonstrated on chest X-ray. Physiotherapy should not be employed for at least 24 h after surfactant instillation.

Antibiotics

Broad-spectrum antibiotics are usually administered to all babies with RDS after superficial and deep cultures have been taken. This is because sepsis/pneumonia, especially group B streptococcal infection, can produce a nearly identical picture. Antibiotics should be stopped once cultures, blood count and ancillary investigations for sepsis are reported as negative.

Appropriate fluid balance

See p. 41.

Blood pressure monitoring

See p. 177.

Minimal handling and nursing in a neutral environmental temperature

See Chapter 9.

Complications

In general, the risk of complications is related to the severity of the underlying RDS. Table 10.2 lists the more common short- and long-term complications.

Prognosis

Most infants who die do so not as a direct result of RDS but rather of a related complication (intraventricular haemorrhage, infection, chronic lung disease). Those weighing 1000 g or below are most at risk. More mature infants, even with severe RDS,

Table 10.2 Short- and long-term complications of RDS

Acute	Subacute	Chronic
Respiratory		
Perinatal asphyxia	Convulsions	Cerebral palsy
Pulmonary air leak	Collapse/ consolidation	Bronchopulmonary dysplasia
	Pulmonary haemorrhage	SIDS
	Prolonged intubation	Subglottic stenosis
Cardiac		
Patent ductus arteriosus	Lung oedema	Chronic neonatal lung disease
Pulmonary hypertension	Cor pulmonale	
Cerebral		
Cerebroventricular haemorrhage	Ventricular dilatation	Hydrocephalus
	Convulsions	Porencephaly
Periventricular leukomalacia	Cysts	Cerebral palsy
Gastrointestinal		
Necrotizing enterocolitis	Bowel obstruction	Malabsorption
	Gut perforation	
Special senses	Retinopathy of prematurity	Visual impairment
	Airway secretions	Conductive/ sensorineural hearing loss

are unlikely to die but may require mechanical ventilation for sometime. Survival figures by birthweight are shown in Table 10.3.

Pneumonia

Pneumonia in the newborn infant is relatively common and may be due to viral, bacterial or other agents. Pneumonia may be contracted *in utero* and be present at birth (congenital) or acquired after birth (nosocomial). Congenital pneumonia may be due to ascending infection with prolonged rupture of membranes, or less frequently due to a transplacental infection (see Chapter 7). The diagnosis is suspected on maternal history, clinical examination and chest radiograph, and confirmed

Table 10.3 Typical incidence and survival rates for infants of different birthweight groups with a diagnosis of RDS

Birthweight categories (g)	Incidence (%)	Survival (%)
<500	100	10
500–999	80	80
1000–1499	55	95
>1499	20	100
Total 500–5000	N/A	94

by bacteriological cultures from blood and tracheal aspirate.

Aetiology

Pneumonia in the newborn is usually bacterial, and the most frequent bacterial pathogens causing congenital and acquired pneumonias are the Gram-negative bacilli (*Escherichia coli*, *Klebsiella*, *Pseudomonas*, *Serratia* spp.), group B β-haemolytic streptococcus and *Staphylococcus* spp.

Rarer bacterial infections include *Listeria monocytogenes* and anaerobic bacilli. Occasionally, pneumonia is due to *Chlamydia trachomatis*, *Mycoplasma pneumoniae* or opportunistic pathogens such as *Candida albicans* and *Pneumocystis carinii*. Viral pneumonitis is rare but occurs with cytomegalovirus (CMV), Coxsackie virus, respiratory syncytial virus (RSV) and rubella.

Clinical features

The early clinical signs and symptoms are often non-specific and may include lethargy, apnoea, bradycardia, temperature instability and intolerance of feeds. At birth it may be difficult to distinguish pneumonia from other forms of lung disease causing respiratory distress. In other cases the typical signs of respiratory distress may be present from birth. The maternal and birth histories may reveal predisposing factors for neonatal infection.

Auscultation of the chest may reveal diminished air entry over areas of consolidation or effusion. Adventitial breath sounds may be heard on inspiration.

Radiology

The appearances are non-specific and pneumonia may be difficult to distinguish radiologically from aspiration syndromes and even TTN. There are usually patchy opacities or more confluent areas of radiodensity through the lung. Lobar pneumonia is rarely seen in the newborn.

Treatment

1 *Antibiotics.* Administer broad-spectrum antibiotics after deep and superficial cultures have been taken. Choice of antibiotics depends on the predominant pathogen causing sepsis and the antibiotic sensitivity pattern for the microorganisms causing early-onset sepsis in a given region (or hospital). Empirical therapy must cover both Gram-positive and Gram-negative organisms. The most frequently used combination is penicillin or ampicillin (or amoxicillin) and an aminoglycoside (frequently gentamycin). After an organism has been identified, the antibiotic therapy should be tailored according to the sensitivities.
2 *Respiratory support* is given according to the severity of signs and symptoms (see Chapter 11).

Thoracic air leaks

This term refers to a collection of gas outside the pulmonary compartment, and a variety of disorders are included in this category, such as
1 pneumothorax – air in the pleural space (Fig. 10.4);
2 pneumomediastinum – air in the anterior mediastinum (Fig. 10.5);
3 pneumopericardium – air in the pericardial sac;
4 pulmonary interstitial emphysema (PIE) – air in interstitial lung spaces (Fig. 10.6);
5 pneumoperitoneum – air in the peritoneal cavity;
6 air embolus – air dissecting into pulmonary veins and disseminating throughout the bloodstream.

The pathophysiology of these conditions is similar in that the alveoli become hyperinflated and rupture. Air then escapes into the lung interstitium

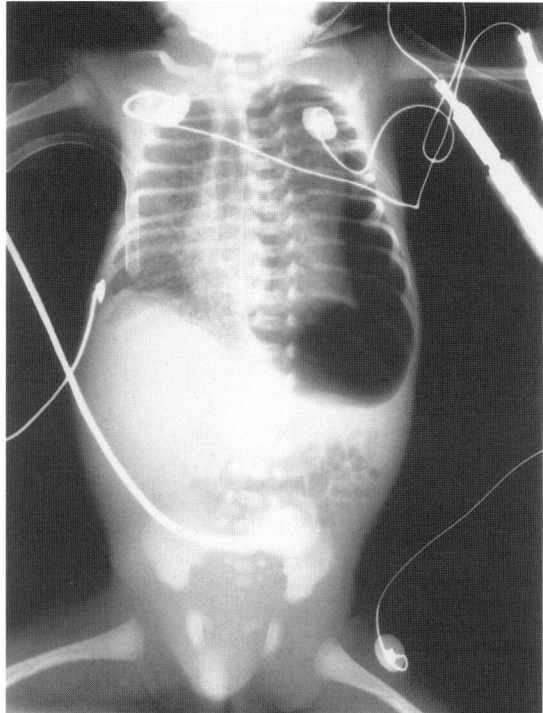

Figure 10.4 Chest radiograph showing left-sided tension pneumothorax.

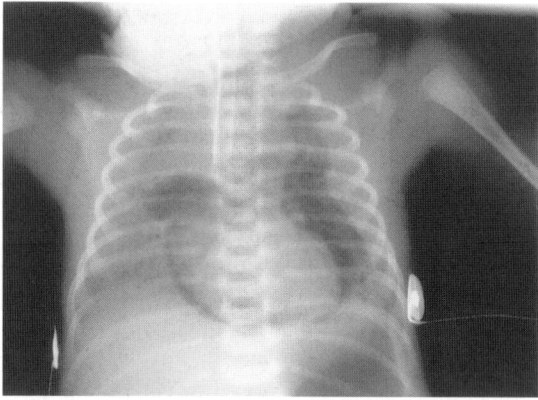

Figure 10.5 Chest radiograph showing pneumomediastinum. The heart and thymus are outlined by gas..

(PIE) and tracks along the perivascular spaces into the mediastinum (pneumomediastinum) through the visceral pleura (pneumothorax), or rarely into the pericardium (pneumopericardium).

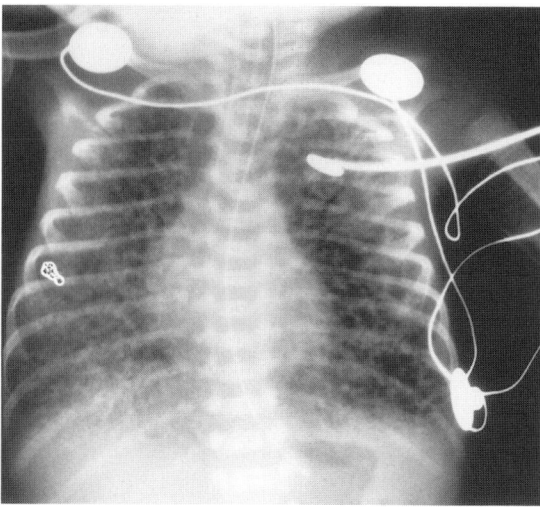

Figure 10.6 Chest radiograph showing extensive PIE. Note the overinflated chest with flattened diaphragm.

Spontaneous pneumothorax occurs in approximately 1% of vaginal deliveries and 1.5% of caesarean sections. Many of these have only minor symptoms, are discovered unexpectedly on a chest X-ray and may not require intervention.

Resuscitation with positive-pressure ventilation makes the occurrence of a pneumothorax far more likely. Surfactant therapy has markedly reduced the incidence of pulmonary air leaks in ventilated infants.

Pneumothoraces commonly occur in the following conditions or situations:

1 Stiff lungs, e.g. hyaline membrane disease.
2 Hyperinflated lungs, e.g. meconium aspiration.
3 Hypoplastic lungs, e.g. Potter's syndrome, diaphragmatic hernia.
4 Mechanical ventilation or CPAP, which predisposes to pulmonary air leaks. Prolonged inspiratory time and high end-expiratory pressures are particularly likely to cause pneumothorax. Active expiration against a ventilator 'breath' (asynchrony between mechanical and spontaneous breaths) is also a probable cause (see p. 116).

Clinical features

Infants with a tension pneumothorax exhibit signs of severe respiratory distress. Frequently a pulmonary air leak occurs in a baby who already has respiratory distress and there may be sudden deterioration, with cyanosis, poor peripheral perfusion and bradycardia. Specific signs of a tension pneumothorax are a shift of the mediastinum to the opposite side, asymmetrical chest expansion, asymmetrical air entry and weak peripheral pulses. A prominent sternum may suggest a pneumomediastinum.

Occasionally, unilateral PIE develops as a result of a ball-valve effect in a main bronchus. The emphysematous lung may cause compression of the more normal lung, thereby further embarrassing ventilation (Fig. 10.7).

Diagnosis

The definitive diagnosis is made by an anteroposterior chest X-ray. To detect a small pneumothorax, an erect film will be required, whereas a lateral film will be necessary to diagnose air in the anterior mediastinum. When a pneumomediastinum is present, the chest X-ray may reveal the sail or spinnaker sign. In the critically ill infant who has a tension pneumothorax, chest transillumination may be used to make the diagnosis. Occasionally, the insertion of a 21G butterfly needle with stopcock and syringes may be life-saving in suspected tension pneumothoraces. This is an emergency diagnostic and therapeutic procedure undertaken when there may be delay in obtaining an X-ray in a critically ill

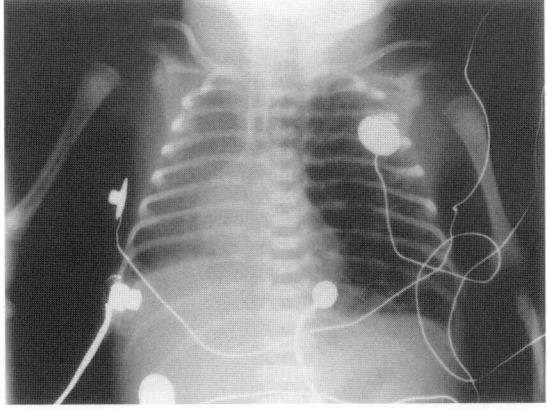

Figure 10.7 Chest radiograph showing left-sided PIE. The mediastinum and right lung are compressed by the overinflated left lung.

infant. Blind needling of the chest may create a pneumothorax and should not be attempted except in an emergency.

Management

A tension pneumothorax will need to be released by an intercostal catheter inserted into the second intercostal space in the midclavicular line and connected to underwater seal drainage or a Heimlich one-way flutter valve (see p. 303). Occasionally, evacuation of the pneumothorax will be incomplete with this catheter, and a catheter sited more posteriorly in the sixth intercostal space in the midaxillary line will be necessary. For non-tension pneumothoraces in full-term infants, nursing in 100% oxygen for up to 12 h may accelerate reabsorption of the pneumothorax. The rare pleural effusion or chylous effusion in the newborn may require thoracocentesis if large.

Generalized management of PIE is focused on reducing or preventing further barotraumas to the lung by decreasing peak inspiratory pressure (PIP) to the minimum required to attain acceptable arterial blood gases. Reduction in positive end-expiratory pressure (PEEP) may also help in decreasing the PIE. High-frequency oscillatory or jet ventilation is a successful means of ventilation for infants with PIE (see p. 118). Localized PIE may resolve spontaneously or may persist for several weeks with a sudden enlargement and deterioration in an infant's condition. Severe unilateral PIE with compression of the other lung can be treated by selectively intubating the more normal lung, thereby allowing the emphysematous lung to collapse. After 24–48 h, and when radiological improvement has occurred, the tube is withdrawn.

Pneumomediastinum is often of little clinical importance and usually does not need to be drained. Pneumopericardium can cause life-threatening cardiac tamponade (compression), which requires pericardiocentesis (needle aspiration via the subxiphoid route). The procedure can be facilitated by transillumination guidance. Pericardial tube placement and drainage (like a chest tube for pneumothorax) may be necessary if the pericardial air reaccumulates.

Meconium aspiration syndrome

Meconium aspiration syndrome (MAS) is a serious and potentially preventable cause of respiratory distress in the newborn. Meconium staining of the amniotic fluid (MSAF) occurs almost always in full-term or post-term infants and is seen in about 13% of deliveries. However, MAS occurs only in 4–5% of newborns born through MSAF. The passage of meconium often indicates fetal distress, but in the breech presentation may be normal. Whether it is a sign of fetal distress or not, the possibility of aspiration into the lungs must be taken seriously. Meconium aspiration most commonly occurs *in utero* and less so at the onset of neonatal respiration. The response of the infant to intrapartum asphyxia is to gasp, and if meconium is present it will be aspirated deep into the bronchi. Once respiration begins, distal migration of the meconium into small airways occurs.

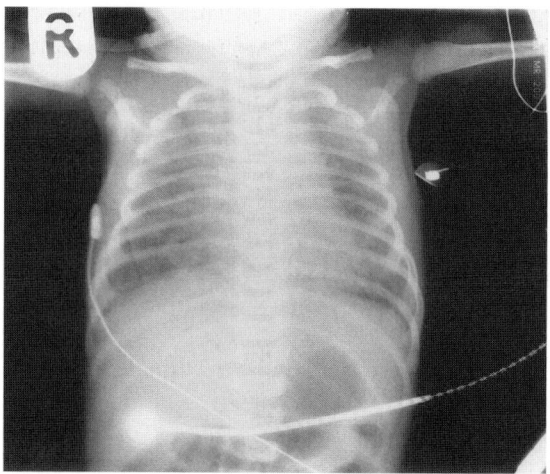

Figure 10.8 Chest radiograph showing meconium aspiration syndrome. There is extensive discrete shadowing throughout both lung fields.

Clinical features

There is a wide spectrum of presentations, ranging from severe birth asphyxia requiring active resuscitation through early onset of respiratory distress to a vigorous baby with no major problems. Typically the infant is born covered in meconium-stained liquor and has meconium staining of the umbilical cord, skin and nails. The chest appears to be hyperinflated and there may be a prominent sternum. Respiratory distress may be mild initially, becoming rapidly more severe after several hours. The baby may also show signs of cerebral irritability.

Pathogenesis and aetiology

Meconium causes a number of anatomical and physiological problems to make lung function worse:
1 Plugging of the airways, with consequent atelectasis. It also causes a 'ball-valve' obstruction with hyperinflation of the lungs and a high risk of pulmonary air leaks.
2 Irritation of the airways, causing a chemical pneumonitis.
3 Antagonism of surfactant production.
4 Possible secondary bacterial infection.
5 In a proportion of infants with severe aspiration syndrome, there is development of marked ventilation/perfusion inequality and right-to-left shunt due to persistent pulmonary hypertension (PPHN, see p. 189).

Radiology

Chest X-rays show hyperinflation (flat diaphragms, widening of rib spaces) with diffuse patchy opacities throughout both lung fields (Fig. 10.8). Pneumothorax or pneumomediastinum may also be seen.

Prophylactic management

Morbidity and mortality from meconium aspiration syndrome can be prevented or minimized by optimal perinatal management. There is controversy as to whether a neonatal paediatrician should attend every delivery where there is meconium staining of the liquor. It is important, however, that an experienced neonatal paediatrician be present for the delivery if *thick* meconium is present.

The following therapeutic interventions have been subject to Cochrane systematic reviews with clear-cut results:
1 Amnioinfusion therapy for thick-consistency MSAF does not reduce the risk of MAS, according to a recent randomized controlled trial (RCT).

2 Intrapartum naso- and oropharyngeal suctioning does not reduce the incidence of MAS (large RCT) and hence is not recommended.

3 Routine endotracheal intubation and suctioning is of no benefit in vigorous infants born through MSAF of any consistency. This should, however, be performed in infants born through MSAF if they are depressed, if they need positive-pressure ventilation, or if they are vigorous initially but develop respiratory distress within the first few minutes of life.

The baby is intubated with a wide-bore endotracheal tube and the trachea is suctioned clear. Suctioning is facilitated by the use of a meconium aspirator. Mouth-to-endotracheal tube suctioning must not be practised. Further suction is applied directly to the endotracheal tube as it is being removed. If a large quantity of meconium is present in the endotracheal tube after extubation, the baby should be reintubated and further tracheal suction applied. The stomach should be aspirated following intubation and, if there is a moderate or large volume of meconium in the stomach, the gastric tube should be left *in situ* for lavage to be performed later. All depressed babies who are born through thick MSAF should be carefully assessed and regularly monitored for signs of MAS.

Treatment of established meconium aspiration syndrome

The treatment will be the same as for respiratory distress (see Chapter 12). Particular emphasis or consideration should be given to the following:

1 Humidification of inspired oxygen.

2 Postural drainage positioning, suctioning of airways and chest percussion, although commonly performed, has never been studied in clinical trials and is of unproven benefit; bolus exogenous surfactant treatment can be used but is of no proven value.

3 Antibiotics are usually given, although the efficacy has not been established.

4 No single approach regarding ventilatory strategies is recommended for babies with MAS requiring mechanical ventilation. Both conventional and high-frequency ventilation can be used with multiple strategies to achieve normal gaseous exchange and prevent complications such as air trapping and air leaks, which are common in such infants.

5 Exogenous surfactant has been used with success in some studies and may reduce the risk of pneumothorax and shorten the duration of mechanical ventilation. It may also reduce the need for subsequent extracorporeal membrane oxygenation (ECMO) therapy. In some centres lavage with surfactant is practised but there are limited data suggesting that this is effective therapy.

6 Inhaled nitric oxide (iNO) therapy.

7 Extracorporeal membrane oxygenation (ECMO) should be considered in infants with concomitant PPHN who are not responding to conventional treatment.

Pulmonary hypoplasia

For adequate fetal lung development the fetus must be able to make breathing movements and move a column of amniotic fluid up and down the trachea and main bronchi. Hypoplasia may therefore be due to

1 failure of fetal breathing (neuromuscular disorders);

2 inability to expand the lungs (diaphragmatic hernia, pleural effusions);

3 lack of liquor (oligohydramnios) due to renal or bladder neck abnormalities or prolonged rupture of the membranes.

Infants with pulmonary hypoplasia may have associated facial abnormalities and limb contractures. The fetal side of the placenta should be examined for amnion nodosum, which is suggestive of severe oligohydramnios, especially Potter's syndrome.

Clinical features

The infant develops severe respiratory distress from birth, with marked hypoxia, hypercapnia and metabolic acidosis. Pneumothorax is a common complication. The lungs are very stiff and there is little chest movement with mechanical ventilation. It may be difficult to diagnose lung hypoplasia on chest X-ray. Severe lung hypoplasia is incompatible with life, and less severe forms contribute towards chronic ventilator dependency and bronchopulmonary dysplasia.

Massive pulmonary haemorrhage

Massive pulmonary haemorrhage has a characteristic clinical presentation in newborn infants, with cardiovascular collapse associated with an outpouring of bloodstained fluid from the trachea and mouth. The condition is usually fatal and occurs in about 1/1000 births. Amongst survivors, there is a high incidence of chronic lung disease. The underlying mechanism for pulmonary haemorrhage can be classified as

1 Haemodynamic – a manifestation of an exaggerated haemorrhagic pulmonary oedema brought about by an acute increase in pulmonary blood flow as in large Patent Ductus Arteriosus (PDA).

2 Haematological due to associated coagulation abnormalities such as in disseminated intravascular coagulation (DIC) associated with sepsis or other coagulopathy. Pulmonary haemorrhage is often associated with bleeding in other organs such as brain or gut.

The incidence of pulmonary haemorrhage is inversely related to the gestational age of the babies. Prematurity, RDS and exogenous surfactant therapy (in combination) are the three most important risk factors. Other antecedent risk factors include severe birth asphyxia, hypothermia, small for gestational age (SGA) infants, coagulation disturbances and congenital heart disease.

The severity and magnitude of clinical signs depend upon the magnitude of haemorrhage and the severity of the underlying condition leading to the episode. The clinical manifestations result from several interrelated pathophysiological consequences of blood loss and haemorrhage into the lung parenchyma and airways.

Treatment

The treatment will be that of respiratory distress (see Chapter 11). However, particular emphasis must be given to

1 Resuscitation of cardiovascular collapse with volume expanders such as plasma protein fraction, blood and sodium bicarbonate.

2 Treatment of pulmonary oedema with frusemide and perhaps morphine.

3 Correction of coagulation disturbances; recombinant factor VIIa (rFVIIa) has been used with success in a limited number of patients.

4 If mechanical ventilation is required, high positive end-expiratory pressures may help to decrease bleeding. Exogenous surfactant improves the respiratory status in infants with pulmonary haemorrhage.

5 Other measures to stop pulmonary haemorrhage include nebulized adrenaline (epinephrine) but experience with its use is limited.

Congenital diaphragmatic hernia (CDH)

The hernia is usually a posterolateral (Bochdalek) type; 80% occur on the left side. This occurs through a defect in the diaphragm as a result of a persistent pleuroperitoneal canal caused by failure of the muscular components to develop. The defect in the diaphragm permits herniation of the abdominal contents into the thorax. Consequently, there is hypoplasia or compression of the lung on the side of the hernia, with displacement of mediastinum to the contralateral side. Sometimes there is hypoplasia of the contralateral lung. Babies with a large diaphragmatic hernia have rapidly progressive respiratory failure after birth, with persistent cyanosis. A less acute diaphragmatic hernia may present in the nursery, with respiratory distress, or occasionally on routine examination a 'dextrocardia' or scaphoid abdomen will be found. On auscultation of the lungs, bowel sounds may be heard on the side of the lesion if gas has entered the gastrointestinal tract. The lungs will not inflate adequately with normal pressure.

Diagnosis

Most cases are now diagnosed *in utero* by routine obstetric ultrasound at 17–19 weeks' gestation or following investigation of polyhydramnios. In view of the poor prognosis of early-onset CDH (see below) termination of pregnancy is offered to many parents, but most choose to continue the pregnancy. The diagnosis of a diaphragmatic hernia is confirmed by chest X-ray, which shows bowel loops in the thorax (Fig. 10.9). If the X-ray is taken shortly after birth, there may be some difficulty in

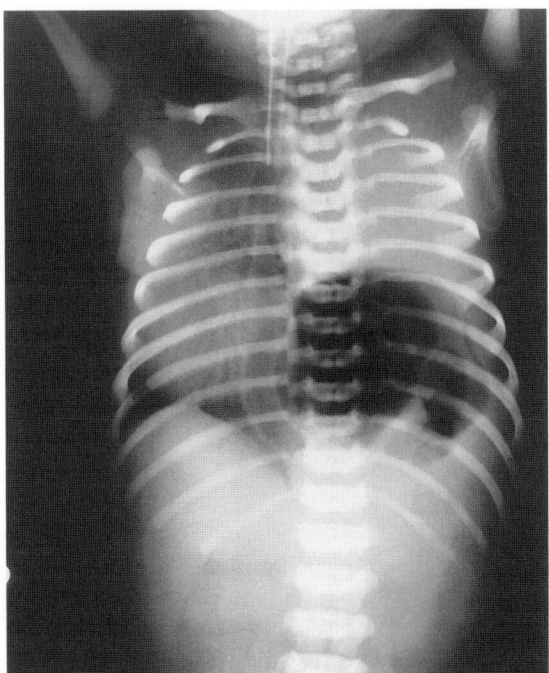

Figure 10.9 Chest radiograph showing a left-sided diaphragmatic hernia.

determining whether the bowel is in the chest, especially if there is little air in the gastrointestinal tract Similarly, diagonsis may be delayed when the liver is in the chest, in cases of right-sided diapharagmatic hernia. The X-ray should be taken with a radio-opaque catheter in the stomach and should include the abdomen, to show a paucity of abdominal gas pattern. A rarer form of diaphragmatic hernia is through an anteromedial defect beneath the sternum (Morgagni type). This typically contains part of the colon. It is usually symptomless and often detected on a lateral chest X-ray. Eventration, which results from a failure of muscle development in the primitive diaphragm, is not a true hernia. CDH can be a part of a syndrome or associated with a chromosomal abnormality.

Treatment

If a congenital diaphragmatic hernia is suspected, an orogastric tube should be inserted and the abdominal contents in the chest aspirated free of gas and secretions. If the baby requires assisted ventilation, it should be performed via an endotracheal tube and never by bag and mask, because of the increasing gaseous distension of the bowel within the chest. Care must be taken to prevent rupture of the contralateral lung, as the baby is almost exclusively dependent on this lung for ventilation. Following initial diagnosis the baby should be stabilized and referred to a paediatric surgeon for operative treatment. Surgery for the more severe cases is often delayed for 3–7 days to enable maximum stabilization, often with high-frequency oscillation ventilation. Surgery consists of reduction of the abdominal contents, closure of the diaphragmatic defect and correction of any bowel malrotation.

Pulmonary hypertension is a common complication of severe diaphragmatic hernia and usually develops after a postoperative 'honeymoon' period of 24–48 h. The infant then develops severe hypoxia with a right-to-left shunt. Infusion of both volume and inotropes may be required to maintain adequate systemic blood pressure in order to maintain adequate tissue perfusion and minimize the right-to-left shunt. Avoid fluid overload. Elective hyperventilation and infusion of sodium bicarbonate to induce alkalosis (pH >7.5), although practised in the past, cannot be recommended. Magnesium sulphate, prostacycline or tolazoline may be tried but are of unproven benefit. Inhaled nitric oxide has no long-term benefits (see p. 119). The continuation of postoperative anaesthesia with muscle paralysis may be necessary on return from the operating theatre in the more severe cases. ECMO has been used to provide stability and for associated PPHN; however, it is of no clear benefit in terms of long-term outcome. The role of fetal surgery is being reinvestigated, with procedures to plug the trachea being performed typically at 23 weeks' gestation.

Prognosis

This depends on the degree of pulmonary hypoplasia and the age at presentation. Infants with respiratory distress in the first 6 h have a high mortality (about 70%), whereas those presenting between 6 and 24 h have a much better prognosis (mortality rates 10–15%). Later presentation is not likely to be associated with pulmonary hypoplasia and the prognosis is very good. Bad prognostic features include polyhydramnios, persistently elevated P_{CO_2} levels with mean airway pressure >20 cmH$_2$O, and hypoxia requiring pulmonary vasodilators.

Oesophageal atresia and tracheo-oesophageal fistula

Oesophageal atresia is a congenital anomaly in which there is usually complete interruption of the lumen of the oesophagus, in the form of a blind upper pouch. This is commonly associated with a tracheo-oesophageal fistula. The commonest variety of this condition is a blind-ending upper oesophageal pouch, with the lower oesophagus arising from the trachea above the carina Fig. 10.10c). A variety of other patterns occur much less commonly (Fig. 10.10).

Clinical features

Maternal hydramnios occurs in 60% of cases and is largely responsible for the high frequency of premature births. The oesophageal atresia is associated with excessive saliva and mucus production, with a high incidence 'of aspiration pneumonia. If the infant is fed, milk accumulates in the upper pouch and spills over into the trachea. The aspiration of gastric contents and bile into the bronchial tree via the fistula results in pulmonary complications, with collapse and pneumonia. Abdominal distension is due to air passing down the fistula into the stomach, and may develop rapidly.

Coexistent congenital anomalies may be present and may be either major or minor. Major anomalies consist of cardiac disease, intestinal atresia, imperforate anus, skeletal anomalies and renal anomalies.

VACTERL association is the term often used to describe these anomalies. This stands for Vertebral, Anal, Cardiac, Tracheal, 'Esophagus', Renal and Limb. The most important aspect of oesophageal atresia is that it should be recognized as soon as possible after birth, preferably prior to the first feed, so that pulmonary complications are less likely to occur. All babies with suspected oesophageal atresia and choanal atresia should have a size 5 nasogastric tube passed down each nostril in turn and into the stomach shortly after birth, preferably before the first feed. If this is not practised, oesophageal atresia is generally diagnosed by excessive secretions or cyanosis and coughing with feeds. The definitive diagnosis is made by the inability to pass a firm radio-opaque no. 10 catheter or a replogle tube into the stomach, as it arrests about 10 cm from the lips. Once the catheter has been passed as far as possible, an X-ray of the neck and upper chest should be taken to confirm that it has become obstructed at this level. The abdominal X-ray should be inspected for gas in the stomach and the chest X-ray assessed for areas of collapse. Air is a useful contrast medium in the upper pouch. It is not usually necessary to put radio-opaque contrast medium into the upper pouch to confirm the diagnosis, but if this is done a non-irritant substance such as metrizimide should be used. For an H-type fistula, which presents with recurrent aspiration or infections, radiological diagnosis may be difficult. A cine contrast swallow will usually confirm the diagnosis.

Treatment

A baby with oesophageal atresia and tracheo-oesophageal fistula should be nursed supine and propped head-up 60° to avoid gastric contents spilling into the lung through the fistula. An intravenous

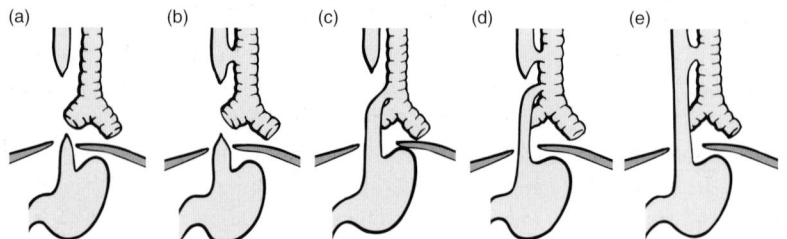

(a) (b) (c) (d) (e)

Figure 10.10 Variants of tracheo-oesphageal fistula with or without oesophageal atresia. Type c accounts for 85% of cases, the others being equally uncommon.

infusion should be commenced and the baby rehydrated with correction of electrolytes and blood glucose disturbances in preparation for surgery. Surgery should be performed by a paediatric surgeon as soon as the baby has been adequately resuscitated and stabilized. Antibiotics will be required if there has been significant aspiration pneumonia. Surgery consists of division of the tracheo-oesophageal fistula and anastomosis of the two segments of the oesophagus if possible. Occasionally, the atretic segment is too long to enable primary anastomosis, and exteriorization of the cervical oesophagus as an oesophagostomy and the stomach as a gastrostomy will be necessary. A definitive operation will be undertaken at a later date.

With a cervical oesophagostomy the baby should be encouraged to practise sucking on a dummy during gastrostomy feedings. Complications and sequelae from surgery are frequent and include a brassy cough, associated with coexistent tracheomalacia, oesophageal stricture, breakdown of the anastomosis with mediastinitis, recurrence of the tracheo-oesophageal fistula and gastro-oesophageal reflux.

Lobar emphysema

Congenital lobar emphysema is a rare anomaly due to a cartilaginous deficiency of the lobar bronchus, most commonly involving the left upper lobe (50%), the right middle lobe (24%) or the right upper lobe (18%), and frequently associated with congenital heart disease (30%), such as tetralogy of Fallot, ventricular septal disease (VSD) or total anomalous pulmonary venous drainage. The onset of respiratory distress is frequently insidious, usually taking 2–3 weeks to develop, and is caused by lung collapse around the hyperinflated lobe. The mediastinum becomes displaced and the chest wall is prominent over the affected area. Breath sounds are diminished and the percussion note is hyperresonant. Once a definitive diagnosis is made, a lobectomy is generally required. Acquired lobar emphysema may be secondary to an extrinsic or intrinsic bronchial obstruction, such as a mucous plug. This type should be treated conservatively with physiotherapy and postural drainage.

Congenital cystic adenomatous malformation

Congenital cystic adenomatous malformation (CCAM) is a rare cystic lesion found more often in males than females, and often diagnosed on antenatal ultrasound. This emphysematous lesion may be associated with polyhydramnios, hydrops fetalis, prematurity and stillbirth. There are three distinct types. Type I CAM (70%) presents as single or multiple large cyst(s) confined to one lobe; type II (18%) is composed of multiple medium-sized cysts and 50% have other anomalies; type III (10%) is a large bulky lesion with evenly distributed small cysts. This is one of the few conditions that is successfully treatable by fetal surgery in selected cases.

Chronic neonatal lung disease

Chronic neonatal lung disease , the severest form of which is also known as *bronchopulmonary dysplasia* (BPD), is a condition that develops in newborns treated with oxygen and mechanical ventilation for a primary lung disorder. It is usually defined as the presence of chronic respiratory signs, a persistent oxygen requirement, and an abnormal chest radiograph at 1 month of age or at 36 weeks corrected age.

The incidence depends on the definition used and the gestational age of the population studied. Although surfactant treatment has improved overall survival of premature infants, the incidence of chronic lung disease (CLD) remains approximately 30–40% (inversely proportional to gestational age at birth). With the use of standardized oxygen saturation monitoring involved in the physiological definition,the incidence may further decrease by as much as 10% (Walsh *et al.* 2004). Table 10.4 lists a classification of chronic neonatal lung disease.

Bronchopulmonary dysplasia

This is usually associated with the healing phase of severe RDS, but occasionally complicates meconium aspiration, pulmonary haemorrhage and severe neonatal pneumonia. This was first described by Northway *et al.* (1967) but since then the characteristics of the disease have changed and it is now essentially a condition seen mostly in babies who

Table 10.4 Classification of chronic neonatal lung disease

Bronchopulmonary dysplasia

Wilson–Mikity syndrome

Chronic pulmonary insufficiency of prematurity

Recurrent aspiration:
   Pharyngeal incoordination
   Gastro-oesophageal reflux
   Tracheo-oesophageal fistula

Interstitial pneumonitis:
   Cytomegalovirus
   Candida albicans
   Chlamydia
   Pneumocystis carinii
   Ureaplasma urealyticum

Chronic pulmonary oedema due to a left-to-right shunt

Rickets of prematurity

are born very premature and require mechanical ventilation (Bancalari *et al.* 2003). The incidence of BPD varies according to the definition used, and recently a physiological definition of BPD has been introduced. The latter facilitates the measurement of BPD as an outcome in clinical trials and comparisons between and within centres over time (Walsh *et al.* 2004).

Aetiology

BPD occurs in about 5% of very low birthweight (VLBW) infants and is multifactorial in origin (known as the 'pulmonary injury sequence'). The incidence relates to the severity of RDS and the degree of prematurity. It has only been described in infants who have received positive-pressure ventilation, and probably relates to barotrauma as measured by the mean airway pressure (this term is used to include inspiratory pressure, expiratory pressure, inspiratory/expiratory ratio and rate) and volutrauma (alveolar overdistension due to excessive tidal volume delivery). Oxygen therapy for prolonged periods of time also appears to be linked with its development. Other probable associations are pulmonary interstitial emphysema and pulmonary oedema. The roles of gastro-oesophageal reflux with recurrent aspiration and infectious agents such as *Ureaplasma urealyticum* are not clear.

Clinical features

Infants who develop BPD have persistent chest retractions, crepitations and rhonchi on chest auscultation, gross hyperinflation of the lungs and an increased anteroposterior chest diameter. Most of these infants also have a patent ductus arteriosus, and after a period of time may develop right heart failure (cor pulmonale).

Radiology

The original description of BPD by Northway *et al.* (1967) staged the radiological appearances in four grades (Table 10.5). The first two are indistinguishable from RDS and are not helpful for descriptive purposes. In the most severe form there is an irregular honeycomb appearance to the lung, with overinflated lung fields, extensive fibrosis and multiple cysts of irregular size (Fig. 10.11).

The majority of infants with BPD now do not develop these gross radiological signs but exhibit a finer, more homogeneous pattern of abnormality, with some dense streaks on chest X-ray.

Management

The prevention of BPD requires careful management of infants receiving mechanical ventilation. Pulmonary interstitial emphysema, pulmonary oedema and patent ductus arteriosus and

Table 10.5 Radiological classification of bronchopulmonary dysplasia

Stage	Days of life	Description	X-ray appearances
1	2–3	Acute RDS	Generalized granuloreticular pattern, air bronchograms or 'white out'
2	4–10	Period of regeneration	Near or total opacification
3	10–20	Period of transition	Small cystic infiltrates, chronic disease
4	>4 weeks	Period of chronic disease	Hyperlucency, strand-like infiltrates, enlargement of cysts

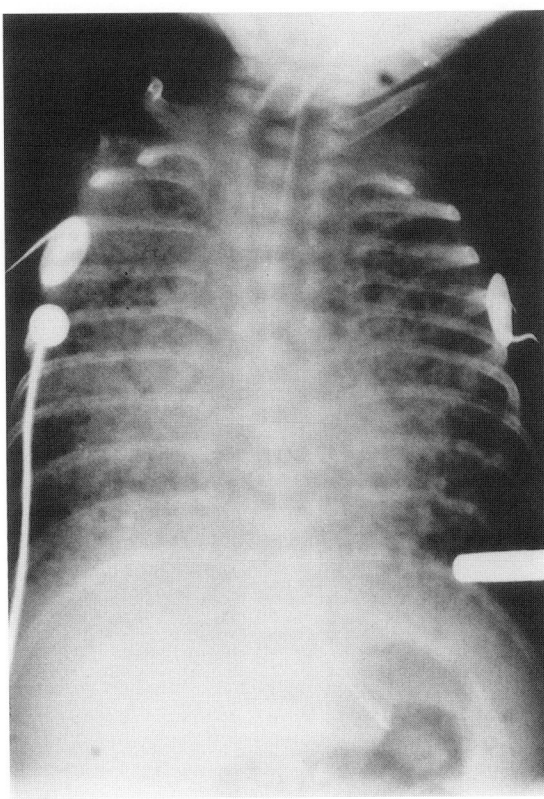

Figure 10.11 Chest radiograph showing severe bronchopulmonary dysplasia.

overhydration appear to increase the risk of BPD developing. Early closure of a patent ductus arteriosus that is producing congestive heart failure, either medically with indometacin or surgically, is desirable. Established BPD is often associated with congestive cardiac failure or cor pulmonale, and under these circumstances fluid restriction and diuretics are used. The following methods of treatment are thought to be of some benefit:

1 *Dexamethasone.* Studies have shown that dexamethasone reduces the oxygen requirements of babies with BPD. It should only be considered after the first 2 weeks of life in infants with severe lung injury who remain ventilator-dependent because of serious neurological side effects including an increased incidence of cerebral palsy. The dose and duration of treatment must be kept to the minimum necessary to achieve the desired effects.

2 *Diuretics.* Diuretic therapy reduces interstitial lung fluid and has been used for acute deterioration associated with pulmonary oedema. However, routine prolonged use is not recommended because of lack of evidence that it improves the incidence or severity of BPD and concern over side effects.

3 *Therapy directed at reducing oxygen toxicity.* Antioxidants such as vitamin E and superoxide dismutase appear to be of no benefit, but vitamin A has been shown to reduce BPD and death in VLBW infants.

Adequate oxygenation throughout all daily activities (O_2 saturation 92–96%) minimizes progressive pulmonary vascular disease. Nutritional supplementation is necessary to obtain optimal growth in the presence of high energy consumption due to the work of breathing. Adequate nutrition is a key aspect of care for the infants with CLD.

BPD spells

Spells refer to episodes where the baby with severe BPD rapidly desaturates and requires resuscitation. On bagging the lungs feel very stiff and it takes a number of vigorous inflation breaths to expand the lungs. These spells usually occur in spontaneously breathing babies who take a large inspiratory breath, and may happen when the baby breathes out of synchrony with the ventilator. It is probably due to bronchomalacia or tracheomalacia. The management is to sedate or paralyse the baby for a number of days and then allow him or her gently to wake but not to become agitated. These spells resolve as the BPD improves.

Prognosis

Mortality figures vary from 0 to 75%, depending on when the diagnosis is made. If stage 4 BPD is diagnosed while the baby is still requiring ventilation, it is unlikely that he or she can be 'weaned' off the ventilator. Most infants with resolving BPD have episodes of wheezing, often associated with a viral infection. The healing stage is associated with continued lung growth and may take 2–3 years. The majority of surviving infants are asymptomatic by 2 years, and chest X-rays are normal by 2–3 years. Respiratory function tests are abnormal for many years, although the child is usually asymptomatic.

Many infants with severe BPD are discharged home on continuous low-flow intranasal oxygen, with intermittent monitoring of oxygen requirement by pulse oximetry.

Children with BPD have been shown to have increased airway resistance and are more likely to wheeze. They also have increased airway reactivity. Episodic wheezing is commonly seen in infants and children who have had BPD in the newborn period. The wheeze may be resistant to sympathomimetic and xanthine drugs, but steroids may be of benefit.

Lower airway infection in the first year of life is a particular risk to children who have had BPD in the neonatal period. Pneumococcal vaccine is now in routine use. Such children appear to be particularly likely to develop respiratory syncytial virus (RSV)-positive bronchiolitis, which may cause very severe respiratory failure. Monoclonal RSV antibody (palivizumab) is used for prophylaxis during the RSV season. Advice must be given to the parents to avoid exposing the baby to the risk of viral infection in the first year or two of life.

PRACTICE POINTS

- Changing from the intrauterine to extrauterine environment requires an effective transition in the cardiorespiratory system, and failure to do so may result in cardiorespiratory disorder of varying severity at birth.
- There are various causes for respiratory distress at birth including prematurity, congenital infections and fetal to neonatal maladaptation.
- Investigating the cause of respiratory distress in newborns requires careful history (including antenatal and birth details), detailed physical examination and relevant investigations including chest X-ray, infection screening and, at times, echocardiography.
- Exogenous surfactant therapy has become the 'standard of care' for treating preterm babies with surfactant-deficient lung disease. Other treatments include supportive measures and artificial respiratory support such as CPAP or ventilation if there is evidence of concomitant respiratory failure. Oxygen therapy should be closely monitored to avoid hyperoxaemia by keeping pulse oximetry below 95% and $P_{a}o_{2}$ between 8 and 10 kPa (60–80 mmHg).

References

Bancalari E, Claure N, Sosenko IRS. Bronchopulmonary dysplasia: changes in pathogenesis, epidemiology and definition. *Semin Neonatol* 2003;**8**:63–71.

Comroe JM. Retrospectroscope: Insights Into Medical discovery. California: Von Gehr, 1977.

Greenough A, Milner AD. Pulmonary disease of newborn; acute respiratory disease. In: *Roberton's Textbook of Neonatology* (ed. JM Rennie), 4th edn, pp. 468–553. Philadelphia: Elsevier, 2005.

Northway WH, Rosan RC, Porter DY. Pulmonary disease following respirator therapy of hyaline membrane disease; bronchopulmonary dysplasia. *N Engl J Med* 1967;**276**:357–368.

Roberton NRC. Developments in Neonatal Paediatric Practice. In: *Recent Advances in Paediatrics 6* (ed. D Hull), pp. 13–50. Edinburgh: Churchill Livingston.

Sinha SK, Moya F, Donn SM. Surfactant for Respiratory Distress Syndrome: Are there important clinical differences among preparations? *Curr Opin Paediatr* 2007; **19**: 150–154.

Walsh MC, Yao Q, Gettner P *et al.* Impact of physiologic definition on bronchopulmonary dysplasia. *Pediatrics* 2004;**114**:1305–1311.

Further reading

Avery GB, Fletcher MA, MacDonald MG (eds) *Neonatology: Pathophysiology and Management of the Newborn*, 4th edn. Philadelphia: Lippincott-Raven, 1994.

Donn SM, Sinha SK. *Manual of Neonatal Respiratory Care*. Philadelphia: Elsevier, 2006.

Rennie JM. *Textbook of Neonatology*, 4th edn. Philadelphia: Elsevier, 2005.

Spitzer AR. *Intensive Care of the Fetus and Neonate*. St Louis: Mosby, 1994.

Yu VYH. *Respiratory Disorders in the Newborn*. Edinburgh: Churchill Livingstone, 1986.

11 Respiratory physiology, respiratory failure and mechanical ventilation

Respiratory distress is a non-specific term referring to a group of clinical signs with multiple causes. The management of infants with respiratory disorders involves careful clinical assessment as well as the evaluation of radiological and biochemical data. The decision to give respiratory support by means of continuous positive airway pressure (CPAP) or mechanical ventilation depends on a number of variables, which are discussed below. Respiratory failure is used to describe the endpoint of a variety of respiratory, neurological and cardiac conditions. If respiratory failure occurs, respiratory support is necessary. This chapter outlines the methods and indications for such support, and aspects of relevant respiratory physiology are reviewed.

Respiratory physiology

Oxygen transport

Oxygen is essential for the production of adenosine triphosphate (ATP), a molecule that stores and releases energy. Severe hypoxaemia greatly reduces the production of ATP and the resultant anaerobic metabolism produces lactic acid. Lactic acid accumulation significantly contributes to the development of metabolic acidosis.

Oxygen diffuses across the alveolar membrane from a higher to a lower concentration. It is carried in the blood attached to haemoglobin, or to a lesser degree dissolved in plasma. The partial pressure of oxygen (Po_2) refers to the amount dissolved in plasma. Delivery of oxygen to the tissues depends on oxygen concentration and tissue perfusion. Oxygen combines with haemoglobin to be transported as oxyhaemoglobin. The saturation of the haemoglobin refers to the percentage of it that carries oxygen. There is not a constant relationship between the oxygen saturation and the Po_2, so that at a relatively low tissue Po_2 larger amounts of oxygen are released than when the Po_2 is higher. The P_{50} is the P_aO_2 at which the haemoglobin is half saturated with O_2; the higher the P_{50}, the lower the affinity of haemoglobin for oxygen. The oxygen dissociation curve for fetal haemoglobin (HbF) is different than that for adult haemoglobin (HbA) in that it is shifted to the left (Fig. 11.1). The fetus lives in a relatively hypoxic environment and the oxyhaemoglobin saturation is greater at lower partial oxygen pressures. This is of benefit to the fetus but is disadvantageous to the newborn infant, who at any given Po_2 level gives up less oxygen to the tissues than older children with HbA. Table 11.1 lists the factors responsible for a shift in the oxygen dissociation curve. A right shift of the curve means a

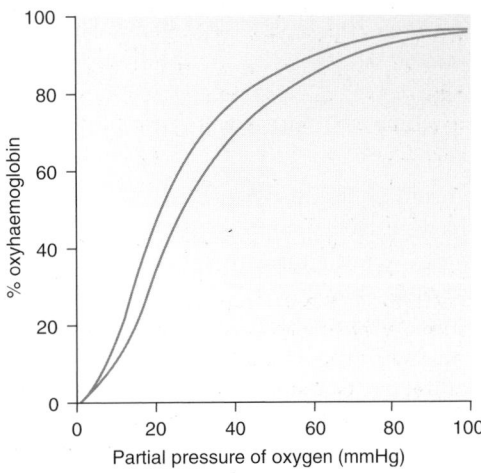

Figure 11.1 Oxygen dissociation curve for fetal haemoglobin (upper line) and adult haemoglobin (lower line).

Table 11.1 Factors that influence the oxygen dissociation curve

Factors producing (L) shift	Factors producing (R) shift
$\downarrow$ Temperature	$\uparrow$ Temperature
$\downarrow$ Basal metabolic rate	$\uparrow$ Basal metabolic rate
$\downarrow P_a co_2$	$\uparrow P_a co_2$
$\uparrow$ pH	$\downarrow$ pH
$\downarrow$ 2,3-DPG	$\uparrow$ 2,3-DPG
$\uparrow$ Fetal haemoglobin	$\downarrow$ Fetal haemoglobin

2,3-DPG, 2,3-diphosphoglycerate.

higher P_{50} (i.e. a higher $P_a o_2$ is required for haemoglobin to bind a given amount of O_2).

Carbon dioxide transport

Carbon dioxide may be transported dissolved in the blood, but is mainly present as bicarbonate ions (HCO_3^-). Carbon dioxide is produced as a byproduct of cellular respiration and is liberated into the blood. It diffuses through the alveoli to be excreted in the expired air. The CO_2 content of the blood is referred to as the partial pressure of CO_2, or $P co_2$.

Acid–base balance

In the presence of the enzyme carbonic anhydrase (CA), carbon dioxide dissolved in plasma forms carbonic acid, which in turn dissociates to H^+ and HCO_3^- ions. This is described in the Henderson–Hasselbach equation:

$$H_2O + CO_2 \overset{CA}{\rightleftharpoons} H_2CO_3 \rightleftharpoons HCO_3^- + H^+ \quad (11.1)$$

As a result of this dissociation carbonic acid can be indirectly excreted through the lungs. Lactic acid must be excreted through the kidneys, and this occurs more slowly.

Buffer systems exist in the body to prevent rapid pH changes. The HCO_3^-/CO_2 relationship is an important buffer system; other buffers include haemoglobin and, to a lesser extent, plasma proteins. Disturbance of the acid–base balance can produce either acidosis or alkalosis, which may be due to either metabolic or respiratory causes.

During aerobic metabolism CO_2 is produced, and in the presence of respiratory disease is less effectively excreted, causing the $P_a co_2$ to rise. As a result the infant becomes acidotic – respiratory acidosis. If the infant with relatively normal lungs breathes or is ventilated rapidly, more CO_2 is excreted and the reaction moves in the other direction to produce a respiratory alkalosis.

Lactic acid, the product of anaerobic metabolism, can only be excreted by the kidneys and, if in excess, the H^+ ions are buffered by haemoglobin, proteins and H_2CO_3. The HCO_3^- can be excreted through the lungs to compensate, thereby leaving an excess of H^+ causing a metabolic acidosis. Persistent vomiting causes loss of H^+, resulting in an excess of HCO_3^- with consequent metabolic alkalosis.

Thus, to keep the blood pH stable, the $P co_2$ will fall in both metabolic acidosis and respiratory alkalosis, and the $P co_2$ will rise in metabolic alkalosis and respiratory acidosis. In practice a simple respiratory acidosis rarely occurs, and in neonatal lung disease there is likely to be impairment of CO_2 excretion, together with production of lactic acid as a result of anaerobic metabolism, leading to a mixed respiratory and metabolic acidosis.

The base excess is derived from the relationship between pH and $P co_2$ using the Siggaard Anderson nomogram. It is the amount of buffer base added to blood, assuming that $P co_2$ is 5.5< kPa (40 mmHg), to correct the pH to 7.40. Thus, it is a direct measurement of the metabolic component of acidosis or alkalosis. Positive values represent excess of base and negative values excess of acid. The base excess is therefore valuable in assigning a predominant metabolic or respiratory component to acidosis or alkalosis.

The acid–base status of the infant can be derived from the blood gases. Normal biochemical ranges for arterial blood in term and preterm infants are shown in Table 11.2.

Specific treatments for various abnormalities of acid–base balance are described below.

Metabolic acidosis

Metabolic acidosis arises when there is tissue hypoxia (inadequate perfusion, hypoxaemia), excessive acid intake (total parenteral nutrition

Table 11.2 Normal biochemical range for arterial blood in term and preterm infants

Parameter	Term	Preterm
P_{O_2} mmHg (kPa)	60–90 (8–12)	50–80 (6.7–10.7)
P_{O_2} mmHg (kPa)	35–42 (4.7–5.6)	30–40 (4–5.3)
pH	7.35–7.42	7.32–7.40
Base excess (BE) (mmol/L)	−2–0	−4–0
Bicarbonate (mmol/L)	22–26	19–24

(TPN)), the production of excessive or abnormal acids (inborn errors of metabolism) or renal inability to excrete the acid load (tubular acidosis). In the presence of normal lungs the pH may be normal but the P_{CO_2} is low, and the base excess may be −8 mmol/L or more. Treatment is directed at the underlying problem.

In addition, metabolic acidosis may be treated by infusion of a molar (8.4%) solution of sodium bicarbonate. A solution containing 8.4% $NaHCO_3$ has 1 mmol of $NaHCO_3$ in 1 mL of solution and is usually infused slowly as a half-strength solution (4.2%). The dose is calculated as follows:

$$\text{Vol. of 8.4\% } NaHCO_3 \text{ (mL)} = \text{base excess} \times \text{weight in kg} \times 0.5 \quad (11.2)$$

The factor 0.5 represents the proportion of extracellular fluid to body weight in infants. The usual dose is 2–5 mmol/kg.

Sodium bicarbonate combines with excess hydrogen ions to produce unstable carbonic acid, which in turn is hydrolysed to CO_2 and H_2O. The CO_2 is excreted by the lungs. For this reason, bicarbonate should not be given in the presence of high P_aCO_2. Under these circumstances, trishydroxyaminomethane (THAM) is preferable to bicarbonate, and this is described in the section on respiratory acidosis.

Metabolic alkalosis

This metabolic derangement usually occurs following excessive vomiting or the overuse of sodium bicarbonate. The pH may be normal or high. The P_aCO_2 is usually raised and the base excess is positive. Treatment is by infusion of normal saline.

Respiratory acidosis

This is due to lung disease and is usually aggravated by a metabolic acidosis as a result of anaerobic metabolism and poor tissue perfusion. If there is a mixed acidosis the pH is low, P_aCO_2 high and base excess strongly negative. Treatment depends on the severity of the lung disease, but if the pH is below 7.25 the infant will usually require mechanical ventilation. Sodium bicarbonate should not be given if the P_aCO_2 is more than 45 mmHg (6 kPa). If the base excess is more than −10 mmol/L and the P_aCO_2 exceeds 45 mmHg (6 kPa), then THAM can be used. The dose is 0.3 M strength, 7 mL/kg infused over 30–60 min. THAM buffers H^+ and binds CO_2, thus lowering the P_aCO_2. It may cause apnoea and should only be used in infants being mechanically ventilated.

Respiratory alkalosis

This is due to overventilation and if it occurs while an infant is receiving mechanical ventilation it is simply treated by reducing the ventilator rate or inspiratory pressure.

Typical examples of acid–base derangements in the newborn, with interpretation and possible causes, are shown in Table 11.3.

Respiratory failure

Respiratory failure is present when there is a major abnormality of gas exchange resulting in hypoxaemia, hypercarbia and acidosis. Hypoxaemia may be due to either respiratory or cardiac abnormalities and, as an isolated factor, is not of great value in predicting the need for respiratory support. Hypercarbia is a much better indicator of respiratory failure. A rising P_aCO_2, particularly in the presence of a falling pH (respiratory acidosis), is an ominous sign. A value for P_aCO_2 of above 60 mmHg (8 kPa), with a respiratory acidosis (pH <7.25), indicates the need for mechanical ventilation. Some infants, particularly if very small, may require ventilation before these criteria are met. Hypercarbia and acidosis are strongly associated with the development of intraventricular haemorrhage in premature infants (see p. 216). The causes of respiratory failure are listed in Table 11.4.

Table 11.3 Examples of abnormal arterial blood-gas results and their interpretation

F_iO_2	P_aO_2 mmHg (kPa)	pH	P_aCO_2 mmHg (kPa)	BE	Bicarbonate (mmol/L)	Interpretation	Possible cause
0.21	75 (10)	7.13	60 (8)	−10	13	Mixed acidosis	Severe birth asphyxia
0.65	53 (7)	7.18	60 (8)	−8	15	Mixed acidosis. Hypoxia	Acute RDS
0.35	53 (7)	7.33	68 (9)	+8	34	Chronic respiratory. acidosis with renal compensation	Bronchopulmonary dysplasia
0.21	83 (11)	7.53	53 (7)	+15	44	Metabolic alkalosis with mild respiratory compensation	Vomiting. Pyloric stenosis

Assisted ventilation

Babies with signs of respiratory failure require artificial respiratory support, which can be given as follows:

1 continuous positive airway pressure (CPAP) administered via a face mask, a single nasal prong, twin nasal cannulas or an endotracheal tube; and
2 intermittent positive-pressure ventilation (IPPV) by means of a mechanical ventilator.

Continuous positive airway pressure (CPAP)

Mechanisms of CPAP

The first published report of the use of CPAP in the treatment of respiratory distress syndrome (RDS) was in 1971 (Gregory *et al.* 1971), and since then the technique has been widely used in the treatment of this condition. Infants with RDS often grunt on expiration because of their own attempts to apply an end-expiratory distending pressure. Exhalation against a closed glottis produces a grunt and maintains a larger functional residual capacity. CPAP mimics and augments this expiratory grunt. Continuous distending pressure maintains expansion of the alveoli and terminal bronchioles on expiration. This ensures a reasonable lung volume with more evenly distributed ventilation and reduces surfactant consumption. CPAP results in increased P_aO_2 but has a variable effect on P_aCO_2.

The introduction of CPAP to a preterm infant with RDS results in a decrease in respiratory rate, expiratory grunt, chest retractions and apnoea, and

Table 11.4 Causes of respiratory failure in the neonate

Poor respiratory effort	Extreme immaturity, CNS depression, postoperative infections, metabolic, neuromuscular disease
Abnormal lungs	Surfactant deficiency – RDS Retained fetal lung fluid –TTN Pulmonary oedema – hydrops, CCF
Abnormal airways	Infections – pneumonia Obstructed airways – meconium, pneumothorax
Hypoplastic lungs	Obstructive uropathy Diaphragmatic hernia
Small thoracic volume	Bowel obstruction, exomphalos/ gastroschisis repair, ascites, chondrodystrophic dwarfism

CCF, congestive cardiac failure; RDS, respiratory distress syndrome; TTN, transient tachypnoea of the newborn.

improves oxygenation, regularity of breathing and, from a physiological viewpoint, dynamic compliance, tidal volume and functional residual capacity.

Applying CPAP

CPAP may be administered in a variety of ways, including via a face mask, but nasal prongs seem to be the most satisfactory (or least unsatisfactory) method. For the most part, newborns are obligatory nose breathers; therefore nasal CPAP is easily facilitated. One or two prongs are inserted into one or both nostrils and attached to a ventilator or other device for delivering CPAP. Binasal (double) prongs are more effective than a single long prong. A binasal device that is claimed to have a 'fluidic flip' when the baby expires through the device is said to reduce the work of breathing, but there are few clinical data to substantiate any superiority over other available devices.

The disadvantages of nasal prongs include obstruction of the narrow-bore tube, gastric distension and pressure necrosis of the nares. Increased nasal secretions and mucus plugs lead to obstructive and mixed apnoea, often delaying the successful removal of CPAP.

CPAP can be given through an endotracheal tube (ETT) for a short period, especially when a baby is being weaned from the ventilator, but an ETT should not be used solely for the purpose of delivering CPAP because the resistance makes it difficult for the baby to breathe effectively for more than a short period.

Indications for CPAP

Respiratory distress syndrome. This is the classic indication in spontaneously breathing babies. For infants less than 1500 g birthweight CPAP is indicated if inspired O_2 exceeds 60%, to maintain Po_2 >60 mmHg (8 kPa). For many infants CPAP will be adequate, but mechanical ventilation may be requried if fractional oxygen (F_iO_2) of more than 0.6 to 0.7 is needed to maintain resonable arterial oxygen saturation. For infants of 800–1500 g birthweight who are vigorous at birth, CPAP may be commenced to maintain airway stabilization and allow time to assess the presence and severity of RDS. Mechanical ventilation is required if F_iO_2 exceeds 0.6, P_aCO_2 exceeds 55 mmHg (7.3 kPa) (particularly if pH <7.25) or the baby has apnoea. CPAP has proved beneficial in facilitating successful extubation in very low birthweight (VLBW) infants in many randomized trials.

The optimal pressure is difficult to predict. Generally CPAP of 4–8 cmH_2O is appropriate, but some infants benefit from higher pressures. This can be assessed by increasing the CPAP to 10 cmH_2O while watching a continuous readout of P_aO_2. The lowest pressure that produces the best arterial oxygenation is the optimal CPAP pressure.

Regular evaluation of P_aCO_2 and arterial pH is necessary to assess the infant's response to CPAP,

and mechanical ventilation may be necessary if deterioration occurs.

Obstructive apnoea. CPAP is beneficial in cases of obstructive apnoea due to floppiness of the posterior pharyngeal wall or collapse of the upper airways, as in premature infants.

Neuromuscular disorders. In conditions where there is reduced lung volume owing to poor fetal breathing movements, CPAP may be of some value.

Skeletal disorders. In certain conditions, such as neonatal rickets, where there is a highly compliant chest wall, CPAP of 4 cmH_2O may be beneficial, by increasing functional residual capacity and thereby reducing the work of breathing.

Chronic pulmonary insufficiency of prematurity. This is a non-specific term to describe chronic ventilatory dependency in very preterm babies due to a combination of factors such as poor respiratory drive and respiratory muscle weakness (low endurance).

Pulmonary oedema. This may be due to congestive cardiac failure, fluid overload or patent ductus arteriosus.

Contraindications for CPAP

CPAP should not be used in the following situations:

1 Severe acute episode(s) of apnoea – he or she should be intubated and ventilated.

2 When ventilation is required because the baby has respiratory failure (inability to maintain normal oxygenation with an F_iO_2 >0.6, a P_aCO_2 >60 mm (8 kPa), and pH<7.25).

3 In cases of upper airway abnormality (cleft palate, choanal atresia, tracheo-oesophageal fistula).

4 Severe cardiovascular instability.

5 Unstable respiratory drive with frequent apnoeas and or bradycardia.

Complications

The possible complications of CPAP are:

1 Pneumothorax or pulmonary interstitial emphysema due to overdistension of alveoli.

Table 11.5 Suggested ventilator settings when initiating ventilation for four different conditions. Changes are made on the basis of blood-gas data and non-invasive monitoring

	RDS (pre-surfactant)	PIE/pulmonary hypertension	Apnoea	Meconium aspiration
Rate	40–60/min	50–60/min	30/min	40/min
*PIP (cmH$_2$O)	25–30	20–25	14–16	30
PEEP (cmH$_2$O)	4–6	4	3–5	4–6
I:E ratio	2:3	1:1	–	2:3
Inspiratory time (s)	0.4	0.4	0.4	0.4
Fio$_2$	0.8	1.0	0.21	1.0

I:E, inspiration:expiration; PIE, pulmonary interstitial emphysema; RDS, respiratory distress syndrome.
*PIP is adjusted to provide a tidal volume delivery of 4–6 mL/kg (normal range for newborns).

2 Gastric distension and vomiting with face mask and nasal prongs.
3 Hypercapnia.
4 Pressure necrosis owing to a tight nasal tube.
5 Cerebellar haemorrhage and skull deformities with a tight face mask.
6 Nasal secretion, mucus plugs.

Initial ventilator settings

The initial intermittent positive-pressure ventilation (IPPV) settings for various indications are shown in Table 11.5.

Mechanical ventilation

Despite widespread use of non-invasive forms of respiratory support such as CPAP, a significant proportion of babies,especially those born under 28 weeks of gestation, require assisted breathing through mechanical ventilators. Since 1971 the standard method of mechanical ventilation has been intermittent mandatory ventilation (IMV), which provides a fixed rate of mechanical ventilation (mandatory breaths), determined by the clinician, and allows spontaneous breathing between mechanical breaths. This mode historically has been called time-cycled, pressure-limited ventilation, and used both during the acute phase of illness (high rates) or during the weaning phase (low rates). Although life saving, IMV has a major disadvantage in that the machine-delivered breaths and the baby's spontaneous breaths may not coincide. This asynchrony between machine and the patient can lead to a number of complications including poor gas exchange, airleaks and intraventricular haemorrhage. This has led to the development of a number of newer ventilatory modalities, collectively called *synchronized ventilation*, in which the machine delivers the breath only when it detects the onset of the patient's own inspiratory effort. This requires placement of a sensor at the proximal endotracheal tube, which should be sensitive to detect changes in airflow (flow sensors) and the capability of the machine to respond promptly by delivering gas to the airways during the inspiratory phase (patient-triggered ventilation). Synchronized ventilation can be accomplished in a number of ways, such as synchronized intermittent ventilation (SIMV), assist/control (A/C), pressure support ventilation (PSV) and proportional assist ventilation (PAV). The salient features of these methods are described below. The last decade has also seen an explosion of other advanced forms of ventilatory support, such as volume targeted modes of ventilation, high-frequency oscillatory ventilation (HFOV), high-frequency jet ventilation and extracorporeal membrane oxygenation (ECMO).

Sedation and paralysis

Mechanical ventilation in immature infants has been shown to be stressful, and many neonatologists sedate babies for at least some of the time that they are ventilated. An opiate (morphine or fentanyl) by continuous infusion is the most widely used sedative drug and also provides analgesia. If sedation without analgesia is required then midazolam or lorazepam is used, also by continuous infusion. These drugs may only be required for the first few days of mechanical ventilation and must be stopped prior to elective extubation for fear of causing respiratory depression.

Some babies on conventional ventilation breathe out of synchrony with the ventilator (this is often termed 'fighting the ventilator') and has been associated with the development of pneumothorax and intraventricular haemorrhage. Sometimes the baby's respiratory pattern can be entrained to that of the ventilator, but if the baby does 'fight' with vigorous out-of-phase spontaneous breaths, paralysis with pancuronium is often necessary. The newer techniques such as trigger ventilation and high-frequency ventilation (HFV) reduce the need for paralysis.

Conventional ventilation

Mechanical ventilation of the newborn has been traditionally accomplished using time-cycled, pressure-limited ventilation. This form of ventilation is designed to deliver a volume of gas using a preset peak inspiratory pressure delivered over a defined cycle time. As a result, the peak pressure at the proximal airway remains constant; however, the tidal volume delivered to the lungs is variable depending upon both the underlying pulmonary and chest wall mechanics. Thus, when the lungs are stiff, tidal volume delivery is lower at the same peak pressure than when the lungs are more compliant. This inconsistency in tidal volume delivery may be undesirable, especially in very preterm infants, as both overexpansion (volutrauma) and underexpansion/collapse (atelectotrauma) are thought to contribute to the pulmonary injury sequence. This has led to the introduction of a number of newer forms of ventilation, which aim to deliver a desired tidal volume automatically, irrespective of the underlying lung mechanics. One such modality is volume-controlled ventilation (VC), also referred to as volume-targeted or volume-limited ventilation, in which the primary gas delivery target is tidal volume, and inspiratory pressure is automatically adjusted from breath to breath depending on pulmonary compliance. Thus, in conditions with low lung compliance (stiff lungs), more pressure is generated to deliver the desired tidal volume. As lung compliance improves with resolution of the underlying pulmonary condition, the pressures generated

are automatically reduced, sometimes referred to as auto-weaning. Both pressure-limited and volume-controlled modes of ventilation can be provided in SIMV and A/C modes (Fig. 11.2).

Synchronized intermittent mandatory ventilation (SIMV)

SIMV is a ventilatory mode in which mechanical breaths are synchronized to the onset of a spontaneous breath and delivered at a fixed rate set by the clinician. Between these set breaths, the patient breathes spontaneously, supported only by the machine's baseline pressure. Thus SIMV offers some improvement over IMV in that it provides synchrony during the inspiratory phase, but because the inspiratory time of the machine-delivered breath and the baby's spontaneous breaths are not the same, this mode provides only partial synchrony.

Assist/control ventilation (synchronized intermittent positive pressure ventilation; SIPPV)

This is a dual mode form of ventilation providing additional improvement in synchronized ventilation compared with SIMV. In assist/control mode, there is delivery of a synchronized mechanical breath each time the machine detects the patient's inspiratory effort (assist), but if the patient fails to breathe (becomes apnoeic) the machine will deliver the breaths at a backup rate set by the operator. Although the spontaneous and mechanical breaths are completely synchronized to the onset of inspiration, again the possibility exists (like SIMV) that dyssynchrony will occur during the expiratory phase because of different inspiratory time (assist/control, time cycled). This problem has been overcome with the introduction of a second signal detection system that determines when the patient's inspiratory effort is about to cease and then synchronizes the termination of the mechanical breath to this signal (assist control, flow cycled).

Pressure support ventilation (PSV)

PSV is also a patient-triggered (synchronized) mode of ventilation in which spontaneous breaths are fully or partially supported by an inspiratory pressure assist ('boost') above baseline pressure to decrease the imposed work of breathing created by the narrow-lumen endotracheal tube and ventilator circuit. The amount of flow delivered to the patient during the inspiratory phase is variable and proportional to the patient effort in this mode. It can be used alone in patients with reliable respiratory drive, or in conjunction with low-rate SIMV. PSV is generally used during the weaning stages of ventilation and is designed in such a way that the patient can breathe as much (because of variable gas delivery) and for as long he or she wants (as it is flow cycled). Thus PSV provides complete synchrony and physiologically resembles a normal breath. It can be confused with flow-cycled, assist/control mode of ventilation, as both provide synchrony during both inspiratory and expiratory phases but the gas flow delivery characteristics of the two methods are different. Being servocontrolled PSV seems to be better suited as a weaning mode.

Proportional assist ventilation (PAV)

In PAV, the ventilator is continuously sensitive to the spontaneous respiratory efforts and adjusts the assist pressure in a proportionate and ongoing fashion. PAV does not by itself initiate breaths, and instead relies on a largely intact functioning of the infant's own breathing mechanism. During episodes of apnoea or hypoventilation, PAV reverts to back-up conventional ventilation, which is automatically withdrawn when the patient resumes spontaneous breathing. This may achieve near-perfect synchrony between the ventilator and spontaneous breathing, resulting in relief from disease-related increased work of breathing.

High-frequency ventilation (HFV)

HFV is conceptually different from conventional ventilation. In HFV, gas exchange is achieved with smaller tidal volumes and pressure amplitude than with conventional ventilation, features that are thought to reduce ventilator-associated lung injury. A comparison of the basic parameters of HFV and conventional ventilation is given in Table 11.6.

There are various ways in which HFV can be accomplished. The most commonly used method is high-frequency oscillatory ventilation (HFOV). Essentially this is a safer way of using 'super' PEEP (positive end-expiratory pressure). The lungs can be inflated to higher mean volumes without having to use high peak airway pressure to maintain ventilation (CO_2 removal). This produces more uniform lung inflation and reduces the risk of air leaks. Nonetheless, as with CV, there is the potential for gas trapping, which can cause overinflation of lungs with potential adverse consequences. Despite putative advantages of HFOV in physiological terms, there is no scientific evidence of its superiority over CV when used as the primary mode of ventilation. However, when used as an early rescue treatment in specific situations such as severe RDS, airleak syndromes and pulmonary hypoplasia, the results are encouraging.

Another method of providing HFV is high-frequency jet ventilation, but this is not practised as widely as HFOV. It works by providing pulses of high-velocity gas (jet-stream) down the centre of the airway, penetrating through the dead space gas. The kinetic energy of the gas emerging from the jet nozzle at high velocity, rather than the pressure gradient, drives gas movement in large airways. Air leak syndrome has been the most commonly treated underlying disorder but jet ventilation has been successfully used in a variety of other respiratory conditions in newborns.

Table 11.6. Comparison of basic parameters of HFV and conventional ventilation

Parameter	HFV	CV
Rate (breaths/mt)	180–1200	0–60
Vt (mL/kg)	0.1–5	4–20
Alveolar pressure (cmH_2O)	0.1–20	5–50
End-expiratory lung volume	High	Low
Minute ventilation	Rate$^{(0.5-1)} \times$ Vt$^{(1.5-2)}$	Rate × Vt

Vt, tidal volume.

Alternative strategies for refractory respiratory failure

Despite the introduction of newer modes of ventilation and strategies such as HFV, a number of babies still fail treatment and require adjunctive treatment. Two such methods, inhaled nitric oxide (iNO) therapy and extracorporeal membrane oxygen (ECMO), are now considered to be a part of the armamentarium of various treatment strategies and have been proven to be of value in selected cases (Cochrane review).

Inhaled nitric oxide (iNO) therapy. This form of treatment of newborns with hypoxaemic respiratory failure and pulmonary hypertension has dramatically changed management strategies for this critically ill group of babies. In 'term' newborns it causes potent, selective and sustained pulmonary vasodilatation (without decreasing systemic vascular tone), and improves oxygenation with dramatic improvement and a reduced need for ECMO. However, the potential role of iNO in 'preterm' newborns is currently controversial and remains under investigation. The recommended starting dose for iNO in term newborns is 20 ppm (parts per million), and the typical duration of therapy is <5 days, which parallels the clinical resolution of persistent pulmonary hypertension. Babies undergoing iNO therapy require monitoring of NO_2 and methaemoglobin. A combination of iNO and HFOV seems to provide the best result in babies with persistent pulmonary hypertension of newborn (PPHN).

Extracorporeal membrane oxygenation (ECMO). This uses an artificial lung circuit to provide 'lung rest' in babies (usually term) with reversible lung disease. Such a period of rest may allow lung recovery and help survival of the infant who has intractable respiratory failure not responding to conventional methods of respiratory support. ECMO circuits are of two types: venovenous (VV), which increases oxygen content; and venoarterial (VA), which increases oxygen content and can also increase cardiac output (pump flow).

For VA bypass, the right internal jugular vein and common carotid artery are used as access points and are often ligated as a part of the bypass procedure. Venous blood is passively drained via the right atrium and passed via a roller pump to a venous capacitance reservoir (bladder box), membrane lung, heat exchanger and arterial perfusion cannula.

For VV bypass, a double-lumen cannula is used to remove and return the blood to the right atrium; the rest of the circuit is the same as in VA ECMO. To prevent thrombotic complications while on ECMO, the infant is treated with systemic heparinization.

A randomized controlled trial of ECMO versus conventional ventilation in term infants with severe respiratory failure showed that ECMO was very effective in reducing mortality compared with conventional respiratory management. The developmental outcome in babies treated with ECMO was also very good.

General management of ventilated infants

The following aspects are of fundamental importance when managing ventilated infants:

1 Regular arterial blood-gas assessment, initially 4-hourly and less frequently as the infant stabilizes. Continuous monitoring of oxygenation with a transcutaneous Po_2 monitor and/or pulse oximetry and CO_2 with a transcutaneous Pco_2 monitor. Most of the newer ventilators now provide online continuous pulmonary graphics that can provide useful information regarding pulmonary mechanics.

2 Regular or continuous blood pressure monitoring with vigorous treatment of hypotension (see p. 178) by volume expansion with normal saline and inotropes such as dobutamine and/or dopamine.

3 Regular bacteriological surveillance and appropriate use of antibiotics.

4 Nutritional care through enteral feeding and/or total parenteral nutrition (TPN).

5 Adequate humidification of inspired gases.

6 Nursing in a thermoneutral environment.

7 Careful assessment of fluid balance.

8 Provision of adequate analgesia and sedation

Assessment of ventilation

The effectiveness of mechanical ventilation is judged by the observation of symmetrical chest wall movement, auscultation of equal air entry to both lungs and arterial blood-gas measurements.

Troubleshooting

If a sudden deterioration occurs during mechanical ventilation, then check ventilator failure, for example tube connection, tube blockage, accidental extubation into the oesophagus and tension pneumothorax.

When hypoxia or hypercapnia occur during ventilation it is essential to check whether a mechanical mishap or medical complication has occurred. If these factors are excluded, it may be appropriate to alter the ventilator settings.

Depending on the clinical circumstances hypoxia would generally be defined as a Po_2 <50 mmHg (6.7 kPa); the clinical response would depend on circumstances and ventilator settings, but would include F_iO_2; PIP; PEEP; inspiratory time.

The concept of permissive hypercapnia (P_aco_2 = 45–60 mmHg) is widely accepted, but a P_aco_2 >60 mmHg would generally necessitate a change in ventilator settings, including rate; PIP; ↑PEEP; ↑dead space if possible.

Complications of mechanical ventilation

The main complications of mechanical ventilation are dealt with in detail elsewhere in the book, as indicated below:

1 Pneumothorax and pulmonary air leak (see p. 99). Reversed inspiratory : expiratory (I:E) ratio and high levels of PEEP are most likely to cause this condition.
2 Intraventricular haemorrhage (see p. 216).
3 Patent ductus arteriosus (see p. 188).
4 Subglottic stenosis (see p. 128).
5 Bronchopulmonary dysplasia (see p. 107).

PRACTICE POINT

- Respiratory disorders constitute the major workload in neonatal intensive care units. Although mostly related to prematurity, these can be associated with a variety of conditions and a significant proportion of affected babies develop respiratory failure requiring artificial respiratory support.
- Moderate degrees of respiratory failure can be treated non-invasively by giving oxygen therapy and/or CPAP, which provides a continuous distending pressure and helps to improve lung volumes.
- A smaller proportion of babies with severe respiratory failure require assisted mechanical ventilation, which can be given by using different ventilatory modalities. Although based on sound physiological principles, these modalities are relatively new and require further scientific validation through clinical trials.
- Despite adequate ventilatory support through conventional methods, some babies may require alternative methods of treatment including high-frequency ventilation, inhaled nitric oxide therapy and extracorporeal membrane oxygenation.
- Whatever method is used, one should always compare the risks and benefits in order to prevent iatrogenic complications such as ventilator-induced lung injury (VILI)

References

Bhuta T, Clark RH, Henderson-Smart DJ. Rescue high frequency oscillatory ventilation vs conventional ventilation for infants with severe pulmonary dysfunction born at or near term. *Cochrane Database of Systematic Reviews* 2001, issue 1. Art. No.: CD002974. DOI: 10.1002/14651858. [Cochrane review of HFOV.]

Finer NN, Barrington KJ. Nitric oxide for respiratory failure in infants born at or near term. *Cochrane Database of Systematic Reviews* 2006, issue 4. Art. No.: CD000399. DOI: 10.1002/14651858. Pub 2. [Cochrane review on iNO.]

Greenough A, Milner AD, Dimitriou G. Synchronized mechanical ventilation for respiratory support in newborn infants. *Cochrane Database of Systematic Reviews* 2004, issue 3. Art. No.: CD000456. [Cochrane review of IMV vs synchronized ventilation.]

Gregory GA, Kitterman JA, Phibbs RH, Tooley WH, Hamilton WK. Treatment of the diopathic respiratory distress syndrome with continuous positive airway pressure. *N Eng J Med* 1971; **284**:1333–1339.

UK Collaborative ECMO Trial Group. UK collaborative randomised trial of neonatal ECMO. *Lancet* 1996; **348**:75–82.

Further reading

Avery GB, Fletcher MA, MacDonald MG (eds). *Neonatology: Pathophysiology and Management of the Newborn*, 4th edn. Philadelphia: Lippincott-Raven, 1994.

Donn SM, Sinha SK. *Manual of Neonatal Respiratory Care*. Philadelphia: Elsevier, 2006.

Goldsmith JP, Karotkin E. *Assisted Mechanical Ventilation of the Neonates*. Philadelphia: Saunders, 2003.

Greenough A, Milner A. *Neonatal Respiratory Disorder*. Oxford: Oxford University Press, Oxford: 2003.

12 Apnoea, bradycardia and upper airway obstruction

Physiology

The onset of breathing begins early in fetal life. It is intermittent, irregular and occurs only during periods of active rapid eye movement (REM) sleep. The function of fetal breathing is not fully understood as it has no role in gas exchange. Lung growth is dependent at least in part on fetal breathing activity, and the fetus who does not breathe is at risk of lung hypoplasia (p. 103).

After birth there is a marked change from intermittent fetal breathing to continuous breathing, but the mechanism by which this happens is not known, although increased P_aO_2 levels after birth are a factor. Although neonatal breathing is continuous, it is irregular, and this is especially the case in the preterm infant. Infants, particularly preterm infants, have less well-developed chemoreceptor responses to hypoxia and hypercapnia. Hypercapnia increases respiratory activity and hypoxia causes an initial increase in respiratory activity lasting several minutes, followed by a decrease in ventilatory frequency.

Breathing patterns in the newborn can be divided into four different types:

1 *Regular*. This is infrequent, when there are nearly equal breath-to-breath intervals.

2 *Irregular*. Unequal breath-to-breath intervals; this is particularly common in preterm infants.

3 *Periodic breathing*. Cycles of hyperventilation alternating with periods of hypoventilation and eventual apnoea lasting about 3 s.

4 '*Apnoea*'. Episodes of respiratory pause lasting 6 s or more. With advancing gestation to term, the proportion of time the infant is breathing regularly increases, and phases of irregular, periodic and apnoeic periods decline. Further maturation occurs in the months after birth.

Apnoea and bradycardia

Clinically significant apnoea is defined as a cessation of breathing (absence of respiratory airflow) lasting for 20 s or more. Apnoea lasting for less than 20 s is also significant if accompanied by colour change (duskiness/cyanosis), or bradycardia of less than 100 beats/min.

Apnoea is most common in more immature babies. It is seen in 25% of infants of birthweight <2500 g, and in over 80% of infants with birthweight <1000 g (Miller & Martin 1992). It is most common at the end of the first week of life, and then tends to become less frequent as the baby matures.

Aetiology of apnoea and bradycardia

In the term infant the aetiology is usually identified, whereas in the preterm infant it is unusual to find a cause. Recurrent apnoea of prematurity is presumed to be due to immaturity of the respiratory centre in the brainstem and immaturity of chemoreceptor responses to hypoxia and acidosis, but still the diagnosis is based on exclusion of other causes, which can be pathological and require treatment (see below).

Types of apnoea

Central apnoea

Central apnoea accounts for 25% of all cases of neonatal apnoea. It is due to factors affecting the respiratory centre in the brainstem or the higher centres in the cerebral cortex. Causes include

1 prematurity;

2 hypoxia/acidosis (e.g. in respiratory distress syndrome (RDS), pneumonia, pneumothorax);

3 drugs (e.g. maternal narcotics, trishydroxyaminonethane (THAM), prostin (PGE1), magnesium sulphate);

4 metabolic (e.g. hypoglycaemia, hypocalcaemia, hypomagnesaemia or hypermagnesaemia);

5 generalized sepsis or specific infection (meningitis, encephalitis): apnoea occurring early in the course of respiratory distress must alert the medical attendant to the possibility of group B β-haemolytic streptococcal septicaemia;

6 intracranial haemorrhage or ischaemia (intraventricular haemorrhage, periventricular leukomalacia);

7 polycythaemia with hyperviscosity;

8 necrotizing enterocolitis;

9 patent ductus arteriosus;

10 convulsions (see p. 57);

11 developmental anomalies of the brain;

12 temperature instability: nursing an infant in an environmental incubator temperature that is too high is an important and common cause of apnoea. In addition, hypothermia, too rapid warming or too rapid cooling may be associated with apnoea.

13 central alveolar hypoventilation syndrome (CAHS) (Ondine curse);

14 idiopathic.

Obstructive apnoea

Babies are obligatory nose breathers and if their nares are obstructed, especially while sleeping, they are prone to severe apnoea. Obstructive apnoea accounts for 15% of cases and occurs with congenital malformations, such as choanal atresia and the Pierre Robin sequence. Preterm infants with small upper airways may have apnoea when in the supine position, especially during active (REM) sleep. Apnoea of this type may be minimized by nursing the infant in the prone position. Presence of milk, mucus or meconium in the upper airway is likely to provoke severe episodes of obstructive apnoea.

Mixed apnoea

Mixed apnoea accounts for the majority (approximately 60%) of cases, but may be difficult to diagnose clinically. Superficially it resembles central apnoea initially, with cessation of respiration, but then the baby makes intermittent respiratory efforts without achieving gas exchange.

Reflex apnoea

Babies may develop reflex apnoea or vagally mediated apnoea due to vigorous suction of the pharynx, passage of a nasogastric tube, physiotherapy or sometimes even in response to defecation. Apnoea associated with gastro-oesophageal reflux may be reflex and/or obstructive.

Investigation of apnoea

All babies who suffer from apnoea must be carefully examined to exclude respiratory or remote disease. Investigations are carried out to determine treatable causes of apnoea and will depend on the prevailing clinical condition. Investigations include

1 full blood count;

2 bacterial culture of blood, urine, cerebrospinal fluid (CSF), tracheal aspirate and other potential sites of infection;

3 chest X-ray;

4 blood glucose;

5 serum electrolytes, including calcium, magnesium and sodium;

6 arterial blood gases and continuous monitoring of oxygen saturation and perhaps P_{CO_2};

7 ultrasound examination of the head;

8 if gastro-oesophageal reflux is suspected, a number of further investigations may be undertaken, including an intra-oesophageal pH probe and/or contrast study (see p. 57);

9 (in special circumstances) further neurological investigations, i.e. electroencephalogram (EEG), polygraphic sleep studies;

10 a polymerase chain reaction (PCR) for the *PHOX2B* gene may identify cases of CAHS.

Apnoea monitoring

A variety of respiratory monitors are available, including a pressure-sensitive pad on which the infant lies, an air-filled plastic blister attached to the abdomen (SIMS Graseby Medical ltd, Watford, UK) and impedance monitors using electrodes attached to the chest wall. None of these will detect obstructive apnoea until the infant stops fighting for breath. The use of an oxygen saturation monitor or an electrocardiogram (ECG) monitor together with an apnoea monitor is recommended in order to recognize bradycardia occurring with an obstructed airway.

Treatment of apnoea

General management

Prevention and early detection

Apnoeic episodes should be prevented whenever possible. This involves careful handling of low birthweight infants and attention to feeding techniques, with avoidance of stomach distension and rapid feeding. The infant's temperature needs to be maintained in the thermoneutral range. Careful suctioning of the airway and positioning of the infant should minimize obstruction.

Treatment of an underlying cause

This depends on the results of the relevant investigations.

Acute episode

A suggested approach to managing an acute episode of apnoea is shown in Fig. 12.1. The following procedures are recommended:

1 Stimulation of the infant. If the episodes are brief and not associated with systemic features, this may be all that is necessary.

2 Suction of the upper airways and repositioning is indicated when obstruction is the likely cause.

3 Manual ventilation with a face mask and bag.

4 Intubation and intermittent positive pressure ventilation will be necessary when the baby fails to respond to bag-and-mask ventilation, or when severe apnoeic attacks occur frequently requiring significant resuscitation.

Recurrent apnoea

This usually occurs in preterm infants and may be very difficult to manage. However, before embarking on extreme forms of treatment, the potential hazards of the therapy must be carefully balanced against the potential for the brain-damaging effects of the apnoeic episode. The following techniques are employed in the management of recurrent apnoea:

1 Nurse in the prone position.

2 Consider altering the feeding regimen, i.e. a continuous milk infusion or transpyloric feeding may be better tolerated than intermittent feeds.

3 If anaemia is thought to be a contributing factor, then it should be treated by blood transfusion, but the lowest acceptable level of haemoglobin may be difficult to determine (see p. 193).

4 Increasing the inspired oxygen in small increments while monitoring the oxygen tension.

5 Specific treatment includes drugs, continuous positive airway pressure (CPAP) and frequent stimulation.

Stimulation

Tactile stimulation by regular stroking of the infant has been shown to reduce the number of apnoeic episodes, but this is not a feasible method for routine use. A variety of rocking mattresses have been devised that gently rock or undulate the baby; these appear to reduce the frequency of apnoeas in some infants.

Drug treatment

This is only indicated when specific causes of apnoea have been treated. Drugs for apnoea are usually continued until the baby is 35–37 weeks of postmenstrual age.

Methylxanthines

Theophylline. This is given orally in a loading dose of 6 mg/kg and a daily maintenance dose of 3 mg/kg/day in two or three divided doses. The half-life of theophylline varies between 12 and 56 h. Serum levels of both aminophylline and theophylline should be maintained between 6 and 13 µg/mL. Levels up to 20 µg/mL may be acceptable if there is a poor clinical response to the lower range. Tachycardia and irritability are the first signs of overdosage.

Caffeine. The neonate methylates theophylline to caffeine, and caffeine appears to be the drug of choice in many centres for treatment of apnoea. The loading dose is 20 mg/kg orally followed by 2.5–5 mg/kg once daily. Serum levels of caffeine are not routinely monitored but should be checked if there are any side effects. Therapeutic range is between 10 and 20 µg/mL.

Aminophylline. This is given intravenously, with a loading dose of 6 mg/kg followed by a maintenance dose of 4.5 mg/kg/day given in divided doses 8- or 12-hourly. Serum levels must be regularly monitored

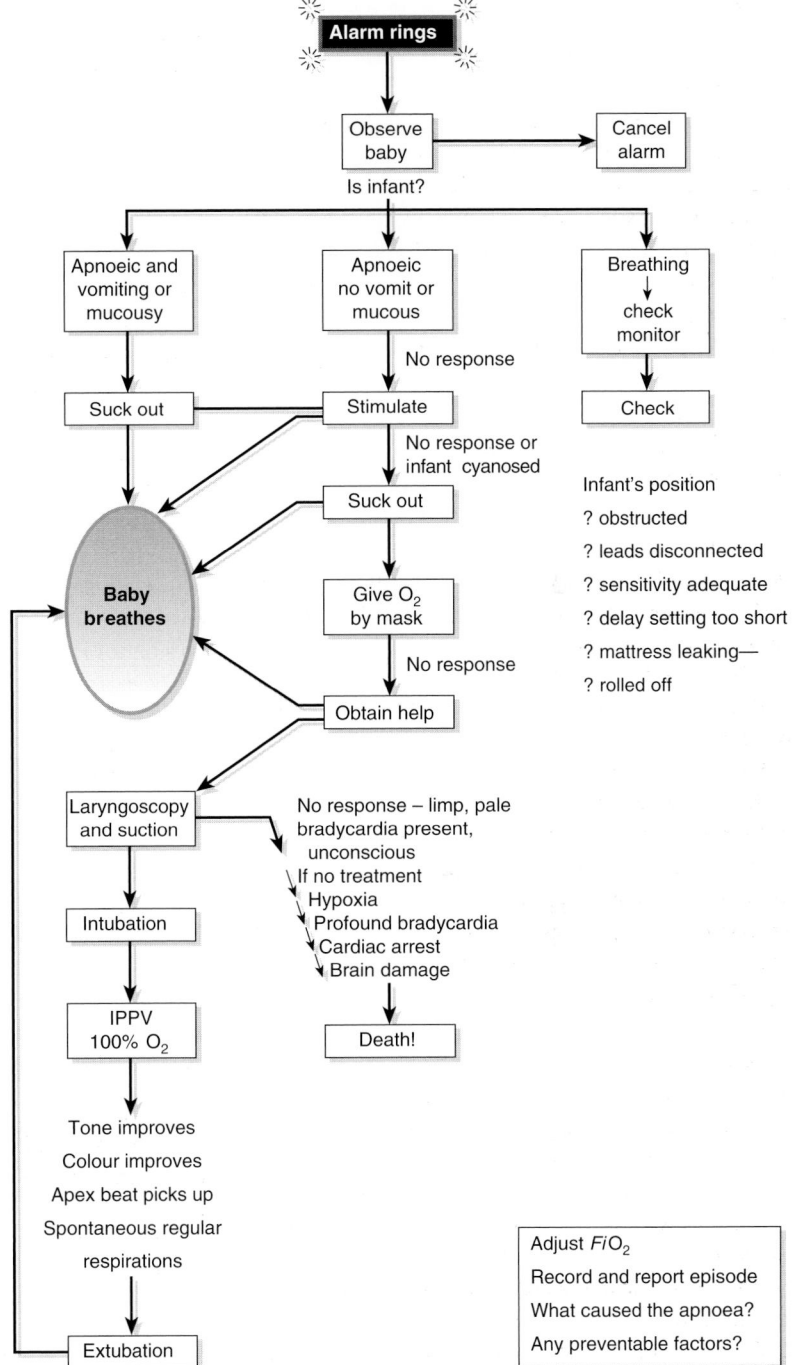

Figure 12.1 Suggested protocol following an apnoea or brady-cardia alarm.

starting 48 h after the loading dose because of the frequent occurrence of side effects.

Doxapram

This is used only in selected infants in whom recurrent apnoea cannot be controlled by methylxanthines. The dose is 0.5–2.0 mg/kg/h by continuous infusion. Extreme jitteriness is a well-recognized side-effect.

Ventilatory support

CPAP may be effective in treating or preventing apnoea. It probably acts in a number of ways, but mainly by splinting open the upper airway structures. It has little effect on central apnoea. The use of nasal prongs to administer CPAP (4–8 cmH$_2$O) may produce additional effects by local stimulation. The administration of CPAP is described in Chapter 11. Theophylline may be more effective for central apnoea, and CPAP for obstructive or mixed apnoea.

In infants who are resistant to CPAP and respiratory stimulants and who continue to have severe apnoeic attacks, intubation and mechanical ventilation are required to avoid major physiological changes associated with the apnoeic episodes. Only minimal pressures and rates are usually required.

Prognosis

With respect to prognosis it is important to distinguish the cause of the apnoea from its effect. There is an association between recurrent apnoea and later cerebral palsy, but this may reflect the common origin of the brain lesion that causes the movement disorder, the prematurity and the resultant apnoea. In general, outcome is related to the underlying cause, and when correction is made for confounding factors, apnoea per se has no additional deleterious effect on outcome.

Recurrent apnoea of prematurity has usually resolved by 37 weeks' postmenstrual age, but in some infants apnoea may persist beyond the expected date of delivery and no cause can be found. In some cases discharge home on methylxanthine drugs is recommended, and home apnoea monitors may be of benefit.

Sudden infant death syndrome (SIDS; sudden unexpected death in infancy, SUDI)

Sudden infant death syndrome (SIDS or SUDI) is the unexpected death of an infant between 1 month and 1 year of age that remains unexplained despite extensive review of the medical records, a postmortem examination and a death scene investigation. To date no exact cause for SIDS has been identified, and it appears likely that it represents a final common pathway for a number of unrelated clinical phenomena.

Neonatologists must be aware of the risk of sudden infant death syndrome (SIDS) in survivors of neonatal care and give appropriate advice to reduce the risk once the baby has gone home. There are a number of risk factors for SIDS that are relevant to the neonatologist. These include
1 maternal smoking or drug abuse;
2 prematurity;
3 low birthweight;
4 multiple births;
5 infant-parent co-sleeping

The incidence of SIDS has fallen in recent years by up to 75% in countries where risk reduction procedures have been widely adopted. These include
1 putting babies to sleep on their backs;
2 avoiding exposure of the baby to tobacco smoke;
3 avoidance of overwrapping the baby and prevention of overheating;
4 breastfeeding, which has been shown to have a protective effect in some countries;
5 additional factors that may be important include early advice about minor illnesses, and discouraging having the baby in the bed with the parents (co-sleeping).

It is important for staff on neonatal units to recognize those babies at high risk and to discuss risk reduction procedures with the parents. Instruction on resuscitation (showing the parents an appropriate video followed by a question and answer session), and for a few the provision of an apnoea monitor for when the baby goes home, is part of this care.

Acute life-threatening events on a neonatal unit

Acute life-threatening events (ALTEs) are sudden unexpected episodes of colour change with limpness, collapse or apnoea in an apparently otherwise well baby. These are very worrying episodes both for the parents and clinical staff. Appropriate investigations must be performed to elucidate a cause, but if no cause is found then anxiety may persist about the risk of a similar event occurring again once the baby has gone home.

The risk of recurrence of ALTE possibly causing SIDS has been much debated, and the subsequent need for monitoring of the baby remains controversial. Recent research has confirmed that there is an association between ALTE and SIDS cases, but when multivariate regression analysis is performed these studies show that the risk is not increased if the data are adjusted for factors such as maternal age, education, smoking, alchohol consumption, social deprivation, tog value of the bedding, co-sleeping with a parent and the baby being placed prone to sleep. Consequently it is believed by some authorities that ALTE do not predict an increased risk of SIDS when the child goes home.

Home apnoea monitors

The parents of prematurely born babies may request apnoea monitors for use at home. There is no evidence that home monitors reduce the risk of a major life-threatening event occurring out of hospital, nor do they prevent death: babies have died despite being monitored.

Many parents whose baby presents with an ALTE demand a home apnoea monitor; but, as described above, there is no evidence that this prevents SIDS. Each case should be considered individually and the parents carefully counselled. In any case where an apnoea monitor is given for home use it is essential that the parents are shown how to apply basic resuscitation skills to their infant prior to giving them an apnoea monitor, in case the baby is found apnoeic or collapsed at home.

Upper airway obstruction

Upper airway obstruction frequently presents in the delivery room or nursery as a result of foreign material in the airway, and can readily be relieved by suction. Upper airway obstruction not relieved by suction is unusual and may be mild, occurring only when the infant is distressed, crying or during feeds. Severe airway obstruction at birth due to anatomical abnormalities may be life threatening.

A spectrum of pathological conditions can affect the neonatal upper airway, and these can be conveniently divided into the following groups according to the site of the lesions:

1 Nasal and nasopharyngeal lesions (choanal atresia, intranasal tumours, nasolacrimal duct cysts).
2 Oral and oropharyngeal lesions (lymphatic malformation at base of tongue, tongue cysts, large tongue)
3 Laryngeal lesions (laryngomalacia, bifid or absent epiglottis, vocal cord paralysis, laryngeal web, subglottic stenosis, laryngeal cleft, subglottic haemangioma, intubation trauma).

Clinical features

Despite the varied pathophysiology, the clinical presentations of these disorders are similar.

1 Stridor. This is the most common symptom. It is mostly inspiratory but there may be an expiratory component if the obstruction is below the glottis (intrathoracic).
2 Suprasternal and sternal retractions. Although chest retractions may be evident, the most marked retractions will be suprasternal.
3 Croupy cough.
4 Hoarse cry.
5 Difficulty in feeding.

With severe increasing upper airway obstruction the baby may develop cyanosis followed by apnoea and bradycardia. Besides looking for the cause of the upper airway obstructon, it is of primary importance to determine the degree of emergency and decide whether the infant needs an artificial airway (endotracheal intubation or tracheostomy). This decision can be made mostly on clinical evaluation.

Causes of persistent stridor include

1 supraglottic – 62% (mostly laryngomalacia, rarely lingual cysts);
2 vocal cord – 15% (nerve palsies, webs, papilloma, foreign body);

3 subglottic stenosis – 14%;
4 tracheomalacia – 9%.

Laryngomalacia (infantile larynx)

The larynx in children with this condition is unusually floppy and narrows on inspiration, with resultant stridor. The stridor is often only present on crying. It is a benign condition that improves with age, but the stridor may not disappear until 6–9 months from birth. Diagnosis is made at laryngoscopy and the parents should be reassured that the condition is self-limiting in the majority of cases. If the condition persists a paediatric ear, nose and throat (ENT) opinion is valuable as in more severe cases, endoscopic laser aryepiglottic fold excision can provide symptomatic relief without the need for tracheostomy. However, for severe cases of laryngomalacia resulting in significant airway obstruction, tracheostomy remains the choice of treatment.

Choanal atresia

This is a developmental anomaly of the nasal airways and can present as an acute emergency at birth. It is caused by failure of the embryonic bucconasal membrane to cannulate, resulting in a bony or membranous obstruction, which is usually unilateral and rarely bilateral. In the latter case recurrent cyanotic and apnoeic spells are a major problem from birth, and the condition requires immediate surgical correction via either a transpalatal or a transnasal approach, with stents left in the posterior nares for up to 6 weeks to prevent the bone overgrowing and closing the posterior nares again. Unilateral atresia rarely requires surgical intervention during infancy. The condition is suspected because of inability to pass a catheter through the nasal passage and worsening of symptoms when baby is fed with a teat in the mouth (as baby cannot breathe). Associated anomalies occur in 20–50% of infants with choanal atresia, such as the CHARGE association, which includes **c**oloboma or other ophthalmic abnormality, **h**eart disease, choanal **a**tresia, **r**etarded development, **g**enital hypoplasia, and **e**ar abnormality with hearing loss.

Subglottic stenosis

This is most commonly an acquired condition, and in the rarer congenital cases the baby often presents early with stridor. Acquired subglottic stenosis is usually related to trauma of the glottic structures by vigorous suction or intubation. More commonly it is related to prolonged intermittent positive pressure ventilation (IPPV) through an endotracheal tube. With modern endotracheal tubes the incidence of this condition has fallen, and it now occurs in only 1% of ventilated infants.

The mechanisms by which stenosis develops are multifactorial, but physical ulceration from the tube, together with the piston action of the ventilator, is a very important causative factor. In addition, poor humidification of inspired gases and local infection may be contributory. The duration of intubation is important, but stenosis has been reported not uncommonly in infants intubated for only a few days.

Most infants with stridor following extubation have some subglottic oedema. If subglottic stenosis is suspected, direct laryngoscopy by an experienced ENT surgeon must be urgently arranged prior to extubating the baby if possible. Those with stenosis usually do not present until after discharge, when an intercurrent upper respiratory tract infection precipitates serious upper airway obstruction. Tracheostomy should be avoided wherever possible as, in many of these children, later closure of the tracheostomy is difficult. Surgical procedures such as repeated dilatation, or cryo- or laser surgery to split the cricoid cartilage anteriorly, may be successful in managing the condition.

Tracheostomy

This is the creation of an artificial airway through the trachea for the purposes of establishing either airway patency below an obstruction or an airway for prolonged ventilatory support. It is used either as an emergency procedure in cases of acute upper airway obstruction (rarely) or as an elective procedure, as in chronic lung disease or neuromuscular diseases, where the infant requires prolonged ventilatory support. Caregivers require training on how to replace the tube if it becomes dislodged or blocked. The tracheostomy can be closed when the underlying pathology improves.

Ex utero intrapartum treatment (EXIT) procedures are performed in selected centres to manage various forms of fetal airway obstruction (congenital high airway obstruction syndrome, CHAOS), unilateral pulmonary agenesis and diaphragmatic hernia. *Ex Utero* Intrapartum Treatment (EXIT) to ECMO has also been successfully reported.

Bronchoscopy

Bronchoscopy is another useful procedure for evaluating upper airway problems. A flexible 2.2-mm or 2.7-mm bronchoscope should be able to pass through a 2.5- or 3.0-mm endotracheal tube and visualize the upper airway structures under light (preferably xenon), producing images that can then be recorded on a video camera. Common neonatal diagnoses amenable to bronchoscopy include

1 Upper airway lesions
   - laryngomalacia;
   - subglottic stenosis;
   - laryngeal haemangioma;
   - laryngeal oedema and/or inflammation.
2 Lower airway lesions:
   - broncho-tracheomalacia;
   - tracheo-oesophageal fistula;
   - tracheal stenosis or web;
   - abnormal tracheal anatomy;
   - tracheal or bronchial granuloma, mucus plugs or blood clots.

PRACTICE POINT

- Apnoea is most common in more immature babies. It is seen in 25% of infants of birthweight <2500 g and in over 80% of infants with birthweight <1000 g.
- Drug treatment for apnoea is only indicated when specific causes of apnoea have been treated. Drugs for apnoea are usually continued until the baby is 35–37 weeks of postmenstrual age.
- CPAP may be effective in treating or preventing apnoea. It probably acts in a number of ways, but mainly by splinting open the upper airway structures. It has little effect on central apnoea.
- Sudden infant death syndrome (SIDS or SUDI) is the unexpected death of an infant aged between 1 month and 1 year that remains unexplained despite extensive review of the medical records, a postmortem examination and a death scene investigation.
- Upper airway obstruction frequently presents in the delivery room or nursery as a result of foreign material in the airway, and can readily be relieved by suction.

References

Miller MJ, Martin RJ. Apnea of prematurity. *Clin Perinatol* 1992;**19**:789–808.

Martin RJ. (ed.) Exploring neonatal apnoea: The journey continues. *Semin Neonatol* 2004;**9**(3):167–244.

Further reading

Jones RAK. Apnoea of immaturity. 1. A controlled trial of theophylline and face mask continuous positive airway pressure. *Arch Dis Child* 1982;**57**:761–765.

CHAPTER 13

13 Jaundice

Neonatal jaundice is the most common problem encountered in the newborn. About 50% of all full-term infants and 85% of preterm infants are visibly jaundiced within the first week of life.

Unconjugated bilirubin, which is elevated in the most common forms of neonatal jaundice, can pass through the blood–brain barrier and cause permanent brain damage with chronic disability (see Kernicterus and bilrubin encephalopathy section in this chapter, p. 138).

Physiology of bilirubin metabolism

Fetal

In the uterus, the fetal liver is relatively inactive. The placenta and maternal liver metabolize the bilirubin from worn-out red blood cells. If there is excessive fetal red cell haemolysis, for example, in rhesus haemolytic disease, the placenta and maternal liver may not be able to deal with the excessive bilirubin load, and the umbilical cord and amniotic fluid will be stained yellow by the bilirubin pigment produced. In addition, the bone marrow and extramedullary organs of erythropoiesis may not be able to keep up with the production of red cells, so that the fetus will become anaemic. Hydrops fetalis, a condition associated with generalized oedema, pleural effusions, ascites and hepatosplenomegaly, is due to a combination of anaemia, intrauterine hypoxia, hypoproteinaemia, a low colloid osmotic pressure and congestive heart failure.

The fetus is capable of conjugating bilirubin in small amounts and when haemolysis occurs *in utero*, as for example, in severe rhesus isoimmunization, bilirubin conjugation increases and high levels of direct-reacting bilirubin may be measured in the umbilical cord blood.

Newborn

The metabolism of bilirubin in the newborn is summarized in Fig. 13.1. Each of the steps in the metabolism of bile will be discussed in turn.

Bilirubin production

Most of the daily bilirubin production comes from senescent red blood cells. The red cells are destroyed in the reticulo-endothelial (RE) system and the haem is converted to unconjugated bilirubin. One gram of haemoglobin will produce $600\,\mu mol$ (35 mg) of unconjugated bilirubin. Haemolysis may be increased by maternal drugs such as salicylates, sulphonamides, phenacetin and nitrofurantoin. Twenty-five per cent of the daily production of bilirubin comes from sources other than the red cells, such as haem protein and free (tissue) haem.

Transport and liver uptake

Most of the unconjugated bilirubin in the blood is bound to serum albumin and is transported as a bound complex to the liver. This binding is extremely important and may be altered by many factors. Factors that decrease albumin binding ability include low serum albumin, asphyxia, acidosis, infection, prematurity and hypoglycaemia.

In addition, there are many competitors for bilirubin binding sites, and these include
1 non-esterified (free) fatty acids produced by starvation, cold stress or intravenous fat emulsion;
2 drugs (sulphonamides, cephalosporins, sodium benzoate (present in diazepam), frusemide and thiazide diuretics).

When bilirubin is bound to albumin it is probably non-toxic, but free unbound unconjugated bilirubin is fat soluble and can be transported across the

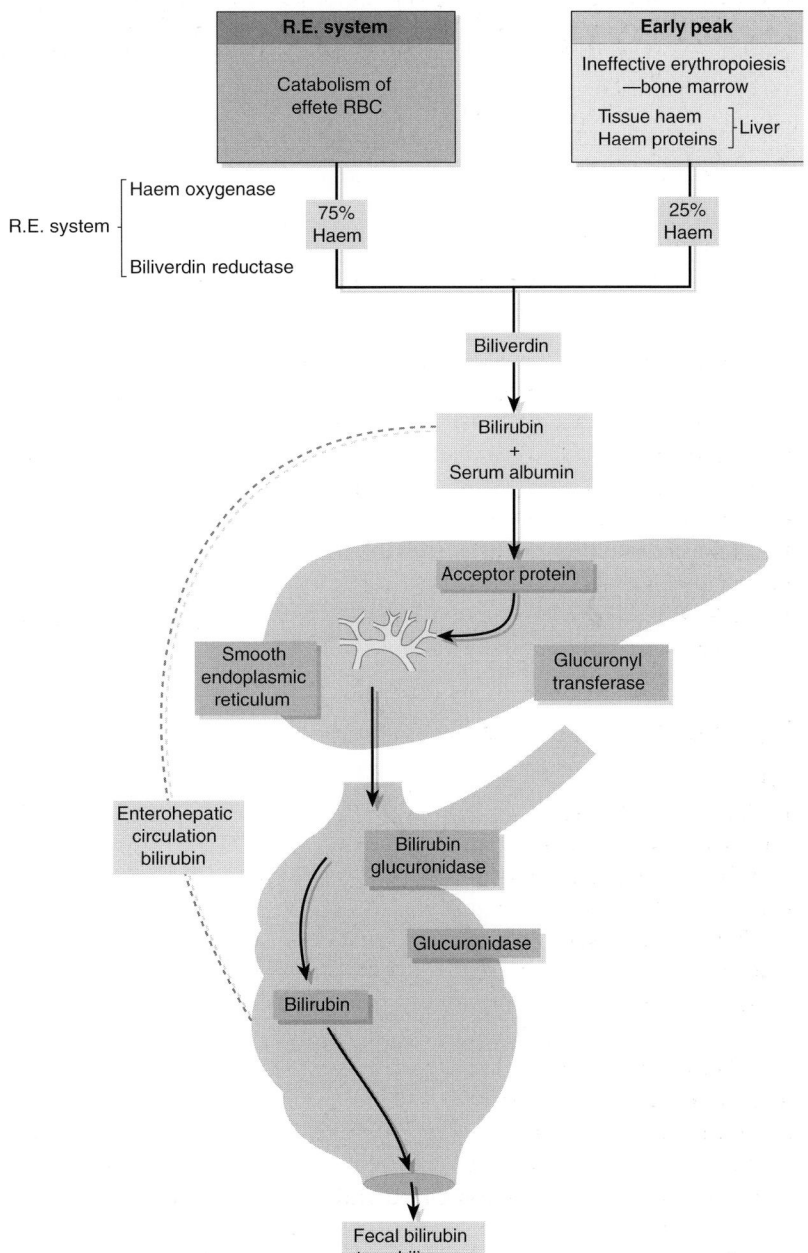

Figure 13.1 Summary of neonatal bilirubin metabolism. (Redrawn with permission from Maisels 1994.)

blood–brain barrier and be deposited in certain neurons, causing kernicterus.

The hepatocytes lining the liver sinusoids are able to extract unconjugated bilirubin from the blood and this is then accepted in the liver cell by the Y and Z proteins (ligandins).

Conjugation and excretion

The unconjugated bilirubin is conjugated in the liver and the reaction involves the conversion of insoluble unconjugated bilirubin to direct-reacting bilirubin (water soluble). Each molecule of bilirubin is conjugated with two molecules of glucuronic acid in a reaction catalysed by the enzyme glucuronyl transferase. The conjugated bilirubin is excreted into the bile, and then into the duodenum and small intestine. In the older child the bilirubin is reduced to stercobilinogen by bacteria in the small bowel, but in the newborn with a relatively sterile bowel and poor peristalsis much of the conjugated bilirubin may be hydrolysed by glucuronidase to unconjugated bilirubin, which enters the enterohepatic circulation for further liver metabolism.

This may be important in pathological situations, and reinforcement of the enterohepatic circulation will increase unconjugated bilirubin levels in prematurity, small bowel obstruction, functional bowel obstruction and pyloric stenosis.

Clinical assessment of the jaundiced infant

Jaundice can be detected in the immediate postnatal period when the serum level of bilirubin is approximately 100 µmol/L. As jaundice is common it is essential to have a clinical method for determining its severity. Proper lighting is important for detecting subtle levels of jaundice.

One clinical method of assessing the degree of jaundice present before investigations are undertaken is the use of Kramer's rule (Kramer 1969). This technique depends on the blanching of the infant's skin with the examiner's finger at standard zones (1–5) and observing the colour in the blanched area (Fig. 13.2). The zones of jaundice reflect the downward progression of dermal icterus.

Other available non-invasive methods used to assess jaundice include transcutaneous bilirubinometry (TcB) and end-tidal carbon monoxide (ETCO) measurements. Both seem to provide a good correlation with total serum bilirubin, but may have certain limitations in specific situations.

In assessing the significance of jaundice in a newborn infant the following guidelines may be useful. Investigations should be carried out under the following circumstances:

1 any infant who is visibly jaundiced in the first 24 h of life;

2 any jaundiced infant whose mother has rhesus antibodies;

3 a preterm infant whose estimated serum bilirubin is greater than 150 µmol/L;

4 a term infant whose estimated serum bilirubin exceeds 200 µmol/L;

5 any infant who has the clinical signs of obstructive jaundice;

6 prolonged hyperbilirubinaemia beyond 1 week in term infants and beyond 2 weeks in preterm infants.

When an infant is considered to have clinically significant jaundice, the assessment must include a thorough physical examination after careful history taking.

The presence or absence of the following features should be noted:

1 extravascular blood, e.g. bruising, cephalhaematoma, purpura, petechiae;

2 plethora or pallor;

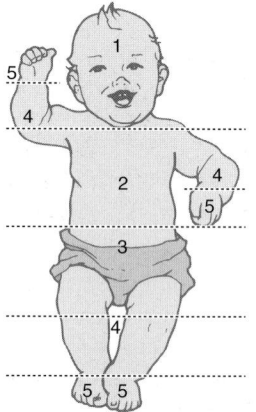

Kramer' s rule		Serum indirect bilirubin (µmol/L)
Zone	Jaundice	Average
1	Limited to head and neck	100
2	Over upper trunk	150
3	Over lower trunk, thighs	200
4	Over arms, legs, below knee	250
5	Hands, feet	>250

Figure 13.2 Kramer's rule for clinical assessment of neonatal jaundice. (Reproduced from Kramer 1969.)

3 hepatosplenomegaly;

4 evidence of intrauterine infection: small for gestational age, cataracts, microcephaly;

5 infection: umbilicus, skin;

6 neurological signs: hypertonia, opisthotonus, fits, abnormal eye movements;

7 abdominal distension: associated with bowel obstruction, bowel stasis or hypothyroidism.

The routine physical examination of a jaundiced neonate should always include a urine test for bile and reducing substance and a description of the stools, that is, whether or not they are pale. Bilirubin in the urine (tested by a 'stick' test) indicates that a component of the serum bilirubin is conjugated. This is an important factor in investigating the cause of jaundice.

Investigations

The investigation of a jaundiced newborn infant must take into consideration the history of the pregnancy, the gestational age and postnatal age of the infant, and the initial physical examination. It is also important to note whether drugs or toxins may have been involved in the production of the jaundice, and the ethnic origins of the parents.

In any jaundiced infant two questions must be answered:

1 Is the unconjugated hyperbilirubinaemia likely to cause neurological damage?

2 Is the bilirubin conjugated?

Conjugated hyperbilirubinaemia is likely to be associated with a more serious cause, which in the case of biliary atresia must be rapidly diagnosed and early surgical treatment undertaken.

Repeated total serum bilirubin estimations should be performed in infants with a rapid and early rise of (unconjugated) bilirubin so that treatment for hyperbilirubinaemia can be instituted. Bilirubin in the urine indicates that the conjugated fraction of bilirubin should be estimated in the laboratory and causes of conjugated hyperbilirubinaemia considered. Table 13.1 lists the possible causes of jaundice presenting at different times in the neonatal period.

A diagnostic approach to neonatal jaundice is shown in Fig. 13.3.

Table 13.1 Possible causes of jaundice presenting at different times in the neonatal period

Day	Unconjugated jaundice	Conjugated jaundice
1	Haemolytic disease assumed until proven otherwise	Neonatal hepatitis Rubella CMV Syphilis
2–5	Haemolysis Physiological Jaundice of prematurity Sepsis Extravascular blood Polycythaemia Glucose-6-Phosphate dehydrogenase deficiency Spherocytosis	As above
5–10	Sepsis Breast milk jaundice Galactosaemia Hypothyroidism Drugs	As above
10+	Sepsis Urinary tract infection	Biliary atresia Neonatal hepatitis Choledochal cyst Pyloric stenosis

Unconjugated hyperbilirubinaemia

Causes

The causes of prolonged unconjugated hyperbilirubinaemia are shown in Table 13.2.

Investigations

Prolonged jaundice requires investigation when present for more than 10 days in a term infant, and for more than 14 days in a premature one. The initial investigation must be to distinguish conjugated from unconjugated causes. Table 13.3 lists investigations for prolonged unconjugated hyperbilirubinaemia.

Management

Box 13.1 summarizes the principles of management of unconjugated hyperbilirubinaemia.

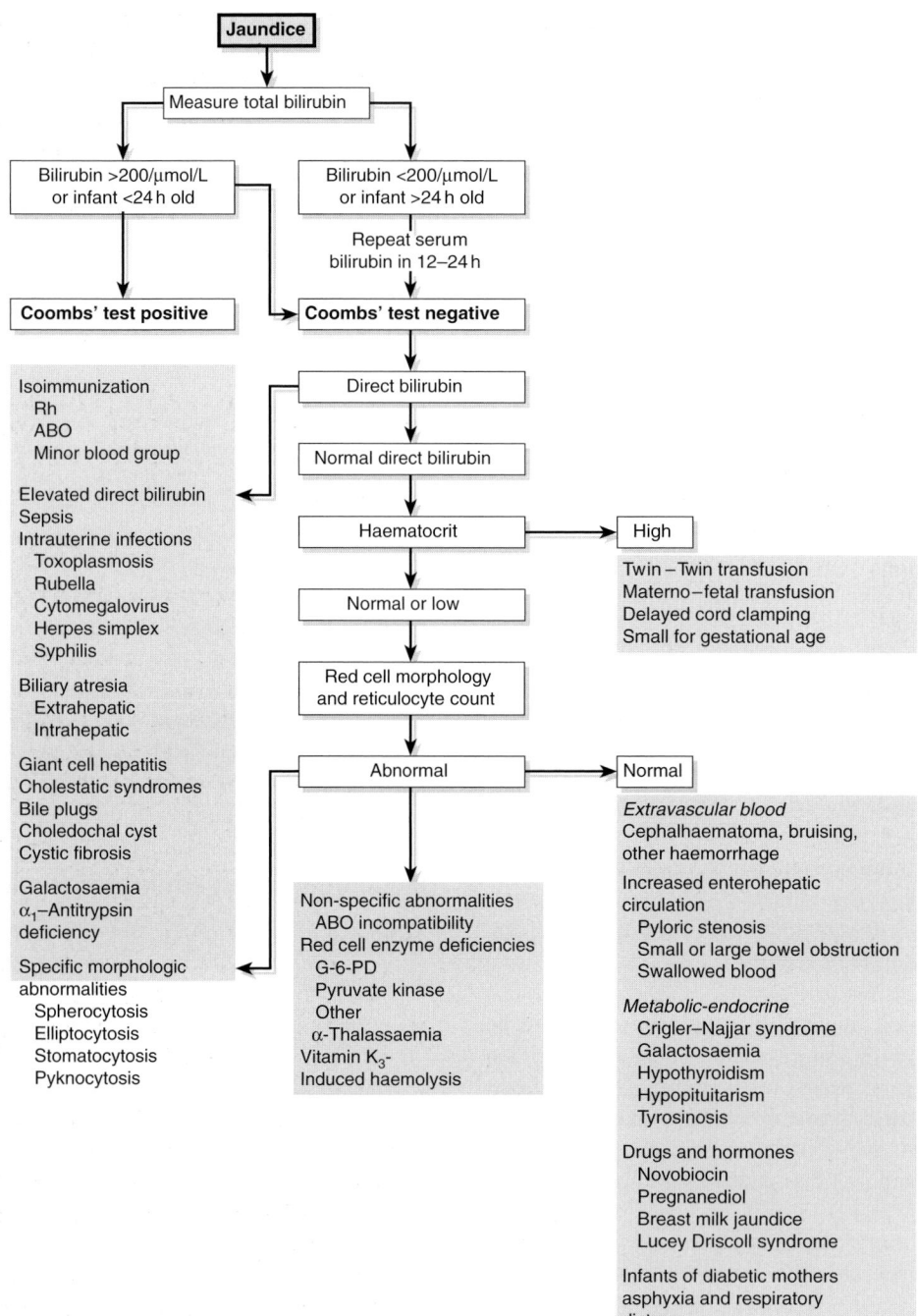

Figure 13.3 Flow diagram showing a diagnostic approach to neonatal jaundice. (Modified from Maisels 1994.)

Table 13.2 Causes of prolonged unconjugated hyperbilirubinaemia

Rhesus and ABO incompatibility
Hereditary spherocytosis
Glucose-6-phosphate dehydrogenase deficiency
Septicaemia and TORCH infection
Extravasated blood and excessive bruising
Twin-to-twin transfusion
Prematurity
Dehydration
Hypothyroidism
Breast milk jaundice
Delayed passage of meconium

Table 13.3 Investigations in an infant with prolonged unconjugated hyperbilirubinaemia

Indirect- and direct-acting bilirubin
Haemoglobin
Blood film for red cell morphology
Maternal and infant blood group
Direct Coombs' test
Maternal haemolysis if ABO mismatch (see p. 197)
Infection screen
Urine-reducing substances
Erythrocyte galactose uridyl transferase activity if
 galactosaemia a possibility
Glucose-6-phosphate dehydrogenase assay
Serum thyroxine and thyroid-stimulating hormone

BOX 13.1 Principles of management of unconjugated hyperbilirubinaemia

Anticipate at-risk infants	Rhesus incompatibility Potential disorder associated with haemolysis (e.g. G6PD)
Observe rise in serum bilirirubin and plot on appropriate chart	Clinical assessment Measurement of unconjugated bilirubin
Investigate cause	
Phototherapy	Indicated on bilirubin chart
Exchange transfusion	Indicated on bilirubin chart
Screen for hearing impairment if severe hyperbilirubinaemia	

Prevention

Early feeding reduces the incidence of jaundice by preventing dehydration and the elevation of free fatty acids. The maintenance of an adequate fluid intake is an essential part of the care of a jaundiced baby. In addition, feeding will overcome bowel stasis and minimize the effects of the enterohepatic bilirubin circulation. Breastfeeding-associated jaundice is minimized by frequent, early breastfeeding in the first 3 days of life.

Phototherapy

This was first used by Cremer in 1958 in the UK and is now widely used. It is particularly useful in preterm infants with non-haemolytic jaundice, and has resulted in a decline in the number of exchange transfusions being performed.

Phototherapy units, which emit light with a wavelength of about 450 nm, are used. Blue or blue/green light is most efficient in photodegradation. A quartz-halogen light source, with a higher radiant flux in the wavelength 425–475 nm, provides more effective photodegradation than fluorescent lights. A recent advance is the use of LED (light-emitting diode) blue light. Light from this source degrades and photoisomerizes unconjugated bilirubin in the skin to non-toxic bilirubin products.

Phototherapy is started after the investigations for the cause of jaundice have been carried out. Once therapy has been commenced serum bilirubin estimates will be necessary to assess the severity of jaundice because the skin colour becomes unreliable. Phototherapy may be used in conjunction with other forms of treatment, such as exchange transfusion. The graphs developed by Cockington (1979) provide guidelines for the treatment of hyperbilirubinaemia in low birthweight (LBW) infants (Fig. 13.4). For term infants over 2500 g guidelines modified after Finlay and Tucker (1978) are recommended (Fig. 13.5).

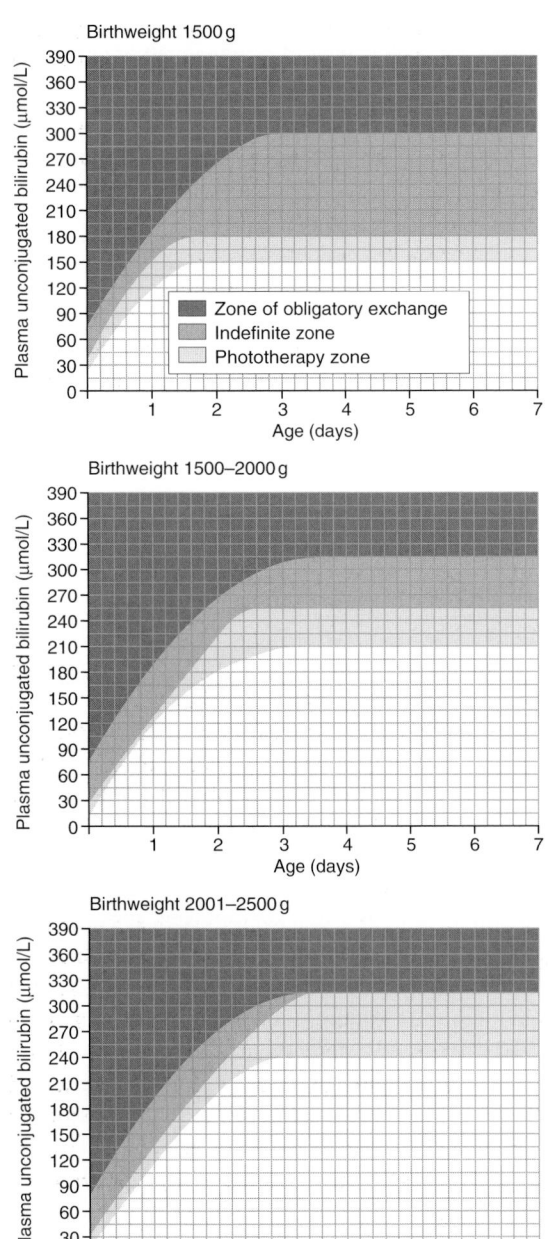

Birthweight 1500 g

Plasma unconjugated bilirubin (µmol/L) vs *Age (days)*

Zone of obligatory exchange
Indefinite zone
Phototherapy zone

Birthweight 1500–2000 g

Birthweight 2001–2500 g

Figure 13.4 Suggested treatment regimen for unconjugated hyperbilirubinaemia by phototherapy or exchange transfusion for different birthweight groups. (Reproduced with permission from Cockington 1979.)

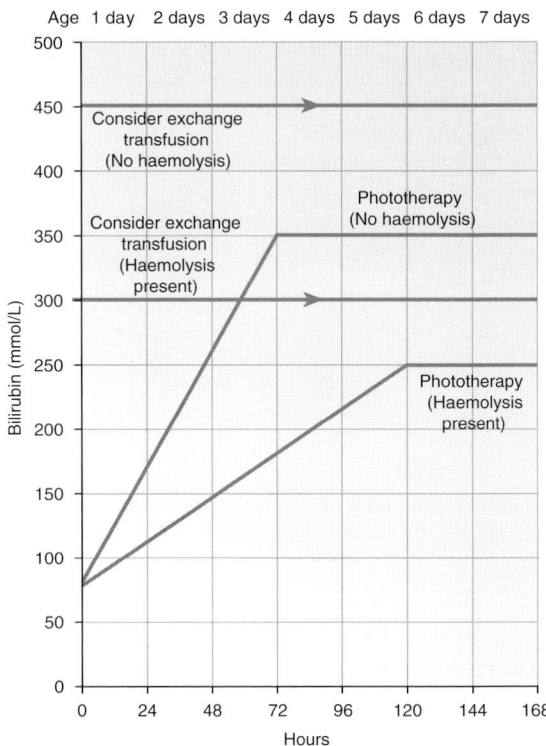

Age 1 day 2 days 3 days 4 days 5 days 6 days 7 days

Bilirubin (mmol/L) vs *Hours*

Consider exchange transfusion (No haemolysis)

Consider exchange transfusion (Haemolysis present)

Phototherapy (No haemolysis)

Phototherapy (Haemolysis present)

Figure 13.5 Bilirubin chart. (Modified from Finlay & Tucker 1978.)

Complications of phototherapy include

1 Temperature instability.

2 Fluid disturbance: the increased insensible water loss may be compensated for by increasing the infant's water intake by 20%.

3 Retinal damage: the eyes are thought to be vulnerable to phototherapy but this has never been proved. It is, however, a wise precaution to protect the infant's eyes from the light by a suitable eye shield.

4 Diarrhoea: phototherapy decreases bowel transit time and induces lactose intolerance; both are important causes of diarrhoea and consequent fluid loss.

5 Bronze baby: this complication may be seen when an infant with obstructive jaundice receives phototherapy.

Early discharge and home management of jaundice

The introduction of early discharge programmes for healthy term infants has resulted in the need for jaundice to be treated at home. The resurgence of kernicterus is probably also related to the combination of early discharge and breastfeeding. This may result in dehydration if the baby feeds poorly and there is a lack of recognition of severe hyperbilirubinaemia. Predicting which infants might require treatment using direct and indirect techniques of measuring serum bilirubin at age 24 h has been suggested, but more research is required to identify sensitive methods. Home treatment has been facilitated by the introduction since 1990 of the BiliBlanket® (MedNow Inc, Eagle, Idaho, USA) using a fibreoptic phototherapy system. The infant is placed on a mat containing fibreoptic strands which flood the body with therapeutic light while the infant is clothed normally.

Exchange transfusion

This form of therapy was first used in 1951 for the treatment of erythroblastosis fetalis (Diamond *et al.* 1951). Exchange transfusions may be required in conjunction with phototherapy for infants with severe jaundice, especially when due to rhesus iso-immunization. The exchange transfusion allows

1 removal of unconjugated bilirubin;
2 removal of immune antibody if present;
3 replacement of sensitized red cells with cells that cannot be haemolysed as easily;
4 restoration of blood volume and correction of anaemia;
5 provision of free albumin for bilirubin binding.

The indications for exchange transfusion depend on the infant's gestational age, postnatal age and state of health. Metabolic compromise with acidosis predisposes to brain damage due to bilirubin toxicity. The level at which bilirubin damages the brain is not known, and the indications for exchange transfusion are therefore arbitrary. Cockington's charts are widely used to decide upon the need for exchange transfusion in LBW infants (see Fig. 13.4). For term infants over 2500 g a chart modified from that used at Hillingdon Hospital is recommended (see Fig. 13.5).

The technique of exchange transfusion is given in Chapter 29.

Complications associated with exchange transfusions include

1 electrolyte disturbance (hypocalcaemia, hyperkalaemia);

2 blood glucose disturbance – initially hyperglycaemia followed by rebound hypoglycaemia, especially in rhesus immunization;
3 infection – viral (cytomegalovirus (CMV), hepatitis B, human immunodeficiency virus (HIV)) or bacterial (*Staphylococcus aureus* and *Streptococcus* spp.) due to contaminated blood;
4 thromboembolism (air or blood clot);
5 necrotizing enterocolitis (NEC);
6 fluid overload or rarely hypovolaemia;
7 acidosis, hypoxia, bradycardia, cardiac arrest;
8 benign intrahepatic cholestasis in severely growth-restricted infants;
9 haemorrhage.

Adjunct therapy

A number of additional treatment methods for jaundice have been described.

Albumin

The administration of 1 g/kg of albumin, either intravenously before the exchange transfusion or added to the donor blood, will increase the efficiency of the exchange by binding more free bilirubin. It is not known whether this will reduce the need for exchange transfusion.

Metalloporphyrins

Haem oxygenase is the rate-limiting enzyme in bilirubin production, and metalloporphyrins inhibit haem oxygenase thereby reducing the production of bilirubin. It has been shown that the intramuscular injection of tin protoporphyrin significantly reduces bilirubin levels in term and near-term infants and may be particularly important in preventing severe jaundice in infants with Glucose-6-phosphate dehydrogenase (G6PD) haemolysis.

Immunoglobulin (IVIG)

There is some evidence (Gottstein & Cooke 2003) that IVIG may reduce the need for exchange transfusion in antibody induced cases of haemolysis (Rhesus and ABO).

Phenobarbitone

This drug improves bilirubin conjugation but is not recommended to treat neonatal hyperbilirubinaemia.

Physiological jaundice

The term 'physiological jaundice' is used by clinicians to describe jaundice that is not severe enough to be treated. It is a diagnosis of exclusion, and if there is any doubt as to the cause, further investigations should be performed. It is presumed to be due to a temporary immaturity of glucuronyl transferase and other factors involved in bilirubin metabolism. Physiological jaundice should not fulfil any of the following criteria:

1 clinical jaundice in the first 24 h of life;
2 total serum bilirubin concentration exceeding 300 μmol/L in a term infant or 255 μmol/L in a pre-term infant;
3 a direct-reacting serum bilirubin concentration exceeding 30 μmol/L;
4 clinical jaundice persisting for more than 10 days in a term infant or for more than 2 weeks in a pre-term infant;
5 an 'ill' infant.

If any of these features are present, full investigation of the jaundice should be undertaken.

Infection

Bacterial infections, particularly septicaemia and urinary tract infections, may cause unconjugated hyperbilirubinaemia. Occasionally severe bacterial infection may cause hepatocellular damage with a conjugated form of jaundice. TORCH (toxoplasmosis, other, rubella, CMV, herpes simplex type II) infections may cause either type of hyperbilirubinaemia, but the conjugated form is most frequently seen.

Breastfeeding and jaundice

Breastfeeding-associated jaundice. This is the term used to refer to the increased bilirubin levels seen during the first week of life in almost two-thirds of infants who are breastfed. It is probably due to calorie and fluid deprivation in the first few days of life and delayed passage of stools, as it can be reduced by an increased frequency of breastfeeding during the first few days of life. The importance of recognizing breastfeeding-associated jaundice lies in the fact that it may rarely cause kernicterus if untreated (Maisels & Newman 1995). In itself it is not a contraindication to breastfeeding.

Breast milk jaundice. This is prolonged jaundice that extends until the first 3 months of life. Characteristically it is a form of non-haemolytic,

unconjugated hyperbilirubinaemia and should be diagnosed primarily by exclusion of other aetiologies in a thriving infant and by its time course. The enzyme β-glucuronidase has been shown to be elevated in some women's breast milk. Excess of this enzyme causes increased enteric absorption of bilirubin, thus increasing the hepatic bilirubin load. In this respect, breast milk jaundice can be thought of as an extension of physiological jaundice, and the greater the consumption of this enzyme in milk, the higher is the concentration of neonatal serum bilirubin. Breast milk jaundice does not require any treatment but babies with high bilirubin levels should be kept under observation.

Delayed passage of meconium

The jaundice is due to increased enterohepatic absorption of bilirubin.

Gilbert's syndrome

This is a common cause of unconjugated hyperbilirubinaemia in young adults, but rarely causes problems in the neonatal period. It is due to a single gene mutation affecting a hepatic bilirubin enzyme uridine diphosphate glucuronyltransferase (UDPGT), and in the newborn is associated with mild unconjugated hyperbilirubinaemia (<85 μmol/L). The prognosis is excellent.

Crigler–Najjar syndrome

This group of conditions have been shown to be due to multiple gene defects and cause very severe hyperbilirubinaemia potentially leading to kernicterus. There is little effective treatment other than prolonged phototherapy. Liver transplantation has been successful in some severe cases; in milder cases phenobarbitone may lower the serum bilirubin.

Complications of jaundice

Kernicterus and bilirubin encephalopathy

Kernicterus, once thought to have disappeared as a cause of disability, is being reported increasingly in Europe and North America. This resurgence is probably due to an increased trend towards early discharge from hospital and inexperienced mothers being left to breastfeed their babies with little support. Dehydration is likely to be a major factor in the development of severe hyperbilirubinaemia.

The classic presentation of kernicterus in the newborn is with progressive development of lethargy, rigidity, opisthotonus, a high-pitched cry, fever and convulsions over a period of 24 h. This is followed by death in 50% of the affected infants. At autopsy there is bilirubin staining and necrosis of neurons, especially in the basal ganglia, hippocampus and subthalamic nuclei. Survivors of kernicterus often demonstrate choreoathetoid cerebral palsy, high-frequency deafness, mental retardation and paralysis of upward gaze (Parinaud's sign). Preterm infants may manifest more subtle bilirubin brain damage consisting of mild disorders of both motor function and cognitive function (minimal cerebral dysfunction) without demonstrating any of the acute clinical features of bilirubin encephalopathy. High-tone frequency hearing loss is the commonest feature of the bilirubin encephalopathy syndrome and is most commonly seen in premature infants.

The levels at which unconjugated bilirubin causes brain damage are not known, and it is probably only free (non-protein-bound) bilirubin that is dangerous, although bound bilirubin has been reported to cross a leaky blood–brain barrier. Acidosis, asphyxia, prematurity and drugs that compete for bilirubin-binding sites predispose infants to kernicterus, possibly by opening the blood–brain barrier to bilirubin molecules, and the indication for exchange transfusion is at a lower level of unconjugated bilrirubin in these babies. By the time that symptoms of kernicterus occur, brain damage has probably already started.

Conjugated hyperbilirubinaemia

Causes

Conjugated hyperbilirubinaemia is much less common than unconjugated jaundice in the newborn, but has a much more serious prognosis. Conjugated forms of neonatal jaundice are due to intra- or extrahepatic obstruction (also called cholestasis). It usually presents in the second week of life or later and is associated with greenish skin discoloration, dark bile-stained urine and pale acholuric stools. Hepatosplenomegaly is commonly present and the infant often fails to thrive. Occasionally, conjugated hyperbilirubinaemia is present at birth as a result of TORCH infections or rhesus isoimmunization. The causes of conjugated hyperbilirubinaemia are shown

Table 13.4 More common causes of conjugated hyperbilirubinaemia (adapted from McKiernan 2002)

Bile duct abnormalities
   Biliary atresia
   Inspissated bile
   Choledochal cyst

Idiopathic

Infection
   Systemic (e.g. septicaemia)
   Hepatic
   TORCH
   Hepatitis B
   HIV

Metabolic
   α_1-Antitrypsin deficiency
   Galactosaemia
   Cystic fibrosis
   Fructosaemia
   Tyrosinaemia
   Alagille's syndrome
   Dubin–Johnson rotor syndrome

Endocrine
   Hypthyroidism
   Hypopituitarism

Toxic
   Parenteral nutrition

in Table 13.4. Many of these are very rare, but neonatal hepatitis and biliary atresia account for 80% of all cases of conjugated hyperbilirubinaemia.

Investigations

The management of obstructive jaundice in the newborn depends on the diagnosis. The diagnostic dilemma is to distinguish biliary atresia from neonatal hepatitis. Table 13.5 lists the investigations that are of value in distinguishing these conditions. Liver biopsy, radionuclide scanning and further management should be carried out in a specialist children's liver centre.

Management

This depends on the cause of the conjugated hyperbilirubinaemia. Antibiotics are appropriate for the rare cases of bacterial infection. In general, supportive

Table 13.5 Investigations to detect the cause of neonatal conjugated hyperbilirubinaemia

Liver enzymes
Alkaline phosphatase
Serial bilirubin levels
α-Fetoprotein
$α_1$-Antitrypsin screen and phenotype
^{123}I Rose Bengal excretion test
Abdominal ultrasound
Sweat test
TORCH serology
Amino acid screen
Percutaneous liver biopsy
Radionuclide (HIDA) scan

HIDA, injection of radioactive hydroxy imino-diacetic acid which is taken up in the liver and excreted in the biliary system.

management is all that is available. Steroids are of no benefit. There is no evidence that cholestyramine or phenobarbitone are beneficial. An elemental diet (Pregestimil, Mead Johnson Nutritionals, Evansville, Indiana, USA) supplemented with medium-chain triglycerides together with parenteral fat-soluble vitamins (A, D and K) are given to prevent deficiencies. Vitamin D may also be necessary.

Neonatal hepatitis

This is a non-specific condition with a variety of causes, which are discussed below; the prognosis depends on the underlying cause. In general, approximately one-third of cases deteriorate and develop hepatic cirrhosis, one-third have evidence of chronic liver disease and one-third recover fully. The prognosis for idiopathic neonatal hepatitis is good and >90% resolve by 1 year of age.

Causes (Table 13.4)
The main causes of neonatal hepatitis are as follows.
1 *Infection.* Most commonly due to TORCH infections contracted in the first trimester, but other viruses may also produce hepatitis (see p. 63). If a mother is positive for hepatitis B, the infant should be protected from infection by immunization (see p. 65).

2 *Metabolic causes.* Fructosaemia and tyrosinaemia may cause severe neonatal hepatitis. Galactosaemia more commonly presents with unconjugated hyperbilirubinaemia, but affected infants later develop cholestasis.
3 $α_1$-*Antitrypsin deficiency.* This is an autosomal recessive condition and causes a relatively common form of conjugated hyperbilirubinaemia. Only infants who are homozygous for the PiZZ type are at risk of neonatal hepatitis. There is no specific treatment, and up to 50% of affected children improve and may recover fully. Death due to liver failure occurs in the other half, and liver transplantation may be life saving in this group.
4 *Severe intrauterine growth restriction.* This results in a benign intrahepatic cholestasis.

Biliary atresia

At birth these infants have absent or atretic bile ductules involving the main bile ducts or the main branches of the bile ducts. The deeper in the liver substance that the ducts are abnormal, the more severe is the condition. The commonest variety is extrahepatic biliary atresia. The onset of jaundice may be delayed by up to 4 weeks from birth. It is a surgically operable condition, but because progressive obliteration of the bile ducts occurs rapidly with advancing age, early diagnosis is essential for successful treatment. If surgery is attempted before 60 days of age, there is an 80% chance of achieving biliary drainage by the portoenterostomy operation, known as the Kasai procedure. Serum bilirubin falls rapidly after successful surgery, but many children develop ascending cholangitis, which is the most serious postoperative complication. Approximately two-thirds of survivors will require liver transplantation by 10 years of age.

Inspissated bile syndrome

High and prolonged levels of unconjugated bilirubin may cause a condition in which the bilirubin produces cholestasis with progressive conjugated hyperbilirubinaemia. Ultrasound scanning may show sludge in the gall bladder. It is usually a self-limiting condition but ursodeoxycholic acid (UDCA) may be an effective therapeutic option.

Dubin–Johnson syndrome

This is a rare and benign condition in which the neonate may develop low-grade conjugated and unconjugated hyperbilirubinaemia.

References

Cockington RA. A guide to the use of phototherapy in the management of neonatal hyperbilirubinaemia. *J Pediatr* 1979;**95**:281–287.

Diamond LK, Allen FH, Thomas WO. Erythroblastosis fetalis VII. Treatment with exchange transfusion. *N Engl J Med* 1951;**244**:39–42.

Finlay HVL, Tucker SM. Neonatal plasma bilirubin chart. *Arch Dis Child* 1978;**53**:90–91.

Gottstein R, Cooke RWI. Systematic review of intravenous immunoglobulin in haemolytic disease of the newborn. *Arch Dis Child Fetal Neonatal* 2003; **88**:F6–F10.

Kramer LI. Advancement of dermal icterus in the jaundiced newborn. *Am J Dis Child* 1969;**118**:454–459.

McKiernan PJ. Neonatal cholestasis. *Semin Neonatol* 2002;**7**:153–165.

Maisels MJ. Jaundice. In: *Neonatology. Pathophysiology and Management of the Newborn* (ed. G.B. Avery), 4th edn. Philadelphia: Lippincott, 1994.

Maisels MJ, Newman TB. Kernicterus in otherwise healthy, breast-fed term newborns. *Pediatrics* 1995;**96** 730–733.

Further reading

American Academy of Paediatrics, Provisional Committee for Quality Improvement and Subcommittee on Hyperbilirubinemia. Practice parameter: Management of hyperbilirubinemia in the healthy term newborn. *Pediatrics* 1994;**94**:558–562.

Milla PJ, Muller DPR. (eds) *Harries' Paediatric Gastroenterology*. Edinburgh: Churchill Livingstone, 1988.

Watchko JF, Maisels MJ (eds) Neonatal jaundice. *Semin Neonatol* 2002;**7**(2).

14 Congenital anomalies: malformations and deformations

Estimates of the incidence of congenital anomalies in all live births vary widely and range from 1% to 7%, depending on the definition of what constitutes an anomaly. Probably about 3% of all babies born have a major congenital anomaly, but the incidence of minor imperfections is about 7% if all skin haemangiomas, preauricular skin tags, etc. are included. The incidence of congenital anomalies is highest in preterm and small for gestational age (SGA) infants. Congenital anomalies are the leading cause of perinatal mortality (20–25% of all perinatal deaths) as well as the leading cause of postneonatal deaths (25–30%). In addition they constitute 25–30% of admissions to tertiary children's hospitals and have major financial costs for society.

Congenital anomalies may be classified into malformations and deformations. *Malformations* result from a disturbance of growth during embryogenesis, for example, congenital heart disease. *Deformations* result from late changes in previously normal structures by destructive pathological processes or intrauterine (extrinsic) forces, for example, talipes, hydrocephalus and bowel atresia. Some defects may arise by one or both mechanisms.

Deformations

Causes

These may be multiple or single. They have many common aetiological factors, which include
1 primigravidity;
2 oligohydramnios;
3 abnormal presentation, e.g. breech position;
4 multiple pregnancy;
5 uterine abnormalities, e.g. fibroids, bicornuate or septate uterus;
6 growth restriction.

Extrinsic forces may cause a single localized deformation, such as talipes equinovarus or a deformation sequence. A *deformation sequence* refers to the moulding effects of intrauterine constraint. Examples are the oligohydramnios sequence, with contractures, facial dysmorphism and pulmonary hypoplasia, or the breech deformation sequence.

Intrauterine contractures that give rise to joint fixation are known as arthrogryposis. The types of problems that lead to prenatal joint contractures are demonstrated in Fig. 14.1.

Malformations

Incidence

Major congenital anomalies are either lethal or significantly affect the individual's function or appearance. Minor anomalies have no functional or major cosmetic importance.

National registers of congenital malformations are available for many countries, but it is difficult to compare overall rates because of reporting differences. Most registers only include abnormalities present at birth. Some do not include data on fetuses terminated after prenatal diagnosis prior to 20 weeks' gestation. There may also be quite large regional variations within the data from a single country.

The incidence of congenital malformations reported for South Australia from 1986 to 2003 was 5.7%, with annual variations from 4.5 to 6.0%. The figures for the UK are similar. The commonest major

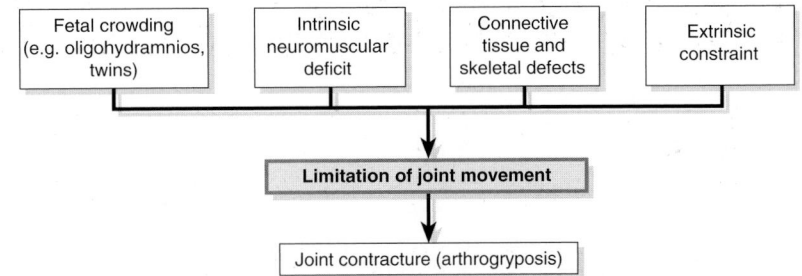

Figure 14.1 The types of problems that lead to prenatal joint contractures.

Table 14.1 Congenital anomalies by major anatomical systems (South Australia 1986–2003)

System	Rate/1000 total births
Nervous system	3.8
Spina bifida 0.9, anencephaly 0.7, congenital hydrocephalus 0.8	
Cardiovascular	12.0
Transposition of great arteries 0.7, hypoplastic Left heart syndrome 0.3, coarctation of aorta 0.6	
Respiratory	1.6
Pulmonary hypoplasia 0.9	
Gastrointestinal	6.4
Cleft lip/cleft palate/cleft lip +palate 2.1, oesophageal atresia ± TOF 0.4	
Congenital	16.4
Hypospadias 3.7, renal agenesis/dysgenesis 0.6, vesico-ureteric reflux 3.1	
Musculoskeletal	16.3
Developmental dysplasia of hip 6.9, talipes equinovarus 2.2, diaphragmatic hernia 0.4, exomphalos 0.4, gastroschisis 0.2	
Chromosomal	3.7
Down syndrome 1.8, trisomy 13 0.2, trisomy 18 0.4	
Metabolic	1.3
Congenital hypothyroidism 0.3, cystic fibrosis 0.4, phenylketonuria 0.1	
Haematological	0.9
Haemolytic anaemia 0.5, thalassaemias 0.1, coagulation defects 0.2	
Others	Total % of births with birth
Non-immune hydrops 0.4, haemangioma/lymphangioma 1.0	defects 5.7%

congenital anomalies involve the central nervous and cardiovascular systems. Table 14.1 lists the incidence of some congenital malformations. Specific congenital abnormalities are discussed in the appropriate chapters.

Teratogenesis

A *teratogen* is an agent (chemical, drug, virus or radiation) that causes a malformation or deformation or affects the wellbeing of the fetus. A *fetotoxin*

Table 14.2 The Australian risk categorization system for drugs used in pregnancy

Category	Description
A	No increase in malformations
B	Human safety data lacking
B1	Animal studies negative. Minimal human exposure suggests safety
B2	Inadequate animal studies suggest safety in humans
B3	Animal studies have shown increased fetal damage of uncertain significance in humans
C	Based on pharmacological effects likely to have reversible harmful effects on fetus
D	Proven or suspected of irreversible harmful effects including malformation and pharmacological effects
X	High risk of permanent fetal damage and contraindicated in pregnancy

Table 14.3 Causes of congenital malformations

Cause	Estimated contribution (%)
Genetic (Mendelian mode of inheritance)	20
Chromosomal	10
Teratogens	
Infection	2–3
Drugs and chemicals (environmental pollutants and insecticides)	2–3
Radiation	<1
Maternal metabolic disease	1–2
Unknown	35–40
Polygenic	25–30

(Teratogens total: 6–9)

is an agent causing damage of any kind to the fetus, and a *mutagen* is an agent that causes a permanent transmissible change in the genetic material. Table 14.2 illustrates a system to describe the risk of drug tetatogenesis.

The critical periods in embryogenic development have been extrapolated from the rubella experience and are likely to affect different organs at different times. Examples of critical periods expressed in days from time of conception are:

Brain   15–25 days.
Eye   25–40 days.
Heart   20–40 days.
Limbs   24–36 days.
Ear   40–60 days.

During the first 2 weeks of development from conception to the first missed period the embryo is resistant to any teratogenic effects of medicines. The critical period of embryonic development begins when development of the organ systems starts at about 17 days post-conception, and extends until this is complete by 60–70 days. In general, exposure to medicines beyond 70 days post-conception is not associated with induction of major birth defects. However, drugs can interfere with functional development of organ systems in the second and third trimesters.

Causes

Congenital anomalies result from a wide variety of mechanisms ranging from genetic (monogenic and polygenic) to environmental factors (teratogenesis), maternal metabolic disease, drugs and chemicals, infectious agents and irradiation (Table 14.3).

Drugs

Drugs may act by interfering with embryogenesis or by exerting their pharmacological actions on developing fetal organs. Adverse effects are influenced by the timing and dose of agent, the efficiency with which the mother metabolizes the agent, placental transfer and the individual susceptibility of the fetus. Table 14.4 lists some of the more common teratogenic drugs.

Vitamin A has for many years been known to be a powerful teratogen in animals, but has only recently emerged as a significant clinical problem, with the introduction of oral retinoids for the treatment of severe acne and psoriasis. Teratogenic effects include spontaneous abortion, cleft palate and severe malformations of the ear, heart and brain.

Fetal alcohol spectrum disorder (FASD)

The term 'fetal alcohol spectrum disorder' is the generic term covering fetal alcohol syndrome, fetal alcohol effects and alcohol-related neurodevelopmental disorders.

Excessive alcohol intake in early pregnancy during the period of fetal organogenesis can result in a

Table 14.4 Drugs as teratogens

Definite	
Hormones	Progestogens, diethyl stilboestrol, male sex hormones
Antipsychotics, hypnosedatives	Lithium, haloperidol, thalidomide
Anticonvulsants	Hydantoins, sodium valproate, carbamazepine, primidone, phenobarbitone
Antimicrobials	Tetracycline, chloramphenicol, streptomycin, flucytosine, amphotericin B
Antineoplastics	Alkylating agents, folic acid antagonists
Anticoagulants	Warfarin
Antithyroids	Iodine, carbimazole, propylthiouracil
Antivirals	Ribavirin
Hypoglycaemics	Biguanides, sulphonylureas
Vitamin A analogues	Isotretinoin, etretinate
Others	Toluene, alcohol, marijuana, narcotics

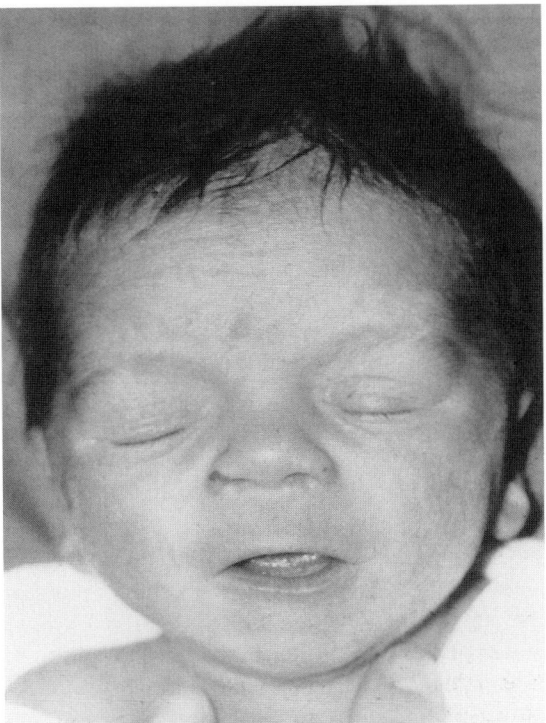

Figure 14.2 A newborn infant showing the facial features of fetal alcohol syndrome.

specific syndrome of facial abnormalities, growth failure, microcephaly, and skeletal and visceral abnormalities. This syndrome was identified in 1973 as the fetal alcohol syndrome (Jones & Smith 1973). The facial features that enable the diagnosis to be made include hypoplasia of the mid-face, with beaking of the forehead and a sunken nasal bridge, a small upturned nose, micrognathia, a prominent philtrum and ear deformities (Fig. 14.2). Growth restriction is usual, with poor postnatal somatic growth. Major abnormalities include cleft lip and palate, and limb, ocular, cardiac and renal malformations. There is usually delayed psychomotor development. Approximately one-third of infants born to chronic alcoholic women develop the fetal alcohol syndrome, whereas others may be growth restricted or demonstrate minor features only. Neonatal withdrawal symptoms, including convulsions, may occur in infants born to alcoholic women.

It is not known whether social drinking of alcohol in pregnancy is associated with intrauterine growth restriction, but in general it is unlikely that the occasional consumption of alcohol during pregnancy will affect the fetus.

There is no laboratory test for FASD. Diagnosis relies on a pattern of abnormalities that makes up the disorder, along with alcohol misuse during the pregnancy and around conception.

Diagnosis is generally made on infants and young children as the features often become more obvious with age. CNS dysfunction and facial dysmorphology is difficult to assess before 2 years of age. As adolescence approaches facial features are less obvious but those that remain for life are microcephaly, short palpebral fissures, indistinct philtrum, thin upper lip and micrognathia.

The 4-Digit Diagnostic Code
A new diagnostic code that uses quantitative, objective measurement scales and specific case definitions has recently been developed. Diagnosis is made using four key diagnostic features:
1 growth restriction;
2 fetal alcohol syndrome facial phenotype;

3 CNS damage/dysfunction;
4 gestational alcohol exposure.

Smoking in pregnancy

Although there is overwhelming evidence of harm to the fetus and mother from tobacco smoking in pregnancy, approximately 25% of pregnant women in developed countries smoke. Maternal smoking has a dose-dependent effect involving decreasing fetal weight owing to impaired uterine perfusion, with structural placental changes, an increase in carboxyhaemoglobin levels and increased fetal erythropoiesis. Passive exposure to smoking by the father has nearly as great (66%) an effect as maternal smoking in reducing birthweight. Complications in smokers compared with non-smokers include infertility, spontaneous abortion, impaired fetal wellbeing, placenta praevia, abruptio placentae, amniotic fluid infection and premature rupture of the membranes. Follow-up of children born to maternal smokers demonstrates increased rates of hyperactivity at 4 years, deficient stature and mental function, and increased risks of sudden infant death syndrome (SIDS) and malignancy. Excessive smoking is not known to be associated with any specific congenital abnormalities.

The drug-addicted infant

A wide variety of drugs are abused during pregnancy, and neonatal withdrawal symptoms have been reported with alcohol, amphetamines, barbiturates, codeine, ethchlorvynol, heroin, pethidine, methadone, morphine and pentazocine. Methamphetamine ('ice') is currently of major concern, but drug-using practices vary according to availability, geography and price. Heroin and methadone are the narcotic drugs most frequently abused during pregnancy. Their illicit use has been associated with increased fetal and neonatal deaths. The mean birthweight of infants born to heroin addicts is only 2500 g owing to an increased incidence of both prematurity and intrauterine growth restriction. About 70% of the infants exhibit withdrawal symptoms. Symptoms usually occur within 48 h of birth, but can be delayed for up to a week. Signs include extreme jitteriness, tachycardia, vomiting, diarrhoea and fever. Convulsions occur rarely. It has been reported that infants born to

drug-addicted mothers may continue to show irritable or restless behaviour for a number of months after birth.

Perinatal cocaine intoxication is a major problem in the USA, and the use of cocaine (or 'crack') in other countries is increasing. This drug is a potent vasoconstrictor affecting the uteroplacental bed as well as the fetal vasculature. It also causes maternal and fetal tachycardia and severe hypertension. The abuse of cocaine in pregnancy results in increased risk of first-trimester abortion, placental abruption and premature birth. Fetal malformations thought to be due to cocaine include hydronephrosis, cryptorchidism, skeletal defects with delayed ossification, exencephaly and eye anomalies. Cerebral artery infarction due to the vasoconstrictive effect of the drug is well described and is most likely to occur in the second and third trimesters.

Management

Infants of mothers who abuse drugs in pregnancy should be carefully monitored in the neonatal period for withdrawal symptoms. These are listed in Table 14.5.

About 30% of infants with drug withdrawal can be managed conservatively without the use of medication. Methods include swaddling, frequent

Table 14.5 Withdrawal symptoms seen in neonates born to drug-abusing mothers

Central nervous system
Irritability and high-pitched cry
Hyperactivity with reduced periods of sleep
Tremors
Increased tone
Convulsions (rare)

Gastrointestinal
Poor feeding
Vomiting
Diarrhoea

Other symptoms
Sweating
Fever
Frequent yawning
Snuffles and sneezing
Tachycardia

feeds, intravenous fluids and decreased sensory stimulation.

If severe signs of withdrawal are present, drug treatment is necessary, but opinions as to the most effective treatment differ. Opiates such as Oramorph, paregoric (0.2 mL 3-hourly), pethidine (1 mg/kg/dose) or morphine sulphate (0.1 mg/kg/dose) may be used. Frequently non-specific sedatives such as phenobarbitone (8 mg/kg/day), diazepam (1–2 mg 8-hourly) or chlorpromazine (2–3 mg/kg/day) are used.

Additional assessments of infants of drug-abusing mothers include screening for hepatitis B and C and human immunodeficiency virus (HIV) infection. When infants are born to mothers with acute hepatitis B in the last trimester of pregnancy or where the mother is hepatitis B surface antigen (HBsAg) positive, hepatitis B immunoglobulin (100 IU) is given as soon as possible after birth. Active immunization with hepatitis B vaccine should be commenced at birth, and repeated at 2, 4 and 6 months.

Prognosis
This depends at least in part on the socioeconomic background of the family. Infants of substance-using mothers exhibit behavioural and physical features reflecting central and systemic dysfunction. These infants may be at increased risk of SIDS, and they and their families require careful follow-up after discharge by medical and community health and social services.

Infections (see also Chapter 7)
Prenatal maternal infections act by causing inflammatory lesions of the embryo or fetus and interfere with cell division. Maternal infections that may cause congenital abnormalities include
1 *definite*: rubella, toxoplasmosis, syphilis, cytomegalovirus, herpes simplex, HIV, varicella, parvovirus B19;
2 *probable*: Coxsackie B, herpes zoster;
3 *possible*: mumps, influenza.

Irradiation
Clinical experience with X-rays and the follow-up studies on pregnant women exposed to atomic bomb irradiation in Hiroshima have confirmed major teratogenic effects, such as microcephaly.

Chemicals
Pesticides and waste products have not been subjected to rigorous teratogenic studies in humans. However, recent experience with the dioxin contaminant in the insecticide 2,4,5-T and its possible association with spina bifida and Potter's syndrome suggest that a much more rigorous surveillance of chemicals is necessary in the future. At present the only environmental chemical for which there is clear evidence of teratogenicity is organic mercury. Long-term prenatal exposure to this chemical has caused neurological damage as a result of disturbed brain development.

Fever
Studies have suggested that it may be the high fever associated with viral infection (e.g. influenza) that causes the malformation. Sauna baths and faulty electric blankets producing very high body temperatures at a critical period of embryogenesis might be teratogenic.

Maternal diseases

Diabetes mellitus. Maternal diabetes, especially with coexisting vascular complications, predisposes to many congenital malformations, including the caudal regression syndrome (sacral agenesis), congenital heart disease, idiopathic hypertrophic subaortic stenosis, hypoplastic left colon and renal vein thrombosis.

If the diabetic woman is well controlled on insulin and her blood sugars remain in the normal range before she becomes pregnant, the risk of congenital malformation is reduced.

Maternal hyperthyroidism (Graves' disease). This disease results in transient neonatal thyrotoxicosis in approximately 10–20% of pregnancies (see p. 169). The best predictors of neonatal thyrotoxicosis are the outcome of previous siblings and assays of thyroid-stimulating immunoglobulin and thyroid receptor-binding inhibitors.

Maternal phenylketonuria. The high phenylalanine levels in a pregnant woman with untreated or inadequately treated phenylketonuria may have a harmful effect on the fetus, resulting in microcephaly, congenital heart disease and mental retardation.

Polyhydramnios. This occurs in 1–2% of all pregnancies. It is usually chronic but may be acute, especially when associated with uniovular multiple pregnancies. Chronic polyhydramnios is often associated with multiple pregnancy, maternal diabetes and a variety of congenital malformations. In a certain proportion of cases no cause can be found. The commonest associated malformations are oesophageal atresia, duodenal atresia and neural tube defects, but many other conditions have been reported.

Prolonged rupture of membranes. Oligohydramnios due to a leak of liquor, as may occur following mid-trimester amniocentesis or prolonged membrane rupture, is associated with lung hypoplasia. An adequate volume of amniotic fluid is necessary for normal lung growth, and any cause of oligohydramnios may be associated with underdeveloped lungs, postural deformities and amnion nodosum of the placenta. Severe renal or bladder outlet obstruction is also associated with oligohydramnios, and produces a similar clinical appearance, referred to as Potter's syndrome (see p. 238).

PRINCIPLES OF MANAGEMENT

- Great care needs to be exercised with drug prescribing during the critical period in embryogenic development, from day 17 to 70 post-conception.
- There is no safe amount of alcohol consumption in pregnancy, and an abstinence approach is recommended.
- There is substantial evidence that tobacco poses a great risk to mother and fetus. Abstinence early in pregnancy has the greatest benefit but cessation at any time is beneficial. Pregnancy is a time when women come into regular contact with health professionals and are motivated to stop smoking.
- Breastfeeding is recommended, where possible, for drug-dependent mothers, with appropriate precautions.
- The health risks of maternal use of drugs such as amphetamines, cannabis and ecstasy in pregnancy have not been clearly established.

References

Batagol R. *Drugs in Pregnancy 2004*. Melbourne: The Obstetric Drug Information Centre, Royal Women's' Hospital, 2004.

Department of Health. *2003 Annual Report of the South Australian Birth Defects Register*. Adelaide: Government of South Australia Department of Health, 2005.

Jones KL, Smith DW. Recognition of the fetal alcohol syndrome in early infancy. *Lancet* 1973;**ii**:999.

Laws PJ, Sullivan EA. Australia's mothers and babies 2004. Sydney: AIHQ National Perinatal Statistics Unit, 2006.

Further reading

American Academy of Pediatrics Committee on Drugs. Neonatal drug withdrawal. *Pediatrics* 1998;**101**: 1079–1088.

Jones KL (ed.) *Smith's Recognizable Patterns of Human Malformation*, 6th edn. Philadelphia: W.B. Saunders, 2005.

McKusick VA (ed.) *Mendelian Inheritance in Man. Catalogs of Human Genes and Genetic Disorders*, 11th edn. Baltimore: Johns Hopkins University Press, 1994.

Online Mendelian Inheritance in Man (OMIM). Baltimore: Center for Medical Genetics, Johns Hopkins University; Bethesda: National Center for Biotechnology Information, National Library of Medicine, 1997 (http://http://www.ccbi.nlm.nih.gov).

15 CHAPTER 15
Genetics and genetic disorders

Genetics is the study of inheritance, part of which is concerned with how diseases are transmitted by parents to their offspring. Terms commonly used in genetics are:

genotype refers to genetic composition;

phenotype refers to the physical expression of the genotype;

karyotype refers to the chromosomal pattern; and

mutation refers to a random but permanent change in the sequence of genomic DNA.

Many diseases, such as diabetes mellitus, have a genetic background (polygenic), but about 3% of all neonates have an abnormality that is due directly to genetic factors. Genetic problems may be classified as chromosomal, inherited single-gene disorders and multifactorial disorders.

Chromosome disorders

Every cell in the body normally contains 46 chromosomes (diploid number) in its nucleus: 44 are autosomal and two are sex chromosomes (females XX or males XY). Half (the haploid number) are derived from each parent at the time of fertilization. During meiosis the chromosomes separate and align themselves around the centre of the cell, and half migrate into each daughter cell. Occasionally, one of the chromosomes does not separate in time (non-disjunction) and stays with its partner in one daughter cell, leaving the other daughter cell with no chromosomes of this type. Sometimes a process known as translocation occurs, whereby part of one chromosome is added to another during the crossover process of meiosis.

Indications for chromosome analysis

Indications for chromosomal analysis include the following:

1 recurrent unexplained abortions;

2 fresh stillbirth with physical abnormalities;

3 a neonate with features suggestive of a chromosomal abnormality; and

4 a neonate with two or more dysmorphic features.

Fetal chromosomes may also be tested during pregnancy (prenatal diagnosis). The most common indications are:

1 advanced maternal age;

2 previous chromosome disorder;

3 parent having a balanced translocation;

4 detection of fetal malformation suggestive of a chromosomal disorder.

Chromosome culture techniques

Various tissues can be sampled or cultured, depending on the timing and urgency of the diagnostic test being undertaken:

1 lymphocytes from peripheral blood (collected in a heparinized tube), ideally from a patient who has not recently ingested alcohol, antibiotics or drugs of addiction;

2 bone marrow: used for rapid diagnosis;

3 skin (fibroblast culture): useful up to 2 days after death;

4 desquamated cells in amniotic fluid: used for prenatal diagnosis;

5 chorionic villus sample: usually at 10–12 weeks' gestation.

Staining

A Giemsa (G) stain gives the overall appearance of the karyotype. G-banding of the chromosomes gives detailed information about more subtle abnormalities. Chromosomes are grouped according to banding characteristics, size of chromosomes and centromere position. The larger chromosomes are designated by the lowest numbers, and each chromosome is divided by the centromere into a short arm (p) and a long arm (q). Karyotype analysis should be available in 24–48 hours but banding can take up to 14 days.

Fluorescence *in situ* hybridization (FISH) allows more careful examination of chromosomes for very small translocations and enables determination of the parental origin of the translocated material.

Classification of chromosome abnormality

With the use of these culture and staining techniques chromosome abnormalities may be classified as numerical abnormalities, structural abnormalities, mosaicism or fragile sites.

Numerical

Aneuploidy is defined as an abnormal number of chromosomes (either too many or too few). One extra chromosome is called *trisomy* and one chromosome deletion is called a *monosomy*. These abnormalities may occur with autosomes or sex chromosomes.

Trisomy.
Autosomal chromosomes: e.g. trisomy 13, trisomy 18, trisomy 21 (Down syndrome) (Table 15.1).

Sex chromosomes: e.g. XXY (Klinefelter syndrome), XYY, triple XXX syndrome.

Monosomy.
Autosomes: usually incompatible with life and cause spontaneous abortion.

Sex chromosomes: e.g. 45,XO (Turner syndrome).

Polyploidy. This is a multiple of the haploid number. For example, the triploidy 69 karyotype usually results in abortion, stillbirth or early neonatal death.

Structural

Deletions
Short arm deletion (p–); e.g. *cri du chat* syndrome (5p–).
Long arm deletion (q–); e.g. 13q– (rare).

Additions
These are rare and only compatible with life if the addition is small.

Translocations
A translocation refers to the breakage of two non-homologous chromosomes with rejoining of the broken pieces in new ways. When there is significant alteration of genetic material (addition or deletion), the translocation is said to be unbalanced and the individual is phenotypically abnormal. Where there is a normal amount of genetic material, the individual has a balanced translocation and is phenotypically normal. Many individuals with a balanced translocation have only 45 chromosomes and convey a considerable risk to their offspring of spontaneous abortion or unbalanced translocation. Alternatively, the infant may inherit the same balanced translocation.

Triplet repeat expansions
Normal people may have a stable number of triplet base pairs and the gene concerned functions normally, but in an affected person the gene has repeated copies of certain base triplets (up to 100), and the greater the number of repeats, the more severely affected is the person. Examples of a triplet repeat expansion disorder seen in neonates include myotonic dystrophy and fragile X syndrome.

Fragile X syndrome. This is a familial form of mental retardation, which has been described in male infants, although one-third of female carriers may be mildly affected. It is the second most common cause of severe mental retardation after Down syndrome, affecting 1/1000 newborn males.

Mosaicism

In this condition there is more than one distinct cell line, one line usually being normal and the other abnormal. Thus, only a percentage of the cells will have the abnormal chromosomes. Approximately

Table 15.1 Specific chromosomal abnormalities

	Trisomy 21 (Down syndrome, Fig. 15.1)	Trisomy 13 (Patau syndrome)	Trisomy 18 (Edward syndrome, Fig. 15.2)	45,XO syndrome (Turner syndrome, ovarian dysgenesis)	XXY syndrome (Klinefelter syndrome)
Incidence	1 in 600 births	1 in 5000 births	1 in 3500 births (females predominate)	1 in 2500 of live female births (however, majority abort in first few prenatal months)	1 in 500 male births
Karyotype	94% result from non-disjunction, 3.5% translocations, 2.5% mosaicism	75% non-disjunction, 20% translocation, 5% mosaicism	85–95% non-disjunction, 5% mosaicism	60% 45,XO. Remainder – great variety including mosaics, deletions	80% XXY, 10% mosaic, 10% XXYY or XXXY
Maternal age	Important. 1 in 1500 incidence with maternal age 15–29 years, 1 in 50 at 45 years	Older maternal age seems to be important. Mean maternal age approx. 31 years	Mean maternal age 32	No apparent influence	Average maternal age slightly increased
Clinical features	These are too numerous to enumerate here refer to larger textbooks. Important are: hypotonia, flat facies, slanted palpebral fissures, small ears, etc. Major congenital abnormalities include congenital heart disease (common A-V canal), duodenal atresia	Large 'onion nose', defects of fusion of eyes, nose, lip and forebrain (holoprosencephaly), polydactyly, microcephaly, single umbilical artery; major congenital abnormalities include congenital heart disease, scalp defects	Triangular face, hooked flexion deformity 2nd finger, rocker bottom feet, single umbilical artery, short sternum; Major congenital abnormalities: heart disease, kidney malformation	Short stature (length), 'shield-like' chest. Widely spaced nipples, neck webbing, lymphoedema of hands and feet. Major congenital abnormalities: coarctation of aorta, horseshoe kidneys	Appear normal male baby. Usually diagnosed at puberty with failure of appearance of secondary sex characteristics; tall stature. Small testes post puberty
Survival	This will depend on associated malformation. Usually good	Majority die in early infancy	Majority die within first 3 months	Normal except for those with serious cardiac and renal problems	Normal
Recurrence risk	Depends on maternal age. Overall approximately 1 in 100 for non-disjunction type. In translocation depends on karyotype of parents	Low in non-disjunction type. Higher in translocation type depending on karyotype of parents	Less than 1 in 100 recurrence risk	No significant risk	No increased risk

2% of Down syndrome babies are mosaics, and these usually have less obvious stigmata and often higher intellectual ability than in the more common trisomy 21.

Clinical features

Table 15.1 gives the more important features of the more common chromosomal abnormalities, and two of these are illustrated in Figs 15.1 and 15.2.

Summary

- Chromosome disorders are complex, but in general aneuploidy is better tolerated than polyploidy.
- Additions are better tolerated than deletions (i.e. trisomy is better than monosomy, p+ better than p–).

- Abnormalities of sex chromosomes are better tolerated than abnormalities of autosomes.
- The higher the chromosome number, the better tolerated is the abnormality.

Inherited single-gene disorders

Many diseases can be inherited from parents by Mendelian modes of inheritance. These are single-gene defects or abnormalities, caused by a defective gene occurring either on autosomes (autosomal disorders) or on sex chromosomes (sex-linked, X-linked disorders). They usually exhibit obvious and characteristic pedigree patterns.

Autosomal disorders

Autosomal dominant (Fig. 15.3)
The features of this group include
1 males and females are affected in equal proportions;

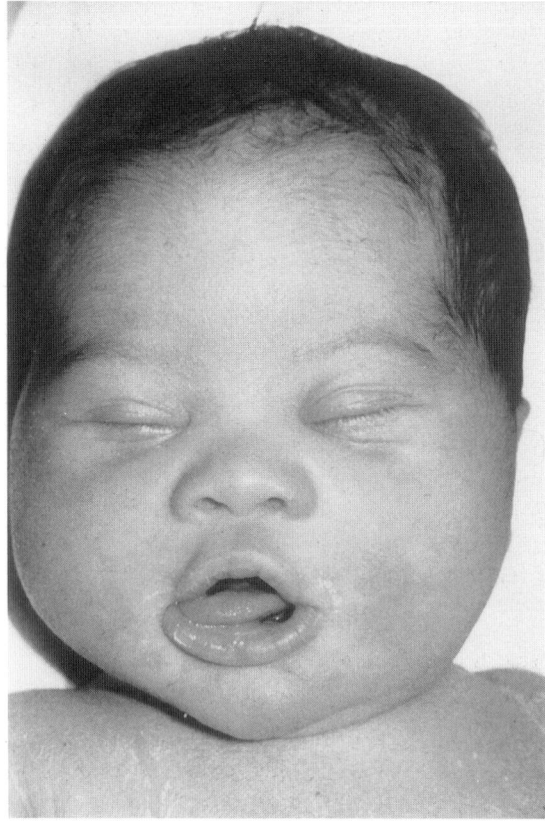

Figure 15.1 Trisomy 21 (Down syndrome).

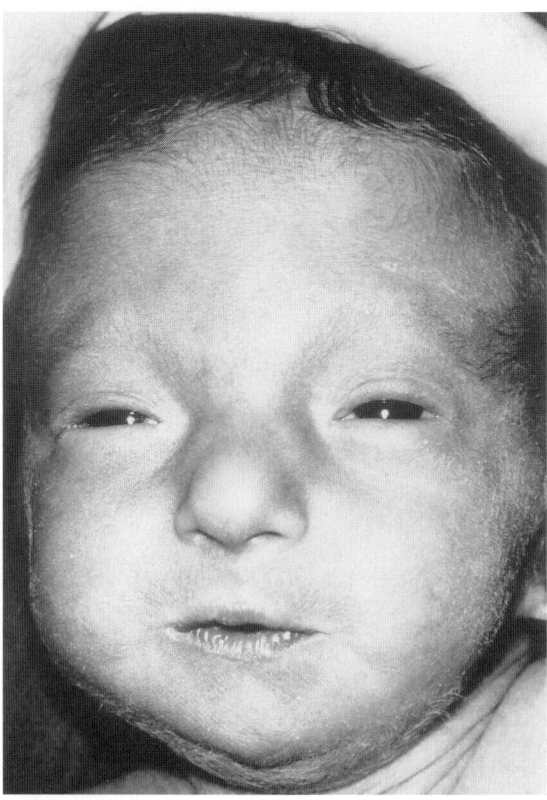

Figure 15.2 Trisomy 18 (Edward syndrome).

2 marked variation in expressivity, e.g. osteogenesis imperfecta may range from blue sclerae or deafness to severe bone fragility;

3 inherited from one parent;

4 half the offspring of an affected parent can be expected to have the disorder;

5 new cases commonly arise as spontaneous mutations, and are more common with advanced paternal age.

The mutation may be present in only one chromosome of a pair (matched with a normal allele on the homologous chromosome) or on both. In either case the cause is a single critical error in the genetic information.

Autosomal dominant disorders include

1 major malformation: polycystic kidneys;

2 minor malformations: finger anomalies – shortening, fusion, additions;

3 central nervous system (CNS) disorders: Huntington's disease, tuberous sclerosis, neurofibromatosis;

4 mesenchymal disorders: osteogenesis imperfecta, achondroplasia, Marfan syndrome;

5 tumours: retinoblastoma, colon polyposis;

6 haematological: hereditary (congenital) spherocytosis.

Autosomal recessive (Fig. 15.4)

The features of this group include:

1 the disorder is inherited from both parents, each of whom is a heterozygote (carrier);

2 the recurrence risk is 1 in 4;

3 males and females are equally affected;

4 if both parents are heterozygous for the condition, two-thirds of the unaffected offspring can be

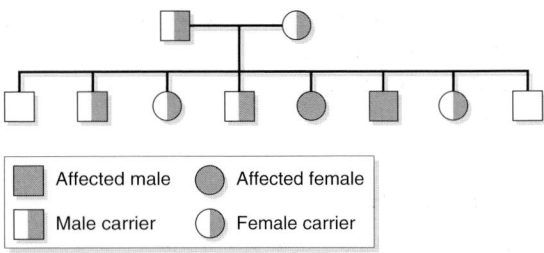

Figure 15.4 A family pedigree showing autosomal recessive inheritance.

expected to be heterozygotes and only one in four of the offspring will be genotypically normal;

5 relatively few recessive disorders arise as mutants;

6 consanguinity increases the likelihood of carriers of rare genes mating, thereby increasing the incidence of affected individuals.

The commonest severe autosomal recessive disease in Europe is cystic fibrosis. The carrier rate in the community of cystic fibrosis is 1 in 25, so that the chance of two carriers mating is 1 in 625. One in four of their offspring will be affected, so that the incidence of cystic fibrosis in the community is 1 in 2500.

Other autosomal recessive disorders include

1 haemoglobinopathies: thalassaemia syndromes, sickle-cell disease;

2 storage diseases: glycogen storage, e.g. type I (von Gierke), type II (Pompe); other, e.g. Hurler syndrome;

3 CNS degenerations: white matter, e.g. metachromatic leukodystrophy; grey matter, e.g. Tay–Sachs, hepatolenticular degeneration (Wilson disease);

4 treatable inborn errors of metabolism: phenylketonuria, galactosaemia, adrenogenital syndrome;

5 neuromuscular: spinal muscle atrophy (Werdnig–Hoffman);

6 other: cystic fibrosis, albinism.

Sex chromosome disorders

X-linked recessive (Fig. 15.5)

An X-linked recessive trait is caused by an abnormal gene on the X chromosome. The pattern of X-linked inheritance depends upon the fact that females have two X chromosomes, whereas males have only one. Thus males are said to be 'hemizygous'

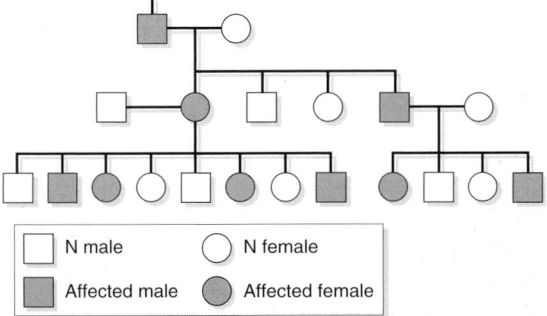

Figure 15.3 A family pedigree showing autosomal dominant inheritance.

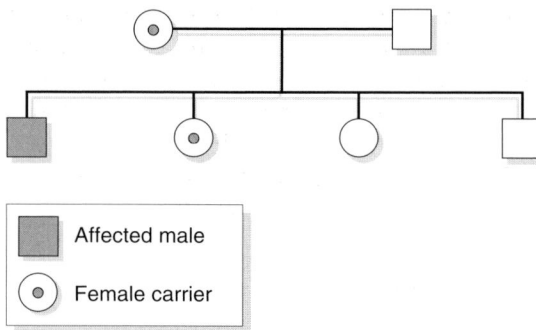

Figure 15.5 A family pedigree showing X-linked recessive inheritance

with respect to X-linked traits, and any gene on the male's single X chromosome is expressed. The 'carrier' female is protected from the effects of the recessive gene by the normal gene on her other X chromosome.

The features of this group are:

1 Predominantly males are affected.

2 The female carries the trait (rarely the female carrier may be mildly affected).

3 Half the male offspring of a female carrier are affected.

4 Half the female offspring of a carrier will themselves become carriers.

5 All the female offspring of an affected male will be carriers.

6 Often expressed as a new mutation, making genetic counselling difficult (probably 33% of all cases of lethal X-linked recessive diseases).

7 Many X-linked recessive diseases are lethal (muscular dystrophy, X-linked agammaglobulinaemia, Lesch–Nyhan syndrome), so that the disorder can only be handed on by the carrier female. However, in glucose-6-phosphate dehydrogenase (G6PD) deficiency and colour blindness the disorder may be passed on by the affected males to daughters but not to sons.

X-linked recessive diseases include

- haemophilia A, haemophilia B (Christmas disease);
- Duchenne muscular dystrophy;
- agammaglobulinaemia;
- G6PD deficiency;
- colour blindness.

The Lyon hypothesis

This refers to the random inactivation of one X chromosome in a female (either maternal X or paternal X) at a stage during cell division. This enables heterozygous females to exhibit some features of an X-linked recessive disease, for example, elevated creatinine phosphokinase in Duchenne muscular dystrophy.

Genomic imprinting

This is the phenomenon in which the expression of certain genes is determined by whether the gene is inherited from the female or male parent. In neonatal practice the best example of this is expression of the Prader–Willi syndrome if the gene is expressed on the paternal allele, or Angelman syndrome associated with expression of the maternal allele.

X-linked dominant inheritance

These conditions are rare, with the only clinically important disorders being vitamin D-resistant rickets, incontinentia pigmenti and pseudohypoparathyroidism. Some X-linked dominant disorders appear to be lethal to the male, so that only females are affected (e.g. incontinentia pigmenti).

Multifactorial or polygenic disorders

Many congenital abnormalities may be caused by the interaction of multiple factors, both genetic and environmental. These disorders do not exhibit the characteristic patterns of Mendelian inheritance, although their recurrence within families is greater than that predicted for the general population.

Such diseases include

- anencephaly;
- spina bifida;
- cleft lip;
- cleft palate;
- cleft palate without cleft lip;
- clubfoot (talipes equinovarus);
- congenital dislocation of the hip;
- congenital heart diseases;
- Hirschsprung's disease;
- pyloric stenosis.

Some diseases that present later in life, such as diabetes mellitus, schizophrenia and hypertension, are probably examples of multifactorial inheritance.

In general, the incidence of conditions associated with multifactorial inheritance is approximately 1/1000 live births. However, once the entity has occurred there is said to be an increased recurrence risk in first-degree relatives of about 1/20–40.

Environmental factors known to cause birth defects include maternal disease, such as insulin-dependent diabetes mellitus, medications taken during pregnancy, and pregnancy infections such as rubella. It is also presumed that vascular accidents during organogenesis can be associated with defects.

Prevention of birth defects

Birth defects are a major cause of perinatal and postnatal mortality and morbidity, which have a significant impact on family life and the community as a whole. It is therefore important to have an approach to preventing such defects and identifying causes when they occur.

Strategies used to prevent birth defects include

1 Preconceptual counselling in mothers with insulin-dependent diabetes mellitus.

2 Prenatal diagnosis using ultrasound, chorionic villus sampling, amniocentesis, maternal serum, fetal blood sampling and fetal biopsy. Early prenatal diagnosis will provide an opportunity for counselling and possibly termination of pregnancy.

3 The administration of folic acid (0.4 mg daily) for at least 1 month before conception in planned pregnancies and in the early months of pregnancy to reduce the incidence of neural tube defects (see p. 208).

4 Rubella immunization of adolescent girls.

5 Avoidance of drugs known to be teratogens (see Table 14.4).

6 Avoidance of maternal exposure to known chemical teratogens and irradiation (see p. 147). There is currently no sound evidence that paternal exposure to environmental chemicals is teratogenic. Theoretically, it is possible that environmentally induced mutations could contribute to the known paternal age-related risk of new dominant mutations, such as for achondroplasia.

7 Community education in the avoidance of harmful practices and the use of potential teratogens, including smoking, alcohol and cocaine during pregnancy.

8 Neonatal screening for the early detection and treatment of diseases or conditions before permanent damage is incurred, for example, phenylketonuria, galactosaemia, hypothyroidism, cystic fibrosis and congenital dislocation of the hip.

9 Genetic counselling where there has been an affected child can prevent recurrence.

Genetic counselling

Genetic counselling aims to provide parents or prospective parents with sufficient knowledge to make an informed decision about their reproduction options and provide information about issues they may have to face.

Indications for genetic counselling include

1 previous stillbirth or multiple miscarriages;

2 previous child with a birth defect, mental retardation or chromosomal abnormality;

3 family history of known genetic disorder;

4 advanced maternal age;

5 exposure to teratogenic drugs, teratogenic chemicals or irradiation during pregnancy;

6 history of neoplastic conditions with genetic implications, e.g. retinoblastoma, colon polyposis.

Molecular genetics

Recent advances in molecular genetics using DNA-based and other techniques have given an added dimension to the diagnosis of genetic disease and counselling. The list of genetic loci and mutations that may cause genetic disease, many of paediatric importance, is ever expanding, and catalogued in Online Mendelian Inheritance in Man (http://www.ncbi.nlm.nih.gov/entrez/query.fcgi?db=OMIM).

A detailed discussion of the causes and types of mutations that may occur is beyond the scope of this book. For further information the reader should refer to specific texts on the molecular basis of genetic disease.

Mutations of developmental genes have been identified as a cause of birth defects. Examples include homeotic (HOX) and paired box (PAX) gene families. HOX genes are involved in the formation of structures developing from specific segments of the embryo; for example, mutation of the *HOXD13* gene is associated with dominant polysyndactyly.

PAX genes are important in eye development; for example, mutant *PAX6* is associated with aniridia.

The types of mutations occurring during DNA replication are complex. Although this is an over-simplification, they may be classified into groups according to the scale of the mutation (a portion of DNA sequence vs entire chromosomes) and the type of mutation (affecting primarily the structure or regulation of the genetic information). Examples of gene structural errors include Duchenne muscular dystrophy, Charcot–Marie–Tooth disease, Hurler syndrome and Crouzon syndrome. Examples of gene function errors include thalassaemia, Beckwith–Wiedemann syndrome and fragile X syndrome. Structural errors of chromosomes involve monosomy (deletion; e.g. Turner syndrome), trisomy (duplications; e.g. Down syndrome) or triploidy (e.g. miscarriages). Function errors of chromosomes occur with uniparent disomy, for instance, Prader–Willi syndrome.

Direct methods involve testing the DNA from an individual, usually using polymerase chain reaction (PCR), to see whether or not it carries a known mutation associated with the suspected disease. For prenatal diagnosis the DNA can be obtained in the first trimester of pregnancy by chorionic villus sampling, or by culturing cells obtained at amniocentesis. Examples of diseases that may be detected in this way include β-thalassaemia, cystic fibrosis and Duchenne muscular dystrophy. In some situations *in utero* treatment may be possible. For example, in cases of congenital adrenal hyperplasia due to 21-hydroxylase deficiency, prenatal diagnosis and treatment of an affected female fetus with dexamethasone may prevent virilization.

Indirect testing (gene tracing) uses closely linked molecular markers in family studies to discover whether or not an individual inherited the disease-carrying chromosome from a parent. An example of this is seen in the preclinical diagnosis of retinoblastoma; 20–40% of cases are hereditary, where the risk for the child is 50%. If the child has inherited the parent's retinoblastoma gene, regular ophthalmological review is mandatory. The same principles apply for adolescent- or adult-onset disease, such as polycystic kidney or polyposis coli.

Diagnostic approach to the dysmorphic neonate

In some instances the suspected cause of dysmorphism in a neonate may be obvious from classic clinical features, such as with Down syndrome. In others the cause may be more subtle, with unusual facies or single and multiple birth defects, some of which may appear unrelated. In all cases a systematic approach to diagnosis, which may aid treatment, is mandatory.

The diagnostic procedure involves

1 A detailed medical history to obtain information about the pregnancy and the possibility of exposure to teratogens. A family pedigree should be obtained when a genetic disorder is suspected.

2 A detailed clinical examination should be carried out and all abnormalities documented.

3 Investigations, which include

(a) chromosomal analysis where two or more dysmorphic features are present;

(b) metabolic studies on blood and urine in suspected inborn errors of metabolism; and

(c) radiology, including head, renal ultrasound and X-rays to distinguish bone dysplasia; autopsy if the infant dies.

4 Database consultation may aid in the diagnosis of multiple birth defects, e.g. OMIM, London Dysmorphology Database.

5 Consultation with specialists: radiologist, geneticist, biochemist, ophthalmologist, neurologist, etc.

Further reading

Cassiday SB, Allanson JE. *Management of Genetic Syndromes*, 2nd edn. John Wiley and Sons, Hoboken, NJ, 2005.

Connor JM, Ferguson-Smith MA. *Essential Medical Genetics*, 5th edn. Oxford: Blackwell Scientific Publications, 1997.

Jones KL (ed.) *Smith's Recognizable Patterns of Human Malformation*, 6th edn. Philadelphia: W.B. Saunders, 2005.

Online Mendelian Inheritance in Man (OMIM) (http://www.ncbi.nlm.nih.gov/entrez/query.fcgi?db=OMIM).

Turnpenny P, Ellard S. *Emery's Elements of Medical Genetics*, 12th edn. Edinburgh: Churchill Livingstone, 2005.

Winter RM, Baraitser M (eds) *London Dysmorphology Database and London Neurogenetics Database* [computer file]. Oxford: Oxford University Press, 1996.

CHAPTER 16

16 Endocrine and metabolic disorders

Glucose homeostasis and its abnormalities

The fetus has a continuous supply of glucose from the mother via the placenta, and consequently fetal blood glucose levels are the same as the mother's. At birth the infant has to switch rapidly to endo-genous gluconeogenesis until feeding is established. At birth the newborn's blood glucose rapidly falls to approximately 75% of the maternal blood glucose level.

Glucose and oxygen are the main metabolic substrates of the mature brain, but in the neonate the brain can use alternative metabolic fuels such as lactate and ketones. Birth at full term is characterized by a vigorous ketogenic response, but this is impaired in preterm infants and infants who experience intrauterine growth restriction (IUGR). This is why the brain can function normally, or near normally, despite very low levels of blood glucose. Profound neurological compromise and irreversible damage occur if the brain is deprived of glucose and alternative metabolic substrates.

Glucose metabolism

Figure 16.1 summarizes the main metabolic pathways involved in gluconeogenesis.

1 *Glycogen production and glycogenolysis.* These occur largely in the liver and muscles, but only if liver glycogen is available for rapid breakdown to glucose.

2 *Gluconeogenesis.* The most important substrates are amino acids (particularly alanine), lactate, pyruvate and glycerol. The points at which these are metabolized are shown in Fig. 16.1.

3 *Lipolysis.* Glycerol is metabolized from adipose tissue and can be directly utilized in gluconeogenesis metabolism. Other products of lipolysis (fatty acids

and triglycerides) are metabolized to ketone bodies, which may be used directly in energy production, particularly by the brain. Ketone body production is stimulated by infant feeding, particularly by breast milk.

These mechanisms are under the control of the endocrine system and are affected by insulin, glucagon, cortisol and growth hormone. Therefore, so that neonates can regulate blood sugar within the physiological range, they must be endowed with adequate liver glycogen, lipid stores and effective metabolic pathways including glycogenolysis and gluconeogenesis, as well as overall endocrine control. Hypoglycaemia will rapidly develop if any of these processes are disturbed.

Measurement of blood glucose

It is essential to measure blood glucose rapidly and accurately in high-risk infants, and a variety of techniques have been developed to give cotside values. Glucose concentrations in plasma or serum are 10–15% higher than in whole blood, and many bedside techniques rely on whole-blood methods, whereas the laboratory techniques are more likely to measure serum glucose levels. In the neonatal unit strip reagents are most widely used, but these are generally unreliable particularly in the presence of low blood glucose, which is the range of most importance in the newborn. Strip tests use glucose oxidase-sensitive blocks, which change colour depending on the blood glucose concentration and are specific for glucose alone. Blood glucose estimation by Dextrostix (Ames, Elkhart, Indiana) is critically affected by the time the block is in contact with the blood, whereas this is less critical with BM stix, (Abbott, Maidenhead, UK). More recently, portable

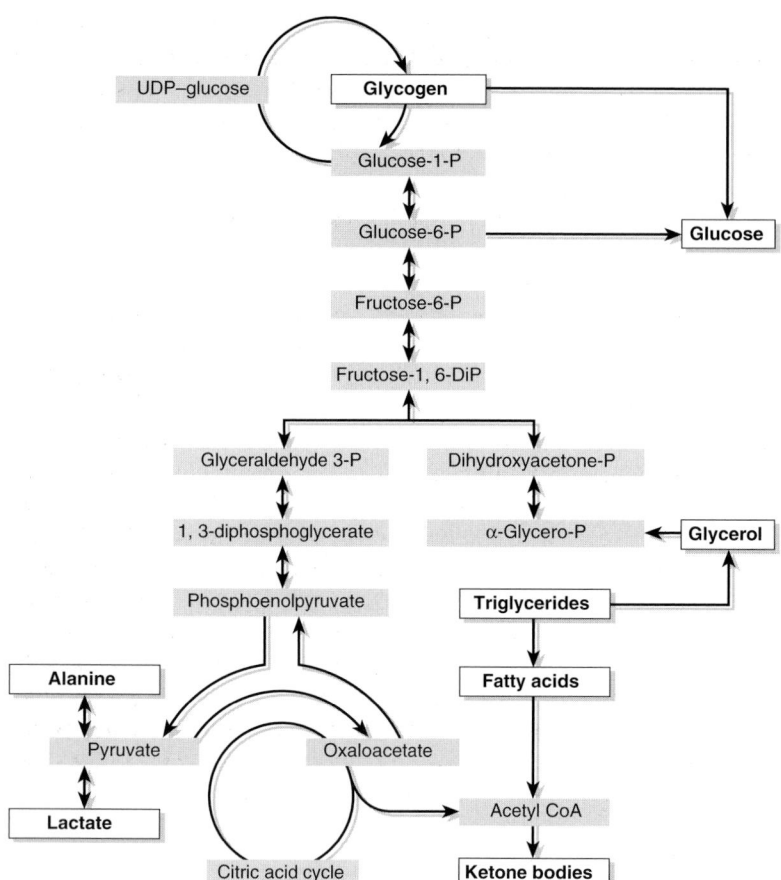

Figure 16.1 Metabolic pathways involved in gluconeogenesis. (Reproduced with permission from Aynsley-Green *et al.* 1981.)

biosensing devices for measuring glucose at or near the cotside have been introduced. These include glucose sensors built into blood gas machines, and these are considerably more accurate than reagent strip testing. Low levels of blood sugar recorded in the nursery should be confirmed by sending a specimen to the laboratory for blood gas analyses.

Hypoglycaemia

The definition of hypoglycaemia has been gradually refined over the last 30 years and higher values for blood sugar are now accepted as normal than was the case in the past. Hypoglycaemia is defined as a blood sugar concentration falling below a predetermined reference value, but this is not usually helpful in a clinical setting. A more important question is what is the lowest acceptable level in an individual

baby before physiological compromise occurs. As discussed above neonatal cerebral function may continue normally despite very low levels of blood sugar because an alternative energy substrate is available.

Attempts have been made to define the level of blood sugar at which cerebral dysfunction occurs and then to set 'normoglycaemia' levels above this. Two important observations have been made in recent years to help determine the lower level of normoglycaemia. In a retrospective study, Lucus *et al.* (1988) found that premature infants (birthweight <1850 g) with blood sugar levels <2.6 mmol/L were at increased risk of lower neurodevelopmental scores, particularly when blood sugar values were below this figure on repeated occasions. It has also been shown that a deterioration in neurological function (measured by evoked potentials) occurred with a blood sugar level <2.6 mmol/L (Koh *et al.* 1988).

As a result of these studies we can define the lower limit of 'normoglycaemia' as 2.6 mmol/L although levels below this do not necessarily mean that damage will occur; however, we recommend maintaining the blood sugar of preterm infants and term infants who are at risk of hypoglycaemia (see below) above 2.5 mmol/L.

Who should be monitored for hypoglycaemia?

The majority of babies who are prone to hypoglycaemia can be predicted on the basis of easily identifiable risk factors (Table 16.1). Careful monitoring of these babies' blood sugar will alert the clinician to the onset of hypoglycaemia and enable management aimed to prevent symptomatic hypoglycaemia.

In babies at risk of hypoglycaemia an early and frequent feeding regimen should be instituted with regular blood sugar monitoring for the first 24 hours. 'At-risk' infants should be fed within 2 h of birth with high-glucose-containing solutions. A suitable regimen would be: glucose 10% or full-strength formula given 2-hourly. Small for gestational age (SGA) infants often tolerate up to 100 mL/kg on day 1 of life. If asymptomatic hypoglycaemia fails to be corrected by early, frequent feeds, an infusion with 10% dextrose will be necessary.

Blood sugar estimates should be made immediately pre-feed, as this is the time when the blood sugar is likely to be at its lowest point. In view of the unreliability of reagent strip tests, it may be preferable to undertake more accurate measurement of blood sugar less frequently: one regimen recommends once or twice daily laboratory measurements starting immediately before the second feed

Table 16.1 At-risk infants for hypoglycaemia

Infants of diabetic mothers
Growth-restricted infants
Premature infants
Birth asphyxia
On rewarming after hypothermia
Infection
Polycythaemia
Beckwith–Wiedemann syndrome

(Deshpande & Ward Platt 2005). More frequent measurements are required in the presence of actual hypoglycaemia. When blood sugar levels are satisfactory, the frequency of heel-prick estimations is reduced before ceasing.

Symptoms of hypoglycaemia

The symptoms of hypoglycaemia in the newborn can be divided into major and minor:
- *Major*. Apnoea, convulsions and coma. Rarely, prolonged hypoglycaemia may cause congestive heart failure or persistent pulmonary hypertension.
- *Minor*. Jitteriness, irritability, tremors, apathy, cyanotic spells and temperature instability.

It is not possible to confidently diagnose neonatal hypoglycaemia clinically as the symptoms are non-specific and similar to those of infection. Hypoglycaemia may remain entirely without clinical signs or symptoms, and this is referred to as asymptomatic hypoglycaemia. It is unusual for a newborn with hypoglycaemia to have a classic autonomic nervous system response, with sweating, pallor and tachycardia, as occurs in adults. A low blood sugar detected by a stick test should be checked by a laboratory blood assay for glucose.

Causes

These can be considered under five major headings, which are summarized in Table 16.2.

Management

The major aim is to prevent hypoglycaemia developing, and this is done by recognizing babies who are at higher risk of this condition and giving early and appropriate feeding (see above).

A baby with symptomatic hypoglycaemia will require a dextrose infusion. An initial bolus dose of dextrose 100 mg/kg is given over 10 min as 1 mL/kg of 10% dextrose. This is usually followed by a steady-state infusion of 10% dextrose at a rate of 80–100 mL/kg/24 h. If the blood glucose estimate is less than 2.6 mmol/L (40 mg/100 mL), the dextrose concentration may need to be increased to 15% dextrose. Up to 12.5% dextrose may be infused via a peripheral intravenous line, but if more than 15% dextrose is required a central intravenous line will be necessary. Where possible oral feeding should be continued, but if hypoglycaemia persists with

Table 16.2 Causes of neonatal hypoglycaemia

Decreased substrate availability
SGA infants (see p. 83)
Premature infants. Second twin, especially if growth
 retarded

Increased glucose utilization
Hyperinsulinaemia
 Infant of a diabetic mother
 Rhesus isoimmunization
 Nesidioblastosis
 Islet cell tumour
 Beckwith–Wiedemann syndrome
Polycythaemia

Inability to utilize glucose
Glycogen storage disease type I
Galactosaemia
Fructose intolerance
Inborn errors of amino acid metabolism

Iatrogenic
Inappropriate infusion of glucose

Miscellaneous
Birth asphyxia
Endocrine deficiencies (e.g. rare types of congenital
 adrenal hyperplasia)
Hypopituitarism

solutions of more than 10% dextrose, feeds should
probably be discontinued.

Resistant hypoglycaemia
Rarely, the above regimen fails to control hypoglycaemia and hyperinsulinaemia should be suspected
(see p. 162). Under these circumstances other forms
of treatment are necessary to control the hypoglycaemia, used in the following sequence:
1 hydrocortisone – 25 mg/kg/day intravenously
(i.v.) or by continuous infusion;
2 glucagon (100 μg/kg/dose) may be useful when
the infant has adequate glycogen stores, e.g. infant
of diabetic mother (IDM);
3 diazoxide – 5 mg/kg/dose, given i.v. every 6 h;
4 somatostatin analogue SMS-201-995 is useful
in the short-term management of neonatal hyperinsulinism;
5 laparotomy and subtotal pancreatectomy when
an insulinoma is strongly suspected;

Investigations

Hypoglycaemia in most infants resolves spontaneously within a few days, but it is sometimes
more severe or fails to resolve rapidly.
Hyperinsulinaemia is suspected clinically when a
baby with severe non-ketotic hypoglycaemia
requires a glucose infusion rate exceeding
10 mg/kg/min to maintain normoglycaemia. These
babies have a very brisk response to glucagon
injections, with the blood glucose increasing to
>1.7 mmol/L above baseline. The definitive diag-
nosis of hyperinsulinism is made by measurement
of serum insulin (>10 mU/mL) during an episode
of hypoglycaemia (<2.2 mmol/L). The plasma
should be separated and frozen immediately after
taking the sample if reliable results are to be
obtained. A screen for inborn errors of metabolism
may be necessary in some cases. An exploratory
laparotomy may be necessary in infants suspected
of having islet cell tumours. Inborn errors of
metabolism or endocrine problems may rarely
cause hypoglycaemia, and if these are considered
to be a possible cause, appropriate investigations
should be undertaken to diagnose or exclude
these conditions.

Prognosis

Severe symptomatic hypoglycaemia carries a
very poor prognosis. Approximately half of these
babies will die and half of the survivors will have
severe neurodevelopmental abnormalities, including mental retardation, convulsions, spasticity
and microcephaly. The prevention of symptomatic
hypoglycaemia is one of the most important factors
in preventing brain damage in the whole of neonatal medicine.

It is widely believed that infants with asymptomatic hypoglycaemia are not at risk of adverse neurodevelopmental outcome, but recent interest in
redefining the level of normoglycaemia is based on
a reassessment of the importance of asymptomatic
hypoglycaemia. At present the data are not clear,
and until a randomized controlled trial is carried
out examining various levels of blood glucose control the question will not be answered. There is currently evidence of neural dysfunction with blood
sugar levels <2.6 mmol/L, and repeated levels below

this may have a cumulative adverse effect on neural function, although the baby may not show clinical symptoms.

Specific causes of hypoglycaemia

Infants of diabetic mothers (IDMs)

Maternal diabetes is classified as follows:
1 pregestational;
2 type I: the basic cause is beta-cell destruction;
3 type II: this is due to insulin resistance with an insulin secretory defect;
4 gestational diabetes.

IDMs have unique problems and require specialized neonatal care. The prognosis for the diabetic pregnancy depends on the severity of the diabetes and the quality of diabetic control during pregnancy.

The two main factors determining whether maternal diabetes will have an effect on the fetus and baby are the vascular complications that the diabetes causes the mother, and the blood glucose control during pregnancy.

1 *Vascular disease*. Mothers with vascular complications as a result of diabetes are much more likely to develop hypertension in pregnancy, which may affect fetal growth and wellbeing.

2 *Glucose control*. The outcome of pregnancy in diabetic women also depends on glucose control both before conception and during gestation. Diabetic women should have their diabetes very carefully managed prior to conception, and combined care through pregnancy by a physician and obstetrician is essential. The blood sugar should be maintained below 8 mmol/L, with soluble insulin if necessary, and hypoglycaemia avoided. On this regimen the complications for the fetus are reduced and may be avoided completely. A variety of congenital malformations are particularly common in women with diabetes, and the risk appears to depend on the mother's pre-pregnancy blood sugar levels.

Clinical features of an IDM

Complications to the fetus are likely to occur in diabetic women in whom glucose control has been less than adequate. The frequencies of complications in

Table 16.3 Frequency of complications (percentages) in infants of diabetic mothers (IDM) and infants of gestational diabetic mothers (IGDM). Complications are related to the quality of glucose control in pregnancy

Complications	IDM (%)	IGDM (%)
Uneventful course	50	80
RDS	30	10
Hypoglycaemia (asymptomatic and symptomatic)	60	16
Symptomatic hypoglycaemia	20	10
Hypocalcaemia	25	15
Polycythaemia	40	30
Hyperbilirubinaemia	50	25
Congestive heart failure	10	Unknown
Congenital abnormalities	10	3

IDM and in gestational diabetic mothers are given in Table 16.3. Complications include:

1 Congenital malformations. The most frequent congenital abnormalities in IDM are:

   (a) congenital heart disease, especially ventricular septal defect, transposition of the great vessels, coarctation of the aorta;

   (b) renal vein thrombosis;

   (c) sacral and coccygeal agenesis (caudal regression syndrome);

   (d) left microcolon;

   (e) hypertrophic cardiomyopathy – this mainly affects the intraventricular septum and may cause ventricular outflow obstruction; it is a transient condition that resolves in the first few months of life; inotropic drugs such as digoxin should be avoided.

2 Stillbirth. There is an increased risk of intrauterine fetal death during pregnancy.

3 Infants born to mothers with diabetic vascular disease are more likely to be SGA.

4 Macrosomia. Insulin is a major trophic hormone influencing fetal growth, and hyperinsulinaemic fetuses become macrosomic. These infants are plethoric, obese and 'Cushingoid' in appearance, and have an enlarged heart, liver and spleen (Fig. 16.2). There is an increased body length and birthweight, but the head circumference and brain weight are appropriate for gestational age. They have excessive fat stores and inhibition of lipolysis and β-oxidation resulting from hyperinsulinaemia.

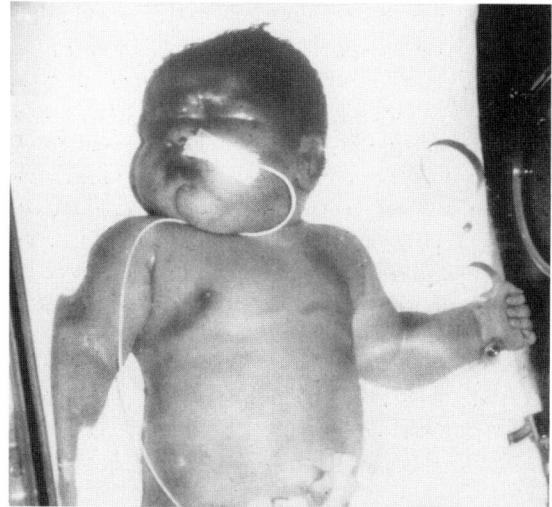

Figure 16.2 Characteristic appearance of the macrosomic infant of a poorly controlled diabetic mother.

The large size predisposes to birth-related problems, including

(a) birth trauma from cephalopelvic disproportion, difficult instrumental delivery and shoulder dystocia; injuries include intracranial haemorrhage, fractured bones and nerve palsies;

(b) birth asphyxia may occur in a poorly controlled diabetic pregnancy and may be related to cephalopelvic disproportion.

5 Neonatal hypoglycaemia. Chronically elevated maternal glucose levels cause hyperplasia of the islet beta cells in the fetal pancreas with fetal hyperinsulinism. Once the baby is born the high circulating insulin causes neonatal hypoglycaemia lasting for several days. There are three common patterns:

(a) transient hypoglycaemia, which lasts 1–4 h, followed by a spontaneous rise in the blood sugar;

(b) prolonged initial hypoglycaemia lasting 24–48 h;

(c) rarely there may be a mild initial hypoglycaemia, followed in 12–24 h by more severe hypoglycaemia, which may be symptomatic.

6 Insulin has an antagonistic effect on surfactant development and hyperinsulinaemic babies are at much greater risk of developing respiratory distress due to surfactant deficiency, retained lung fluid or polycythaemia, even at full term.

Management
Careful control of diabetes during pregnancy decreases many of the complications. Management of the pregnancy involves obsessional diabetic control, planned delivery in a suitably equipped hospital, examination for congenital abnormalities and screening for anticipated complications, especially hypoglycaemia.

Prognosis for IDM
This depends on the quality of glucose control in pregnancy. The risk of insulin requiring diabetes melitis by 20 years of age is seven fold greater than for babies born to non diabetic women. Published studies give perinatal mortality rates of about 30/1000 for diabetic pregnancies.

Congenital hyperinsulinism
This is due to a group of disorders in the regulatory function of pancreatic beta cells resulting in unregulated secretion of insulin and severe neonatal hypoglycaemia. Specific gene defects have been identified as the cause in 50% of cases. The term nesidioblastosis was previously used to describe congenital hyperinsulinism, but the histological features of it are seen in the normal pancreas and the term is no longer used. Congenital hyperinsulinism should be considered in infants who require glucose infusion exceeding 15 mg/kg/min to prevent hypoglycaemia and confirmed by showing high levels of insulin during hypoglycaemia (see p. 160). Few ketone bodies are produced during the hypoglycaemic episodes.

Severe resultant hypoglycaemia can be temporarily reversed by glucagon (1 mg i.m.) and/or octreotide, an analogue of somatostation. The main drug used in the long-term management of this condition is diazoxide. Those who fail to respond to medical therapy will require surgery. Occasionally the hyperinsulism is due to a localized insulinoma, and full excision of this is curative. More commonly the pancreas is diffusely abnormal, requiring near-total pancreatectomy with removal of up to 95% of the pancreas.

Beckwith–Wiedemann syndrome

This refers to the association of macroglossia, umbilical hernia (or exomphalos) and macrosomia. The infants almost invariably show a crease or fissure in their earlobes. There is often hyperinsulinaemia due to beta-cell hyperplasia. Hypoglycaemia occurs in the neonatal period in about a third of cases. Later malignant disease occurs in about 6% of cases.

Iatrogenic hypoglycaemia

This occurs most commonly in infants at risk of hypoglycaemia in whom low blood sugar is detected and aggressive treatment started. Treatment with rapid intravenous injection of concentrated (25% or 50%) dextrose will cause a rapid increase in blood glucose, and in the presence of hyperinsulinism there may be a rebound hypoglycaemia. When the blood glucose is next measured, hypoglycaemia is found as a result of this rebound effect, and another rapid infusion of concentrated dextrose is given with similar effect.

The management of hypoglycaemia is discussed on p. 159. Rapid or concentrated injections of dextrose are rarely necessary and should be avoided if possible. When absolutely necessary, they should be followed by a continuous infusion to avoid rebound hypoglycaemia.

When insulin is used to treat hyperglycaemia or hyperkalaemia, hypoglycaemia may be induced. Regular blood glucose measurements must be performed on all infants receiving insulin.

Hyperglycaemia

Hyperglycaemia is usually defined as a blood sugar concentration greater than 9 mmol/L, at which level glycosuria may occur. Hyperglycaemia frequently occurs in the preterm infant who is receiving 10% dextrose intravenously, or in any infant receiving parenteral nutrition.

Usually hyperglycaemia responds to a reduction in the glucose concentration or the infusion rate. Hyperglycaemia must be considered to be a sign of septicaemia. A full infection screen should always be performed on neonates with high glucose levels or glycosuria. Glycosuria induces an osmotic diuresis and may cause electrolyte imbalance. Very severe hyperglycaemia (>40 mmol/L) is rarely seen, but an increasing number of case reports have shown this to be due to inadvertent infusion of large volumes of dextrose solution or incorrectly made up parenteral feed regimens. If a baby has a blood sugar of >20 mmol/L then immediately change all the baby's infusions to 5% glucose solution and check all the solution formulations and pumps that were used on discovery of the hyperglycaemia.

Rarely insulin is required to treat hyperglycaemia. Soluble insulin 0.1 U/kg should be given intravenously and repeated as necessary to keep the blood sugar below 9 mmol/L.

Transient neonatal diabetes mellitus

This is very rare and occurs in severely growth-retarded infants. Non-ketotic hyperglycaemia develops as a result of inadequate insulin production by the pancreatic beta cells. Treatment is by correction of electrolyte disturbances and the administration of insulin (0.1 U/kg) intravenously. Later, chlorpropamide can be substituted for insulin until normal pancreatic function develops (Kuna & Addy 1979).

Disorders of calcium, phosphate and magnesium metabolism

The metabolism of these three electrolytes is interrelated and not completely understood.

Calcium. Half the total serum calcium is in ionized form and half is protein bound. Ionized calcium is the most physiologically active. Fetal calcium levels are higher than maternal levels but drop rapidly, reaching a low point 18–24 h after birth, largely as a result of calcitonin. This fall in serum calcium stimulates parathormone, with resultant bone resorption and an increase in serum calcium to approximately adult levels.

Phosphate. Most inorganic phosphate is in ionic form (PO_4) or complexed as either HPO_4 or H_2PO_4 ions.

Magnesium. Half the total body magnesium is in bone and most of the rest is intracellular.

Neonatal levels are higher than maternal levels. Low levels of magnesium inhibit parathyroid hormone secretion, and hypomagnesaemia is commonly found together with hypocalcaemia.

Parathormone (PTH).   This is secreted from the parathyroids in response to low ionized calcium levels. PTH increases serum calcium and lowers serum phosphate levels by the following actions:

• increases the reabsorption of calcium and phosphate from bone;

• increases tubular reabsorption of calcium and reduces the reabsorption of phosphate;

• stimulates the production of renal 1,25-dihydroxy-vitamin D.

Vitamin D.   This compound requires skin, liver and renal metabolism. Oral cholecalciferol is converted in the liver to 25-hydroxyvitamin D and then further metabolized in the kidney to 1,25-dihydroxy-vitamin D. 1,25-Dihydroxyvitamin D increases the intestinal absorption of calcium and phosphate. Low maternal vitamin D levels cause the fetus to be born with relatively low levels.

Calcitonin.   This hormone is produced in the thyroid and is secreted in response to a high ionized calcium level. Calcitonin reduces serum calcium and phosphate levels.

Hypocalcaemia

Hypocalcaemia is usually defined as a serum calcium concentration less than 1.8 mmol/L (7.5 mg/dL). It is the ionized fraction that determines whether symptoms occur, but few laboratories routinely measure ionized calcium. Some neonatal intensive care units (NICUs) have blood gas analysers that measure ionized calcium along with other electrolytes. Furthermore, acidosis causes more calcium to be ionized and alkalosis decreases ionized calcium. For these reasons, infants may exhibit few or no symptoms of hypocalcaemia despite low serum calcium levels, provided ionized calcium is normal. This is particularly common in hypoproteinaemic states.

Hypocalcaemia may present early or late.

Early hypocalcaemia.   This occurs within the first 72 h of life, although the reasons for this are not fully understood. It is most liable to occur in the following cases:

1 prematurity;

2 associated with respiratory distress syndrome (RDS);

3 birth asphyxia;

4 IDM;

5 neonatal sepsis.

Persistent hypocalcaemia is due to hypoparathyroidism. This is a rare condition and may be inherited in either an X-linked or an autosomal recessive manner. It also occurs in the DiGeorge syndrome. Hypocalcaemia is associated with hyperphosphataemia and requires lifelong vitamin D treatment.

Late hypocalcaemia.   This is often referred to as neonatal tetany and occurs after the first week of life. It was associated with an unmodified cows' milk diet, but is now rarely seen with adapted infant milk formulas.

Rarely, late hypocalcaemia is due to maternal hyperparathyroidism. Maternal hypercalcaemia causes fetal hypercalcaemia with suppression of the fetal parathyroid. This predisposes the infant to hypocalcaemia in the second or third week of life. It is a transient condition.

Iatrogenic hypocalcaemia.   This may occur following exchange transfusion with citrated blood or as a result of inadequate vitamin D supplementation.

Clinical features

Low ionized calcium levels produce neuromuscular irritability. Tremors, tetany, jitteriness and convulsions may occur. Seizures may be identical to those due to hypoglycaemia or other cerebral causes. Occasionally, bradycardia and apnoea may be due to hypocalcaemia.

Diagnosis

Serum calcium and magnesium levels should be measured in 'at-risk' or symptomatic infants. An electrocardiogram (ECG) will show a prolonged Q–T interval (this needs to be corrected for heart rate).

Management

1 *Asymptomatic hypocalcaemia.* The low serum calcium should be corrected with oral calcium gluconate supplements, or if there is an intravenous

line *in situ* by i.v. calcium gluconate (dose is 300 mg/kg/day).

2. *Abnormal movements or apnoea* due to hypocalcaemia should be corrected by a slow infusion of 10% calcium gluconate (100 mg/kg) over 20 min, with ECG monitoring.

Severe and resistant hypocalcaemia, as occurs in congenital hypoparathyroidism, may require vitamin D supplementation in the form of 1-α-vitamin D.

Some cases of hypocalcaemia will not respond to calcium gluconate infusion and require magnesium sulphate (see below).

Prognosis

Most children with neonatal hypocalcaemia recover completely with no adverse neurodevelopmental sequelae (compare hypoglycaemia). Severe enamel dysplasia is seen in the primary dentition of some infants with tetany due to hypocalcaemia.

Metabolic bone disease (rickets of prematurity)

This condition, also referred to as osteopenia of prematurity, was formally known as rickets of prematurity. Rickets implies a deficiency or abnormality of vitamin D metabolism, which is now known not to be an important factor in metabolic bone disease, hence 'rickets' is a term that is no longer appropriate.

In the late 1980s, metabolic bone disease was reported to occur in over 40% of very immature babies, but it is now a very rare condition as a result of more appropriate feeding regimens in very low birthweight infants. Copper and zinc deficiency causes a condition indistinguishable from the osteopenia due to phosphate deficiency.

The diagnosis is made on radiography of a long bone (Fig 16.3). The main feature of this condition is bone undermineralization (osteopenia), which is seen on X-ray. Skeletal deformities involving the rib cage or alteration in head shape may occur and, in its most severe form, fractures and frank rickets may be present, but these latter abnormalities are now uncommonly seen radiographically. The most sensitive biochemical abnormality is hypophosphataemia with no phosphorus present in the urine.

The key to this condition is its prevention. Metabolic bone disease can be avoided by appropriate dietary intake of phosphorus. All enterally fed preterm infants should receive 2 mmol/kg/day of phosphate. A baby on full milk feeds of an adapted low birthweight formula will receive this intake. Premature babies exclusively fed with breast milk will become phosphorus deficient and, in these, supplementation with phosphorus is necessary. This is most easily done with a powdered breast milk fortifier (p. 50). Additional phosphate supplementation is recommended for the first 6 months of life if the baby remains on breast milk alone.

Babies on total parenteral nutrition also need phosphate supplementation. Enhancement to 1.9 mmol/kg/day of calcium and 2.4 mmol/kg/day of phosphorus is associated with a reduction in the incidence of hypophosphataemia (Ryan 1996).

The treatment of established metabolic bone disease is to increase phosphate intake so that serum phosphate levels are normal and phosphorus is excreted in the urine. In some cases additional calcium will also be required. There is no need to give more than 1000 IU/day of vitamin D (cholecalci-ferol) unless there is evidence of liver disease.

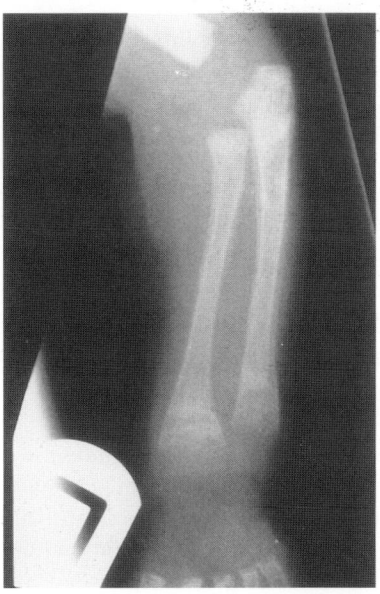

Figure 16.3 Radiograph of an infant's forearm and wrist showing the metaphyseal flaring of neonatal rickets.

Hypercalcaemia

Hypercalcaemia is defined as a serum calcium concentration greater than 2.75 mmol/L (11 mg/dL). This is often iatrogenic due to the excessive use of calcium gluconate in intravenous fluid therapy. Other rare causes include renal failure, inappropriate antidiuretic hormone secretion, hyperparathyroidism, vitamin D intoxication and Williams syndrome (idiopathic hypercalcaemia with elfin facies and often supravalvar aortic stenosis or peripheral pulmonary stenosis).

Disorders of magnesium metabolism

Hypomagnesaemia

Hypomagnesaemia is defined as a serum magnesium concentration less than 0.6 mmol/L (1.5 mg/dL). It is always associated with hypocalcaemia. Sometimes hypocalcaemia will not respond to calcium gluconate infusion, but serum calcium levels rapidly increases following magnesium sulphate injections. The dose is 50–100 mg/kg of a 50% magnesium sulphate solution by deep intramuscular injection or intravenous infusion over 1 h with ECG monitoring.

Hypermagnesaemia

Hypermagnesaemia is defined as a serum magnesium level greater than 1.5 mmol/L, and it may be associated with hypotonia, bradycardia and apnoea. It may occur as the result of magnesium sulphate administration to the mother for severe maternal pre-eclampsia or to the baby for pulmonary hypertension.

Disorders of sodium and potassium metabolism

Sodium metabolism

The full-term newborn infant requires 2–3 mmol/kg of sodium per day. Preterm infants have greater requirements because of the immaturity of renal tubular reabsorption. Requirements in these infants are in the order of 5–6 mmol/kg/day in the first week of life.

Table 16.4 Causes of neonatal hyponatraemia

Maternal hyponatraemia following excessive administration of 5% dextrose or oxytocin in labour

Inadequate sodium intake

Vomiting and diarrhoea

Inappropriate excess of intravenous fluids

Inappropriate antidiuretic hormone secretion (see p. 42).

Congestive cardiac failure (e.g. patent ductus arteriosus)

Diuretic treatment

Indometacin (due to increased intravascular volume)

Renal failure

Sepsis

Cystic fibrosis

Bowel obstruction

Congenital adrenal hyperplasia (salt-losing variety)

Hyponatraemia

The lower limit of normal for serum sodium is 133 mmol/L, and severe hyponatraemia is defined as a serum sodium concentration less than 125 mmol/L, which may cause apnoea and convulsions. The causes of hyponatraemia are listed in Table 16.4, and are discussed in detail elsewhere in this book. Care must be taken in the interpretation of serum sodium, as red cell haemolysis may lower the apparent serum level.

In the assessment of infants with hyponatraemia, serum potassium, creatinine and osmolality should be measured as well as urinary sodium and osmolality (or specific gravity). A careful fluid input and output chart should be kept for these infants.

Treatment
Treatment depends on the cause. If hyponatraemia is due to haemodilution (inappropriate antidiuretic hormone secretion or excessive intravenous water) then water restriction is necessary. If it is due to sodium loss, then carefully replace with hypertonic saline according to the equation:

$$\text{Na required (mmol)} = 135 - \text{actual Na} \times \text{weight (kg)} \times 0.5$$

$$(16.1)$$

where 0.3 represents the 'Na space', which may vary between 0.3 and 0.7 depending on birthweight, gestation and postnatal age.

Hypernatraemia

Hypernatraemia is defined as a serum sodium concentration greater than 150 mmol/L. Newborn infants, particularly those born preterm, rapidly become dehydrated and hypernatraemic if fluid intake is reduced or abnormal losses occur where water loss exceeds sodium loss. There are two main causes of hypernatraemia:

1 Reduced renal excretion. The newborn kidney is less efficient at excreting excess salt than water, and so hypernatraemia is more likely in very immature infants than in older children.

2 Excessive water loss. The lack of keratin in the skin of very tiny babies causes excessive transepidermal water loss. Phototherapy and radiant warmers aggravate this loss.

With hypernatraemia the serum osmolality is high and this may be associated with intra-cerebral haemorrhage. The causes of hypernatraemia are:

1 mismanaged intravenous fluids;
2 dehydration;
3 vomiting and diarrhoea;
4 bowel obstruction: necrotizing enterocolitis (NEC);
5 osmotic diuresis: hyperglycaemia;
6 excessive use of sodium bicarbonate;
7 congenital hyperaldosteronism;
8 faulty technique in making up formula feeds.

Treatment

The serum sodium is reduced by slow infusion of dextrose solution. Too rapid a reduction in hypernatraemia may be deleterious, resulting in cerebral fluid shifts and convulsions.

Potassium metabolism

Hyperkalaemia

This is defined as a serum potassium concentration greater than 6.5 mmol/L, and it may cause life-threatening ventricular dysrhythmias if levels exceed 7.5 mmol/L. Spurious hyperkalaemia occurring with haemolysis during blood sampling should not be confused with true hyperkalaemia.

Pathological causes include renal failure, acidosis, shock, hypoxia and blood transfusion. It is particularly likely to occur spontaneously in very ill, premature infants within 72 h of birth.

Treatment

The underlying cause should be corrected wherever possible.

1 Calcium resonium enemas when the potassium exceeds 7.5 mmol/L.
2 Salbutamol infusion (4 μg/kg over 20 min) has been shown to reduce serum potassium by 1 mmol/L in the first hour after starting the infusion.
3 Insulin infusion started when the potassium is over 8.0 mmol/L, or in the presence of dysrhythmias. Give 0.1 U soluble insulin per kg bodyweight at the same time as starting an infusion of 1 g/kg of glucose intravenously.

The prognosis for severe hyperkalaemia is very poor in terms of both mortality and morbidity. This reflects the fact that hyperkalaemia is most likely to occur in the sickest and smallest of babies, as well as the fact that high levels of potassium may provoke spontaneous cardiac dysrhythmias.

Hypokalaemia

This is defined as a serum potassium concentration less than 2.5 mmol/L (depends on laboratory standards). The causes are:

1 diuretic treatment;
2 alkalosis;
3 inadequate intake of potassium;
4 vomiting and diarrhoea;
5 congenital adrenal hyperplasia.

Treatment

If the hypokalaemia is due to dietary potassium deficiency, it can be replaced orally by adding it to the milk. The normal requirements are 2–3 mmol/kg/day.

Intravenous potassium replacement must only be given in the presence of known and adequate renal function, according to the formula:

$$K \text{ required (mmol)} = (3.5 - \text{actual K}) \times \text{weight (kg)} \times 0.3$$

(16.2)

This is given by slow intravenous infusion up to a maximum of 0.5 mmol/kg/h under ECG control.

Endocrine gland disorders

Disorders of thyroid function

Hypothyroidism

Untreated hypothyroidism is associated with severe intellectual impairment and as such is an important cause of subsequent disability. Because early recognition and effective treatment offer an excellent outcome in the majority of cases, the early detection of congenital hypothyroidism is essential.

The incidence of congenital hypothyroidism in the UK and Australia is approximately 1/3500 live-born infants. Causes of hypothyroidism can be subdivided as shown in Table 16.5.

Screening tests
The aim of screening is to detect all infants with clinically significant congenital hypothyroidism at an early stage in order to effect appropriate treatment to avoid brain damage. Screening is performed on heel-prick blood obtained at the same time as the Guthrie test. In the UK and Australia, thyroid-stimulating hormone (TSH) is assayed. Deficiency of circulating thyroid hormone causes the pituitary to release more

Table 16.5 Causes of hypothyroidism in the neonate

Primary, affecting the thyroid gland (90%)	
Dysgenesis (75%)	Ectopic thyroid (30%) Absent thyroid (30%) Hypoplastic thyroid (15%)
Dyshormonogenesis (20%)	Multiple causes involving biochemical defects in thyroid gland function. These are usually associated with a goitre at birth and are autosomal recessive in inheritance
Isoimmune (5%)	Occurs as the result of transplacental antibodies and may cause permanent or transient hypothyroidism
Secondary, affecting the pituitary or hypothalamus (10%)	
Transient neonatal hypothyroidism	This is the cause of 10–20% of all positive screening tests

TSH to stimulate the thyroid. TSH assay is more sensitive in screening for hypothyroidism than thyroxine assay, but fails to detect the rare cases due to pituitary/hypothalamic failure. It does not detect deficiency of thyroid-binding globulin. If TSH levels are high (>40 mU/L), the infant is urgently referred for definitive investigations of thyroid function. A borderline assay (15–40 mU/L) requires a repeat Guthrie card screen. The median age of notification for congenital hypothyroidism in Scotland following a screening programme is 10 days (Donaldson 1998).

Clinical features
Most infants detected by a screening programme will be clinically normal. The classic signs of severe or untreated hypothyroidism include poor feeding, constipation, abdominal distension, umbilical hernia, mottled skin, coarse puffy facies with a large protruding tongue, hypotonia, hypothermia, failure to thrive, persistent jaundice and both growth and developmental retardation.

Transient hypothyroidism. This refers to babies who have a positive screening test but whose thyroid function subsequently normalizes without treatment. Prenatally acquired causes include maternal thyroid deficiency, antithyroid drugs and thyroid antibodies acquired transplacentally. In the neonatal period the most common transient abnormality is due to topically applied iodine-containing antiseptics. Elevated TSH levels are related to the surface area swabbed and the frequency of skin swabbing.

Investigations
Once a positive screening test has been notified, the following investigations are required:
1 serum thyroxine and TSH;
2 thyroid autoantibodies in mother and baby;
3 radioisotope scan to localize the position of an ectopic or hypoplastic thyroid;
4 ultrasound scan of the thyroid gland;
5 X-ray for bone age – this is delayed in hypothyroidism;
6 enzyme assays may be required in the investigation of inborn errors of thyroid metabolism.

Treatment
Treatment consists of L-thyroxine 7–10 µg/kg/day initially. Monitoring of the dose will be by growth

assessment, bone age, physical appearance and thyroid function tests. Treatment is lifelong in all but transient cases.

Prognosis

The outcome for congenital hypothyroidism depends on the severity of intrauterine hypothyroidism and the delay in establishing effective treatment after birth. The pretreatment venous thyroxine level is the best predictor of eventual IQ (Donaldson 1998); in those with high levels, even with effective treatment after birth, mild educational, motor and behavioural problems are likely at 10 years.

If diagnosis and treatment are delayed until 3–6 months of age, only 50% of treated children achieve an IQ greater than 90. If diagnosis and treatment are commenced by 3 months, 75% will achieve an IQ greater than 90.

Neonatal hyperthyroidism

This is a rare condition that occurs in about 1–10% of infants born to women with Graves' disease. Women suffering from thyrotoxicosis (or who have been treated with subtotal thyroidectomy) may have circulating TSH-receptor-stimulating antibodies that cross the placenta. Neonatal hyperthyroidism secondary to maternal antibodies usually remits after 2–5 months when the maternal antibodies have disappeared.

Clinical features

The infant is usually growth restricted and often has a small goitre at birth and develops irritability and diarrhoea, with failure to gain weight despite feeding well. The most important feature is tachycardia, which may not be present at birth but develops rapidly within 48 h. This may be severe enough to precipitate cardiac failure. In some cases symptoms can be delayed for up to 6 weeks after birth.

Management

All infants born to thyrotoxic women should be carefully monitored for tachycardia for the first 48 h of life. If symptoms develop, propranolol (2 mg/kg/day) is the treatment of choice. The condition is self-limiting and it should be possible to stop treatment by 2–3 months.

Abnormalities of the adrenal gland

Neonatal adrenal disorders fall into the categories of hyperplasia and hypoplasia.

Congenital adrenal hyperplasia

Congenital adrenal hyperplasia (CAH) is a rare but important autosomal recessive disorder of adrenal function with an incidence of 1/10 000; 95% of cases are due to 21-hydroxylase deficiency. Figure 16.4 shows the metabolic pathway for adrenal hormones. An enzyme block causes failure of cortisol production, which results in central overstimulation of the adrenal by adrenocorticotropic hormone (ACTH). This leads to the overproduction of adrenal hormones produced downstream to the enzyme block, and it is the effect of this overproduction that produces the clinical features of CAH.

Clinical presentation

Deficiency of 21-hydroxylase presents in one of two ways:

1 *Virilization.* This is usually most obvious in male infants, who may be born with hypertrophic,

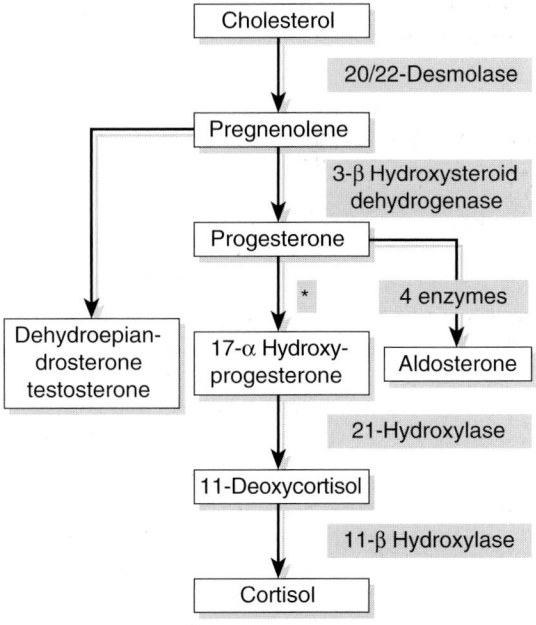

Figure 16.4 A simplified diagram to illustrate the synthesis of adrenal hormones. The asterisk represents the enzyme 17-α-hydroxydehydrogenase.

pigmented genitalia. Female virilization may be missed, as on cursory examination the virilized clitoris may be mistaken for a penis.

2 *Salt-losing.* This is due to an excessive aldosterone effect on the renal tubules and occurs in 75% of cases. Hyponatraemia does not usually become obvious until the second week of life, and is associated with a high serum potassium. Symptoms of vomiting and poor feeding precede shock in these babies.

The other forms of CAH are extremely rare but may present with poor virilization and hypertension (Table 16.6).

Investigations

Plasma 17-α-hydroxyprogesterone is markedly raised in the common 21-hydroxylase deficiency type of CAH. Biochemical abnormalities for the other enzyme defects are shown in Table 16.6. Countries with a high incidence of this condition may screen the entire population of newborn babies.

Treatment

Emergency. Intravenous fluid replacement, electrolyte correction and mineralocorticoids (fludrocortisone) and hydrocortisone (three times a day).

Long term. Medical management consists of replacement therapy with fludrocortisone and other corticosteroids, usually under the supervision of a paediatric endocrinologist. Surgical treatment may be required for the enlarged clitoris in virilized females.

Prenatal therapy

It is now possible to determine whether a fetus is affected by 21-hydroxylase deficiency where there is a family history of this condition. Diagnosis may be made by identifying the gene mutation on tissue obtained at chorionic villus biopsy, or by assay of hormones in amniotic fluid. Dexamethasone given to the mother from 10 weeks of gestation inhibits ACTH overstimulation and reduces the extent of fetal virilization.

Adrenal hypoplasia

This is a rare condition and may arise as primary adrenal failure or secondary to pituitary hypoplasia (as occurs in anencephaly), but may occur in infants with an otherwise normal brain. Adrenal hypoplasia is most often suspected by unrecordable oestriol estimation performed during pregnancy. The infant of any such pregnancy should have his or her adrenal function carefully assessed postnatally. There are also X-linked and autosomal recessive forms of adrenal hypoplasia.

At birth the infant may show hyperpigmentation and hypoglycaemia. Alternatively, symptoms may be delayed until later in infancy. Severe metabolic collapse with profound hypotension may be the first feature of this condition. Adrenal hypoplasia may be confused with CAH, but virilization is not seen and salt loss rarely occurs.

Table 16.6 Clinical and biochemical features of enzymatic defects in congenital adrenal hyperplasia

Enzyme defect	Virilization	Under-virilization	Salt loss	Hypertension	Urinary 17-ketosteroids	Plasma 17-OH progesterone
20/22-Desmolase	−	+	++	−	↓	↓
3-β OH steroid dehydrogenase	+	+	+	−	↑	Normal or ↑
17-α OH steroid dehydrogenase	−	+	−	+	↓	↓
21-Hydroxylase	+	−	+ −	−	↑	↑ ++
11-β-Hydroxylase	+	−	−	+	↑	↑

Infants with a family history or low oestriols during pregnancy should have short and long Synacthen tests to investigate the cortisol response to stimulation. Treatment involves life-long replacement with cortisol and possibly aldosterone.

Inborn errors of metabolism

The term inborn error of metabolism was intro-duced by Garrod in 1896 to describe a group of genetically determined biochemical disorders caused by specific defects in the structure or func-tion of protein molecules. Some of these have no clinical manifestation, such as histidinaemia, whereas others have major clinical sequelae, for example, phenylketonuria (PKU). The majority are inherited as autosomal recessive disorders but some are sex linked, including Hunter syndrome, Lesch–Nyhan disease, Menkes syndrome and ornithine transcarbamylase deficiency.

Metabolic disorders may be understood if the hypothetical biochemical reaction shown in Fig. 16.5 is considered. This reaction may be inter-fered with at the following sites:

1 Failure of substance A to cross into cells, e.g. Hartnup disease (failure of tryptophan to enter cell).

2 Deficiency of enzyme a. This may cause disease by the accumulation of precursor A, as happens in galactosaemia with the build-up of galactose-1-phosphate (see p. 174).

3 Alternatively, a deficiency of enzyme a may be associated with the build-up of alternative meta-bolic products derived from the metabolites of high levels of precursors of A. An example of this is phe-nylketonuria, with the production of high levels of phenylketones (see p. 173).

4 Deficiency of end-metabolic products as occurs in albinism, where there is failure to produce melanin (C in Fig. 16.5).

5 Failure of positive feedback control. This occurs when the end product of metabolism is required to switch off a hormone-controlled loop system. CAH is an example of this condition (see p. 169). Failure of cortisol production by an enzyme block results in failure to inhibit ACTH, with consequent

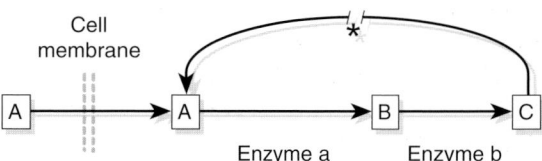

Figure 16.5 Representation of metabolic pathways with a negative feedback loop.

adrenal hyperplasia. This is represented by the asterisk in Fig. 16.5.

The inborn errors of metabolism may be diag-nosed clinically, in either an asymptomatic phase or an acute early symptomatic phase. Preferably they are diagnosed by screening programmes for the newborn.

Newborn screening

There are many important principles inherent in newborn screening. The following criteria should be satisfied:

1 the disease is a significant health problem;

2 the disease has a latent or asymptomatic phase;

3 there is a commonly accepted and successful therapy;

4 the natural history of the disease is understood;

5 the test is suitably sensitive (few false negatives) and specific (few false positives);

6 the screening programme is cost effective;

7 the test sample is acceptable to the patient and easily obtained;

8 adequate facilities for diagnosis and therapy exist;

9 there is a commitment to careful follow-up.

The incidences of diseases that have been consid-ered for newborn screening are given in Table 16.7. Screening programmes that have been adopted in parts of Europe, Australia and the USA include

1 Phenylketonuria (p. 173).

2 Hypothyroidism (p. 168).

3 Galactosaemia (p. 173).

4 CAH (p. 169).

5 Cystic fibrosis. Neonatal screening by elevated immunoreactive trypsin on a dried blood spot detects 90% of cases with severe disease. Positive cases can then be screened by analysis for the δF508 mutation, which accounts for 80% of cases of cystic

Table 16.7 Incidence of diseases considered for newborn screening

Specific metabolic disease	Approximate incidence
Cystic fibrosis	1/2500
Hypothyroidism	1/3500
Phenylketonuria	1/15 000
MCAD deficiency	1/15 000
Hartnup disease	1/18 000
Histidinaemia	1/18 000
Galactosaemia	1/30 000
Homocystinuria	1/150 000
Maple syrup urine disease	1/250 000

fibrosis. Widespread screening for this condition is now available in the UK. Evidence shows that those babies with the disease do better if the diagnosis was made early by screening rather than presenting later in life.

6. Medium-chain acyl-CoA dehydrogenase (MCAD) deficiency. This condition is as common as phenylketonuria and presents with collapse (implicated in some cases of sudden infant death syndrome (SIDS)) and severe hypoglycaemia. If the condition is recognized, hypoglycaemia can be avoided by careful attention to carbohydrate intake, and the prognosis is excellent. Screening using a dried blood spot from a newborn infant is possible using a tandem mass spectrometer, and screening may be adopted in the near future once this new technique is more widely available. The availability of tandem mass spectrometry in many countries has expanded the range of metabolic disorders that can be screened on the day 3–5 blood spot.

Presentation in the acutely ill child

Inborn errors of metabolism as a group are very rare and may present in a number of different ways. In the newborn, presentation is usually dramatic and the infant is very ill. Inborn errors of metabolism must always be considered in the differential diagnosis of an acutely ill infant when there is no obvious alternative diagnosis.

In considering infants with possible inborn errors of metabolism, particular attention should be paid to the following:

1 *Family history.* Most such conditions are inherited as an autosomal recessive disorder, hence consanguinity should be asked about. A family history of unexplained stillbirths or neonatal deaths is important.

2 *Onset of illness related to feeds.* Some of the disorders only become manifest when the infant ingests milk (e.g. galactosaemia).

3 *Is there a characteristic smell?* Infants with isovaleric acidaemia smell of sweaty feet, and in maple syrup urine disease the baby smells of curry.

4 *Dysmorphic features.* Peroxisomal disorders (e.g. Zellweger syndrome) show characteristic facial features. Cataracts are features of galactosaemia.

Diagnosis

Affected infants present in a variety of ways, but the most frequent are:

1 *Encephalopathy.* Symptoms include convulsions, apathy, coma and profound hypotonia. Early onset of severe seizures suggests pyridoxine deficiency and non-ketotic hyperglycinaemia.

2 *Hypoglycaemia.* This is seen particularly in the organic acidaemias and type I glycogen storage disease. Ketonuria in the absence of hypoglycaemia suggests an organic acidaemia.

3 *Acid–base disturbance.* This is seen frequently in any sick baby and is usually not related to inborn errors of metabolism. Calculation of the anion gap may be helpful:

$$\text{Anion gap} = \text{serum } (Na^+ + K^+) \text{ mmol/L} - \text{serum } (Cl^- + HCO_3^-) \text{ mmol/L}$$

$$(16.3)$$

If the anion gap is >25 mmol/L then the patient is likely to have a specific organic acidaemia.

4 *Hepatic failure.* Rapidly progressive liver disease with rising levels of conjugated bilirubin suggests galactosaemia, α_1-antitrypsin deficiency or tyrosinaemia.

If an inborn error of metabolism is suspected, the following investigations should be undertaken as a matter of urgency:

1 amino acid concentrations in blood and urine (freeze all additional urine specimens for more detailed subsequent examination);
2 organic acid analysis;
3 plasma ammonia;
4 serum lactic acid level;
5 urine for ketone estimate.

Management

Definitive treatment depends on the precise underlying condition. While awaiting a diagnosis the following management points are important:

1 stop all milk feeds;
2 treat metabolic acidosis with infusions of sodium bicarbonate;
3 prevent catabolism by giving 10–15% dextrose infusions, together with insulin if necessary;
4 removal of toxic waste products by peritoneal dialysis (see p. 312);
5 if there is hyperammonaemia (>600 μmol/L), give sodium benzoate 250 mg/kg as a loading dose followed by an infusion of 250 mg/kg/day;
6 megavitamin cocktail – some of the inborn errors of metabolism are responsive to large doses of vitamins; the megavitamin doses are shown in Table 16.8.

Phenylketonuria

Phenylketonuria (PKU) is an autosomal recessive condition and, in its classic form, is caused by a deficiency of the enzyme phenylalanine hydroxylase, which converts phenylalanine to tyrosine. Absence of the enzyme results in the accumulation of phenylalanine and its metabolites (see Fig. 16.6). In untreated patients the accumulation of phenylalanine and phenylketones produces a clinical picture of neonatal convulsions, later mental impairment, epilepsy and eczema. Affected children usually have fair hair and skin with blue eyes, owing to a relative lack of melanin, which is metabolized downstream from tyrosine.

Malignant hyperphenylalaninaemia has recently been described and is due to a deficiency of biopterin in the liver. This is required as a cofactor for the enzyme phenylalanine hydroxylase.

Diagnosis

This may be suspected from screening tests and confirmed by definitive investigations.

Screening

Screening for phenylketonuria was formerly based on the Guthrie test, which is a bacterial inhibition assay on blood absorbed onto blotting paper from a heel-prick sample. The infant needs to be on an adequate milk diet for 48 h prior to testing. This is particularly important in preterm and ill infants. Antibiotic treatment of the infant may inhibit the bacteria that produce the Guthrie reaction. Now most screening laboratories use a radioimmunoassay for phenylalanine.

Definitive diagnosis

This involves recalling the infant for definitive biochemical investigations of blood phenylalanine and tyrosine levels, together with urinary phenylketones.

Table 16.8 Megavitamin dosages for infants with suspected inborn errors of metabolism

Vitamin	Dose (mg/day)
Vitamin B_{12}	1.0
Biotin	100
Thiamine	50
Riboflavin	50
Nicotinamide	600
Pyridoxine	100

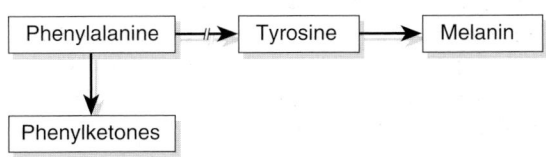

Figure 16.6 Metabolism of phenylalanine. The broken arrow represents the enzyme defect in phenylketonuria.

Treatment

This consists of a diet low in phenylalanine and tryptophan instituted within 20 days of age.

With early treatment the prognosis is good, provided careful control is maintained. The diet should probably be lifelong, but sustained at least into the early adolescent years. In the rare cases of malignant hyperphenylalaninaemia, treatment with biopterin will be necessary.

Such conditions are best managed in specialized metabolic clinics.

Maternal PKU

Undiagnosed maternal PKU may cause the infant to be brain damaged owing to the passage of toxic phenylpyruvate products across the placenta. All women with seizures or low IQ should be tested at booking in the antenatal clinic for urinary phenylketones by means of a simple stick test (Phenistix, Ames Ltd). Women known to have PKU should be well controlled on their diet before conception in order to prevent neurological compromise of the fetus.

Galactosaemia

This rare autosomal recessive condition has many variants, but only classic galactosaemia presents early in the neonatal period. Classic galactosaemia is due to a deficiency of the enzyme galactose-1-phosphate uridyl transferase. It presents with severe illness in the first week of life, with vomiting, encephalopathy, jaundice, failure to thrive, cataracts, hepatomegaly and a coagulation disorder. If treatment is not started the infant will die.

Diagnosis

If galactosaemia is suspected clinically, the urine should be tested for reducing substances. If the urine is positive on Clinitest tablet testing, but negative for glucose on a glucose oxidase stick test, then assay of galactose-1-phosphate uridyl transferase should be performed. A proportion of children with galactosaemia do not show reducing substances in their urine, and an enzyme assay should be performed if the condition is suspected.

Treatment

This consists of careful dietary control using galactose-free milk (see p. 51).

Prognosis

Unlike other inborn errors of metabolism early diagnosis does not appear significantly to improve outcome, as the fetus has been damaged prior to birth. Most have significant developmental delay despite adequate dietary management.

Screening

Outcome is not markedly improved by early diagnosis, which weakens the argument for screening all newborns.

Ambiguous genitalia

The subject of ambiguous genitalia is complex and one where the neonatologist, the paediatric endocrinologist and the paediatric surgeon must work together to achieve the optimal physical and psychological result for the child and family.

The neonate with ambiguous genitalia may represent a medical emergency. Assessment and subsequent gender assignment must consider the future physical and sexual development of the child.

Parents are informed of the medical concern and the baby is examined in their presence. Terms such as 'underdeveloped' or 'overdeveloped' should be used, and 'intersex' and 'pseudohermaphrodite' avoided. The naming of the baby should be delayed until the definitive sex of rearing has been determined.

Clinical assessment

The following are useful guidelines that should be followed.

1 Is the baby a female who has been virilized?
2 Is the baby a male who is undervirilized?
3 Are gonads palpable in the inguinogenital region? If gonads are present it is almost certain that they are testes.

A diagnostic flow chart can be based on these observations (Fig. 16.7).

Discussion of the various conditions and their individual treatment is beyond the scope of this text. CAH has been discussed above.

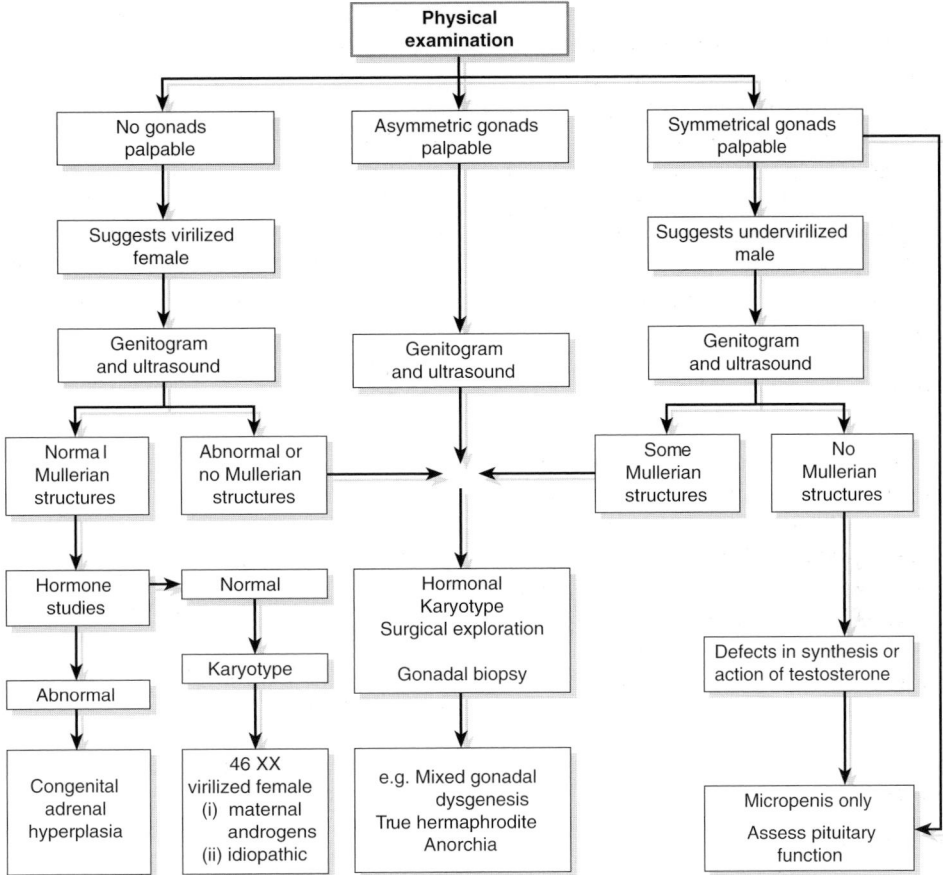

Figure 16.7 Flow diagram showing a scheme for investigating infants with ambiguous genitalia.

References

Deshpande S, Ward Platt M. The investigation and management of neonatal hypoglycaemia. *Semin Fetal Neonat Med* 2005;**10**:351–62.

Donaldson MDC. Neonatal screening for congenital hypothyroidism. *Semin Neonatol* 1998;**3**:35–47.

Koh TH, Aynsley-Green A, Tarbit M, Eyre JA. Neural dysfunction during hypoglycemia. *Arch Dis Child* 1988;**63**:1353–1358.

Kuna P, Addy DP. Transient neonatal diabetes mellitus. *Am J Dis Child* 1979;**133**:65–66.

Lucus A, Morley R, Cole TJ. Adverse neurodevelopmental outcome of moderate neonatal hypoglycaemia. *Brit Med J* 1988;**297**:304–1308.

Ryan S. Nutritional aspects of metabolic bone disease in the newborn. *Arch Dis Child* 1996;**74**:F145–F148.

Further reading

Brook CGD, Clayton PE, Brown RS (eds) *Brook's Clinical Paediatric Endocrinology*, 5th edn. Oxford: Blackwell Scientific Publications, 2005.

Lippe BM. Ambiguous genitalia and pseudohermaphroditism. *Paediatr Clin N Am* 1979;**26**:91–106.

Hawdon JM, Modder J (eds) Glucose control in the perinatal period. *Semin Fetal Neonat Med* 2005;**10**(4).

Visser HK. Sexual differentiation in the fetus and newborn. In: *Scientific Foundations of Paediatrics* (eds J.A. Davis & J. Dobbing), 2nd edn. Oxford: Butterworth-Heinemann, 1981.

CHAPTER 17

17 Disorders of the cardiovascular system

Physiology

The cardiovascular system undergoes major changes in the hours and days after birth. The transition of the circulation from fetal to neonatal is described in Chapter 2. Failure of organ perfusion is a major part of many neonatal disorders, and an understanding of cardiovascular physiology is important in analysing what are the most appropriate management strategies.

Cardiac output

Cardiac output is the total amount of blood ejected from both ventricles, but in the neonatal period reciprocal changes occur in the two ventricles. Pulmonary vascular resistance falls rapidly after birth, with a consequent reduction of right ventricular afterload, whereas systemic vascular resistance gradually increases, resulting in an increasing left ventricular afterload; this leads to a doubling of left ventricular stroke volume with no significant change in right ventricular stroke volume. This means that neonatal cardiac output increases after birth with cardiac performance near the upper limit of its range.

Cardiac output (CO) is dependent on stroke volume (SV) and heart rate (HR):

$$CO = SV \times HR$$

Stroke volume

This is a complicated function that is dependent on the stretch undergone by individual heart myofibrils.

$$SV \sim preload + afterload + contractility$$

- *Preload*. This represents the passive stretching of the resting heart prior to ventricular filling, and is largely influenced by vascular volume. The myocardium contracts most efficiently at a certain preload volume. Underfilling (reduced preload) or overfilling (increased preload) causes the contraction to be less efficient.
- *Afterload*. This is the resistance to ventricular contraction distal to the ventricles, and a variety of factors are involved, including peripheral vascular resistance and the viscosity of the blood.
- *Contractility*. This refers to the metabolic state of the heart muscle itself and is largely independent of both preload and afterload.

Cardiac output can be increased by increasing myocardial contractility (inotropy) or increasing the heart rate (chronotropy). These changes are mediated through adrenergic receptors, either α, β or dopaminergic. These effects include the following:

- β_1 *stimulation* increases myocardial contractility and heart rate;
- β_2 *stimulation* increases pulmonary and systemic vasodilatation;
- α_1 *stimulation* causes arteriolar constriction;
- *dopaminergic stimulation* causes vasodilatation in vascular beds such as the kidney, brain and gut.

Hypotension

Blood pressure is the product of flow and resistance according to the formula:

$$Blood\ pressure = blood\ flow \times peripheral\ resistance$$

Hypotension is a common and important complication of the sick newborn infant, but blood pressure in itself is not the critical physiological function in which the clinician is interested. It is the maintenance of organ perfusion that is essential, because once this falls below a critical limit, organ function will fail. The clinical measurement of blood flow and vascular resistance is not possible, and so blood pressure is the physiological measurement that is used to monitor physiological integrity. Failure to perfuse an organ normally will cause that organ system to fail, and clinical features of this failure may be evident. Such features include

1 Increasing metabolic acidosis, which may indicate tissue hypoxaemia.

2 Reducing urine output. Failure adequately to perfuse the kidneys will cause a reduction in urine production and this may indicate a low cot state.

3 Poor skin perfusion. This can be assessed by blanching the skin over the chest to see how long it takes to recover its colour (capillary refill). Reperfusion within 3 s is normal.

Normal range

Blood pressure varies normally with gestational age and postnatal age, and both may need to be considered when deciding whether a baby needs treatment for low blood pressure. The normal range for blood pressure is shown in Fig. 17.1.

Zone A represents the mandatory need for treatment because the blood pressure is critically low.

Zone B represents possible hypotension and is a level of uncertainty, as the baby may either cope without support or show signs of failing organ perfusion. If clinical signs are present, such as metabolic acidosis, decreasing peripheral perfusion, poor capillary return, poor colour and low peripheral temperature, then treatment should be given.

Zone C represents satisfactory blood pressure and treatment is only required if there are obvious and overriding clinical signs of poor perfusion.

A widely used rule of thumb is to maintain the minimum mean arterial blood pressure (MABP) above the infant's gestational age in weeks + postnatal age in days up to 4 days of age. Therefore, a 27-week infant on day 2 of life should have a MABP no lower than 29 mmHg.

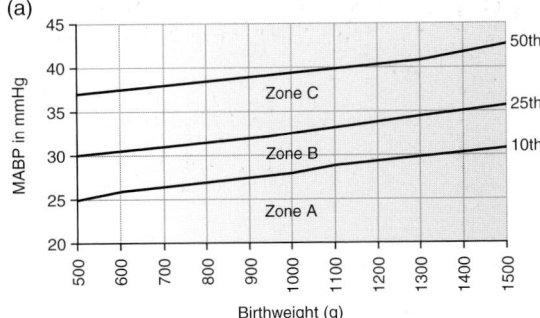

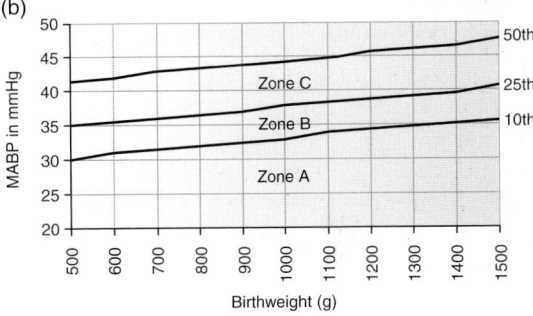

Figure 17.1 (a) Range of mean arterial blood pressure (MABP) measurements in very low birthweight infants less than 36 h of age and (b) more than 36 h old. Zone A: Hypotension requiring treatment (see Fig. 17.2). Zone B: Possible hypotension requiring clinical assessment. Zone C: Blood pressure unlikely to require treatment but clinical signs should be assessed.

Management

There are two important factors to consider:

1 What is the cause of the hypotension? This must be identified and the underlying cause treated.

2 What is the best therapeutic option in restoring adequate blood pressure? In considering the first-line management of hypotension it is important to think through the possible physiological mechanisms:

(a) preload – is the vascular compartment adequately filled?

(b) afterload – should vascular resistance be increased?

(c) contractility – is the myocardium working to maximum advantage?

(d) heart rate – is the heart rate fast enough to maintain adequate cardiac output?

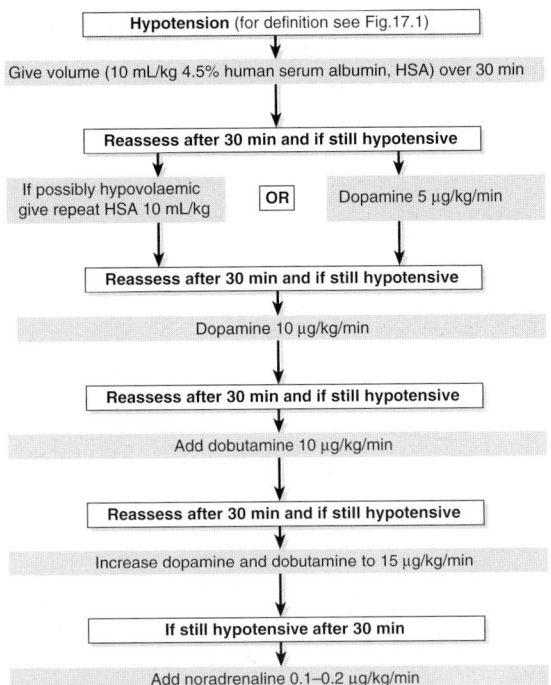

Figure 17.2 Flow diagram showing a suggested graded management response to neonatal hypotension.

Figure 17.2 illustrates the incremental management of neonatal hypotension.

Volume replacement

Many ill premature infants are hypovolaemic. It is difficult to measure circulating blood volume, but serum electrolytes, urinary specific gravity (SG) and weight changes may be helpful in determining this factor (p. 42). If the baby is thought to be hypotensive due to volume depletion, an infusion of either a crystalloid or a colloid fluid should be given (10 mL/kg, repeated once if necessary). There is considerable controversy as to what fluid should be used. Traditionally, human serum albumin was given but because of questions regarding safety, normal saline currently is the first-line volume expander. If the vasculature is 'leaky' both crystalloid and colloid will be rapidly lost into the tissues, which will cause a further loss of fluid from the vascular compartment owing to an osmotic effect.

Giving fluid to a baby who already has increased preload may precipitate further cardiac output decompensation, and positioning a central venous pressure line by inserting an umbilical venous catheter into the right atrium may be useful in the further assessment of some babies in cardiac failure where uncertainty exists about whether they remain fluid depleted.

Inotropic agents

Dopamine acts in a complicated way depending on its dosage. In low dose (1–5 µg/kg/min) it has primary dopaminergic actions and vasodilates the renal, coronary and possibly the cerebral circulation. In higher dose (5–10 µg/kg/min) it stimulates β_1 receptors, enhances myocardial contractility and increases heart rate. At yet higher dosage (10–20 µg/kg/min) the main effects are α-adrenergic, with an increase in peripheral vascular resistance and a reduction in renal blood flow.

Dobutamine (5–20 µg/kg/min by continuous infusion) has mainly β_2 effects, and increases blood pressure by increasing myocardial contractility with some reduction in systemic resistance, thereby reducing afterload, which may be valuable in the failing heart. There is little effect on heart rate.

Noradrenaline (norepinephrine; 0.1–0.2 µg/kg/min by continuous infusion) is sometimes used once dopamine and dobutamine have been given in maximum dosage. It has both α and β effects, causing an increase in contractility, tachycardia and vascular resistance.

Hypertension

Neonatal hypertension is not a rare phenomenon in sick newborn infants. It is rarely due to essential hypertension and is associated with congenital malformations such as coarctation of the aorta and endocrine disorders or acquired conditions such as renal artery thrombosis from umbilical artery (UA) catheter, bronchopulmonary dysplasia (BPD), extracorporeal membrane oxygenation (ECMO) or steroid therapy. Table 17.1 lists the commoner causes of neonatal hypertension.

Management is directed at the underlying cause of the condition, and includes renal or aortic surgery where appropriate. At present there is no evidence that thrombolysis is useful in the treatment of renal artery thrombosis.

Table 17.1 Causes of neonatal hypertension (Adapted from Adelman 1988)

Vascular
  Renal artery thrombosis
  Coarctation of the aorta

Renal
  Renal dysplasia
  Obstructive uropathy
  Polycystic/multicystic disease

Drugs
  Steroids
  Theophylline

Endocrine
  Congenital adrenal hyperplasia (rare forms)
  Phaeochromocytoma

Miscellaneous
  Bronchopulmonary dysplasia
  Intracranial hypertension

Essential

Table 17.2 Contribution of the commoner congenital heart malformations to neonatal congenital heart disease

Ventricular septal defect	25%
Patent ductus arteriosus	15%
Atrial septal defect	15%
Pulmonary stenosis	10%
Aortic stenosis	5%
Coarctation of the aorta	5%
Transposition of the great arteries	5%
Tetralogy of Fallot	5%
Tricuspid atresia	1%
Other individually rare conditions	14%

The medical management of hypertension is largely empirical. Drugs include frusemide (1–2 mg/kg), chlorothiazide (20–40 mg/kg), propranolol (0.5–5.0 mg/kg), hydralazine (0.5 mg/kg 8-hourly) and captopril (0.1–1.6 mg/kg/day).

Congenital heart disease

Congenital heart disease (CHD) refers to an abnormality in the structure or function of the heart that is present at birth. Many congenital cardiac abnormalities remain asymptomatic and undetected in the neonatal period, only to be diagnosed weeks or years later. The incidence of CHD based on the definition given above is therefore higher than previously reported, when only lesions diagnosed at birth were included. The generally accepted incidence is 4–10/1000 births, and represents the commonest form of major congenital abnormality in developed countries. Table 17.2 lists the frequency of different congenital cardiac anomalies.

With advances in second trimester ultrasound examination for diagnosis of congenital malformations, 70% of major congenital heart lesions are diagnosed antenatally.

Aetiology

The aetiology of CHD is multifactorial and depends on the type of abnormality, but overall 75% have no identifiable cause. There is an increased incidence with the following factors:

1 Chromosomal disorders. These account for approximately 5% of all children with CHD:
  (a) Down syndrome – 30% have CHD, most commonly atrioventricular defects, ventricular septal defect (VSD) and atrial septal defect (ASD);
  (b) trisomy 18 – 90% have major cardiac defects;
  (c) trisomy 13 – 80% have major cardiac defects;
  (d) Turner syndrome – 10% have coarctation of the aorta.

2 Single-gene defects. These account for approximately 3% of children with CHD. The following are the most common:
  (a) Syndromes:
    • Noonan syndrome (pulmonary valve abnormalities are particularly common);
    • Marfan syndrome (aortic valve and aortic dissections);
    • Holt–Oram syndrome (VSD and ASD);
    • Goldenhar syndrome;
    • Williams syndrome;
    • Cornelia de Lange syndrome.
  (b) Associations:
    • VACTERL – Vertebral, Anal, Cardiac, Tracheal, Esophageal, Radial, Renal, Limb;
    • CHARGE – Coloboma, Heart, Atresia choanal, Retarded growth, Genital, Ear.

3 Polygenic factors. These are poorly understood but are probably the most important factors in the development of CHD, which may recur in successive generations.

4 Infection – rubella infection in the first trimester may cause a patent ductus arteriosus (PDA) or pulmonary artery stenosis. Coxsackie B and influenza A may cause myocarditis.

5 Drugs – maternal lithium is associated with tricuspid valve anomalies. Amphetamines, antimetabolites and anticonvulsants have been associated with CHD.

6 Alcohol – 30% of infants with fetal alcohol syndrome have CHD.

7 Maternal diabetes – transposition of the great vessels, VSD, coarctation and idiopathic hypertrophic subaortic stenosis.

Familial incidence

In a family with one child who has CHD there is a 2–5% risk of recurrence in siblings. There is a 5–10% risk of an affected individual transmitting the condition to the next generation, reflecting the polygenic nature of the condition.

Mode of presentation

Cardiac disease in the newborn presents in the following ways:

1 cyanosis – this may be due to either cardiac or respiratory causes, which can usually be easily distinguished;

2 congestive cardiac failure;

3 murmur heard on routine examination;

4 circulatory maladaptations at birth;

5 dysrhythmias.

Investigations

Investigations are triggered by symptoms or abnormal signs such as a cardiac murmur. In many centres where there is no direct access to paediatric cardiologists, it is necessary to undertake basic investigations in order to determine which babies require referral to a paediatric cardiologist for further evaluation. These basic investigations include chest X-ray, electrocardiography and nitrogen

washout test. Modern echocardiography has supplanted the need for many of the investigations that were formerly performed, but this technique requires considerable expertise, which is not readily available in many centres.

Chest X-ray

This is used to assess

1 Heart size. This is assessed by measuring the cardiothoracic ratio. The widest cardiac diameter is measured and compared with the maximal internal thoracic diameter of the chest, usually at the costophrenic angles. In the newborn a ratio of up to 0.6 is normal. CHD may exist in the presence of a normal heart size.

2 Abnormal heart shape, e.g. egg on side for transposition of the great arteries (TGA), boot shaped for tetralogy of Fallot.

3 Lung field vascularity. This may be difficult to interpret in the newborn, especially if the film is not correctly exposed or, if taken on day 1 of life, due to residual fetal lung fluid. If there is increased vascularity (pulmonary plethora) then there is a left-to-right shunt, and if reduced vascularity (oligaemia) there is obstruction of right-sided flow to the lungs. Often shunt vessels can be differentiated from Kerley B lines of congestive heart failure.

4 Situs inversus (stomach gas bubble on the right) may indicate serious underlying heart disease. Vertebral anomalies may also suggest cardiac anomalies.

Electrocardiograph (ECG)

This may be helpful in elucidating the nature of a cardiac abnormality prior to transfer to a cardiac centre for full assessment. In infants it is necessary to record from the V4R position (over the right nipple) as well as the traditional chest leads V1–V6. Normal values for various ECG variables are shown in Table 17.3.

Heart rate. The heart rate normally varies with gestational and postnatal age. Normal heart rates for premature and full-term infants are shown in Table 17.4.

Axis. The mean QRS axis in neonates is further to the right than in older children, but moves to the

Table 17.3 Normal range for P–R interval, R and S waves for various postnatal ages (Scott 1981)

Age	P–R Interval (s)	R wave (mm) V1	V6	S wave (mm) V1	V6
0–24 h	0.07–0.13	7–20	2–7	3–27	2–10
1–7 days	0.07–0.13	9–27	2–13	5–19	0.8–10
8–30 days	0.07–0.17	4–20	2–21	3–13	0.6–9
1–3 months	0.07–0.17	4–18	4–13	2–17	0.8–6
3–6 months	0.07–0.13	6–17	5–16	2–12	0.6–5

Table 17.4 Range of normal heart rates for premature and full-term infants at different postnatal ages

Age	Premature infants (Moss & Adams 1968)	Full-term infants (Scott 1981)
0–24 h	109–173	94–145
1–7 days	134–200	100–175
8–30 days	133–200	115–190
1–3 months	128–203	124–190
3–6 months	—	111–179

left within the first month of life. The QRS vector is markedly abnormal in tricuspid atresia (left axis – 45°, i.e. maximal positive QRS deflection in the direction of aVL). The axis is also vertical (–90°) in endocardial cushion defects.

P wave. The P wave precedes atrial contraction. A tall P wave exceeding 3 mm in lead II indicates right atrial hypertrophy, and a broad P wave suggests left atrial hypertrophy but is rarely seen in the newborn.

P–R interval. This measures the time from the onset of atrial contraction to the onset of ventricular contraction. A prolonged P–R interval indicates a degree of heart block (Table 17.3).

Right ventricular hypertrophy (RVH). This is estimated from the right chest leads. The criteria for diagnosis of RVH are:
1 upright T wave in V4R or V1 with dominant R after the first 5 days of life;
2 the voltage of R or S in V1 or V6 exceeds the normal range (see Table 17.3);

3 Q wave in V1;
4 right axis deviation.

Left ventricular hypertrophy (LVH). This is diagnosed according to the following criteria, but left axis deviation on its own does not necessarily indicate LVH:
1 tall R waves in V6 and deep S waves in V1 above the normal range (see Table 17.3);
2 a combined voltage of R in V5 or V6 and S in V1 exceeding 30 mm;
3 inverted T waves in the left chest leads – this suggests ischaemia, but digoxin may also cause this appearance.

Nitrogen washout test

This may be helpful in distinguishing congenital cyanotic heart lesions from respiratory pathology. Blood-gas estimations are performed before and after the infant has been breathing 100% oxygen for 10 min. In normal babies the P_aO_2 should rise to 80 kPa (600 mmHg). With intrinsic lung disease the P_aO_2 increases to 20–53 kPa (150–400 mmHg), depending on the severity of disease. In the presence of cardiac abnormalities with a right-to-left intracardiac shunt there is little increase in P_aO_2.

There is a potential danger in this technique if the patient is dependent on maintaining right-to-left mixing through a PDA. Hyperoxia may cause the ductus to close, thereby seriously compromising the infant. Prostaglandin E_1 (PGE$_1$) (see p. 187) should be available during this procedure.

More specialized investigations

In specialist centres a definitive diagnosis can be made in most cases using echocardiography. More rarely cardiac catheterization is required for diagnosis or therapy in cardiac isomerism, TGA, total anomalous pulmonary venous drainage (TAPVD) or critical aortic stenosis (p. 185).

Echocardiography

The investigation of CHD has been revolutionized by the introduction of high-resolution, real-time, two-dimensional (2D) echocardiography. This allows the heart to be scanned in a number of standard planes, giving fine detail of anatomical structure.

Most lesions can be diagnosed using this technique alone, and increasingly cardiac abnormalities are recognized on prenatal ultrasound assessment.

The heart can be studied in a number of planes that highlight anatomical structures:

1 parasternal long-axis view shows the left-sided structures, including left atrium, mitral valve, ventricles, septum, aortic valve and ascending aorta (Fig. 17.3a);

2 parasternal short-axis view shows the structure of the aortic and pulmonary valves and the main pulmonary artery (Fig. 17.3b); and

3 the apical four-chamber view shows all four chambers simultaneously – the atrioventricular (a-v) valves are particularly well seen (Fig. 17.3c).

Most abnormalities can be readily recognized by an experienced cardiologist using ultrasound.

Cardiac Doppler with colour flow imaging is also very helpful in highlighting cardiac function and blood turbulence through small lesions.

Cardiac catheterization

This is only undertaken in a specialist children's cardiac unit. Cardiac catheterization in the newborn has an approximately 1–2% mortality rate and a significant morbidity rate, including infection and necrotizing enterocolitis (NEC).

Cyanotic heart disease

Persistent central cyanosis in the newborn infant is usually due to respiratory or cardiac disease, but rarely may be due to persistent pulmonary hypertension, methaemoglobinaemia or shock. Central

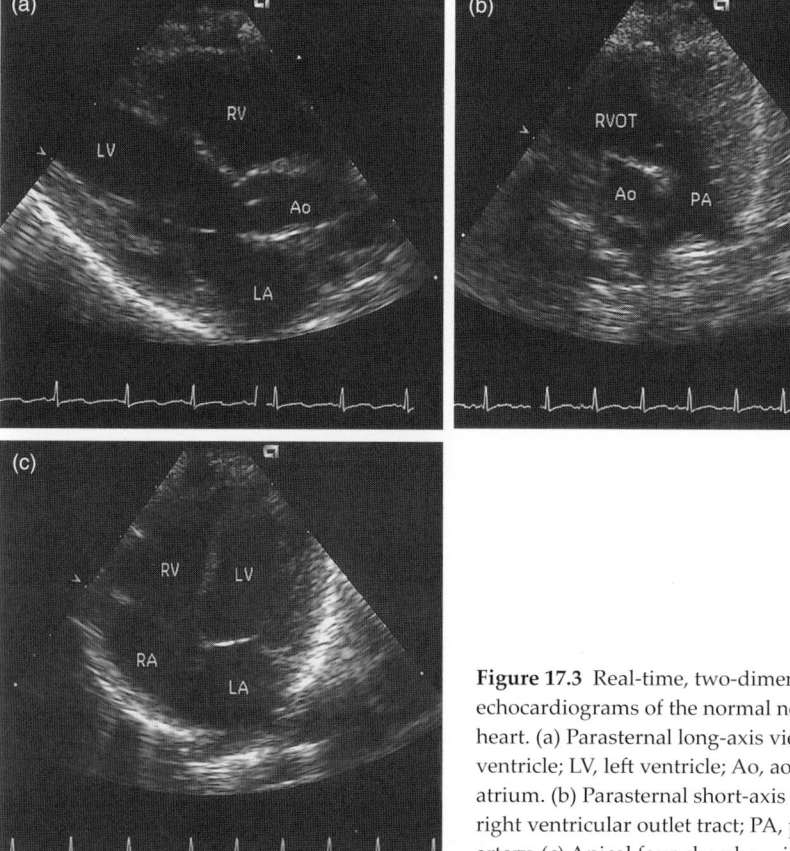

Figure 17.3 Real-time, two-dimensional echocardiograms of the normal neonatal heart. (a) Parasternal long-axis view. RV, right ventricle; LV, left ventricle; Ao, aorta; LA, left atrium. (b) Parasternal short-axis view. RVOT, right ventricular outlet tract; PA, pulmonary artery. (c) Apical four-chamber view, RA, right atrium.

cyanosis occurs when there is more than 5 g/dL of deoxygenated haemoglobin in the blood. This must be distinguished from peripheral cyanosis with a poor circulation due to cold, shock or polycythaemia with hyperviscosity.

Most neonates presenting with cyanotic heart disease do not pose a diagnostic problem as they show central cyanosis with little or no respiratory distress. However, if there is difficulty distinguishing pulmonary disease from cyanotic CHD, a hyperoxia test or nitrogen washout test (see above) should be performed. The causes of cyanotic CHD are shown in Table 17.5. An approach to the diagnosis of cyanotic CHD is shown in Fig. 17.4.

Some causes of cyanotic heart disease rarely present in the neonatal period because cyanosis does not develop for several months (see 'Tetralogy of Fallot' below).

Transposition of the great arteries

Transposition of the great arteries (TGA) is the commonest congenital heart defect presenting with

Table 17.5 Causes of cyanotic CHD

Transposition of the great arteries
Tricuspid atresia
Pulmonary atresia or pulmonary stenosis
Hypoplastic right heart syndrome
Tetralogy of Fallot with severe pulmonary stenosis
Ebstein's anomaly
Total anomalous pulmonary venous drainage
Truncus arteriosus

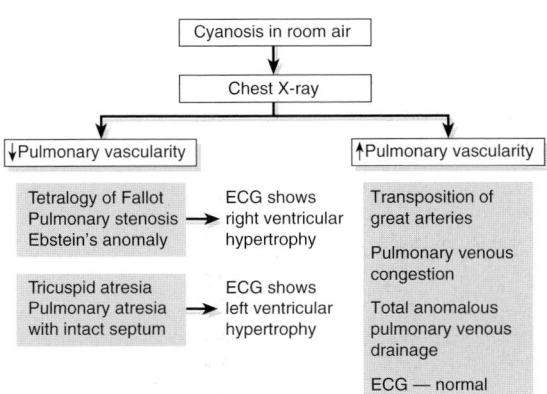

Figure 17.4 A diagnostic approach to cyanotic CHD.

cyanosis in the fetus or newborn. It affects 1 in 3500 births. The aorta arises from the right ventricle and the pulmonary artery from the left, with the aorta lying in front of the pulmonary artery. The degree of cyanosis depends on the mixing of pulmonary and systemic blood. If a VSD is present a murmur may be heard, but in TGA murmurs are usually absent.

Investigations
There is a characteristic chest X-ray appearance with a narrow pedicle (an egg on its side). The lung markings may be normal but are often increased. The ECG shows right axis deviation and RVH.

Treatment
Metabolic acidosis may be severe due to tissue hypoxaemia and should be corrected with bicarbonate. Maintaining the ductus arteriosus open with PGE_1 infusion may be life-saving prior to elective surgery. In cases where oxygenation does not improve with PGE_1 therapy, the foramen ovale is enlarged by a balloon atrial septostomy (Rashkind procedure). Many cardiologists prefer to perform a balloon septostomy before the switch operation so that PGE_1 can be discontinued and surgery performed more electively. The treatment of choice for simple transposition is the arterial switch operation. In experienced hands this has a mortality of <5% for uncomplicated TGA and involves a full anatomical correction by switching the two major arteries and reconstructing the insertion of the coronary arteries. This procedure should be performed within 5–14 days of birth. High-risk patients are of low birthweight (LBW) and/or have additional cardiac lesions (coarctation, dextrocardia) and abnormal insertion of the coronary arteries. Previously the condition was treated by atrial septostomy (Rashkind procedure), with definitive surgery (Mustard's repair or Senning's procedure) carried out at 9–12 months, but this produces a less satisfactory anatomical correction than the switch procedure.

Tricuspid atresia

In tricuspid atresia (TA), which affects 1 in 5500 births, there is obstruction at the level of the right atrium to ventricle, often with hypoplasia of the right ventricle. Pulmonary stenosis commonly accompanies TA, together with a VSD. Pulmonary blood flow is often poor and the pulmonary arteries small. A systolic murmur is usually heard and the infant is severely cyanosed. Pulmonary blood flow is from the left ventricle via an open ductus arteriosus.

Investigations
On a chest radiograph there is pulmonary oligaemia but no cardiomegaly. The ECG shows left-axis deviation and LVH. There are usually tall P waves in lead II. Echocardiography should confirm the diagnosis.

Treatment
Maintaining the ductus open with infusion of PGE_1 may keep the infant relatively pink in the hope that growth will occur until a palliative shunt operation can be performed. When the child is older a further procedure will be necessary. The long-term results of surgery are reasonably good and up to 90% will survive over 10 years, and many into adult life.

Pulmonary atresia (PA) or pulmonary stenosis (PS)

These conditions occur in 1 in 5000 births and involve a number of different anomalies of pulmonary valve. TGA is present in 30% of cases of PA. The symptoms depend on the associated cardiac abnormalities. More than 90% of babies with PA have an associated VSD. Pulmonary atresia or stenosis with VSD is very similar to Fallot's tetralogy but usually presents with cyanosis earlier. Rarely the ventricular septum is intact: the right ventricle is then hypoplastic and the prognosis is very poor.

Investigations
The heart is not enlarged on X-ray but the lung fields are oligaemic. There is right-axis deviation with right atrial and right ventricular hypertrophy if there is a coexistent VSD. Left ventricular hypertrophy is seen in PA without VSD.

Treatment
PGE_1 infusion may be of value in the acute stages to maintain the ductus arteriosus open and allow

pulmonary perfusion. Later a shunt operation may be of value in relieving cyanosis.

Tetralogy of Fallot
Affecting 1 in 3500 births, this does not classically present with cyanosis in the newborn period, but a murmur may be detected early and on investigation some infants are found to be cyanosed. Rarely there may be severe obstruction to pulmonary blood flow necessitating PGE_1 infusion and systemic to pulmonary shunt or complete repair. After the age of 1 month it is the commonest cause of cyanotic heart disease. Treatment is initially with a Blalock–Taussig or central shunt, and later total repair. The long-term prognosis following successful surgery is excellent.

Ebstein's anomaly
In this condition, affecting 1 in 25 000 births, there is downward displacement of the tricuspid valve into the right atrium with obstruction to right ventricular ejection, and diminished pulmonary blood flow. In some children presentation occurs in the first days of life with intense cyanosis and cardiac failure. The tricuspid valve is regurgitant resulting in marked right atrial enlargement, cardiomegaly and congestive heart failure (often occurring *in utero*).

Investigations
The chest X-ray shows a very large heart ('wall to wall') with oligaemic lung fields. The ECG is often pathognomonic, with complete bundle branch block and right atrial hypertrophy (very tall P waves).

Management
Medical management aims to support the neonate and decrease PVR with PGE_1 infusion, high F_iO_2 and inhaled nitric oxide (iNO) through the transitional circulation. Neonatal mortality is contributed to by pulmonary hypoplasia (massive cardiomegaly). Further complications *in utero* arise from supraventricular tachycardia (SVT) and Wolff–Parkinson–White syndrome in 30%.

Total anomalous pulmonary venous drainage
In this disorder, affecting 1 in 15 000 births, the pulmonary veins drain either directly or indirectly

into the right atrium rather than the left atrium. If the drainage is obstructed, little oxygenated blood enters the right atrium and the infant is cyanosed. There is also pulmonary congestion, and the infant often shows features of cardiac failure with respiratory distress. This condition may be very difficult to distinguish from primary lung disease and may require extensive investigation.

The anomalous pulmonary veins may be :
- supracardiac (usually right-sided superior vena cava (SVC));
- cardiac (right atrium or coronary sinus);
- infracardiac (portal system);
- mixed drainage.

Investigations
Chest X-ray shows a normal-sized heart with pulmonary oedema, which may be so severe as to be confused with respiratory distress syndrome (RDS). The ECG usually shows RVH. Echocardiography may be diagnostic, but the diagnosis may require cardiac catheterization. With severe obstruction pulmonary veins may be small and difficult to visualize even with colour flow Doppler.

Medical support with PGE_1, ventilation and extracorporeal membrane oxygenation (ECMO) is often necessary.

Treatment
Urgent surgery is necessary but carries a high mortality.

Prostaglandin treatment
PGE_1 causes the ductus arteriosus to open and can be given as an emergency to any severely cyanosed infant in an attempt to improve pulmonary blood flow. If successful and the ductus opens, the infant rapidly 'pinks up' as soon as the infusion is started. Dosage is 0.01–0.05 µg/kg/min by intravenous infusion, preferably through a vein draining into the SVC. Oral therapy is usually unsuccessful and if prolonged is associated with cortical bone proliferation. PGE_1 may also be life-saving in left-sided obstructive lesions, such as hypoplastic left heart and critical coarctation of the aorta, when systemic blood flow

is achieved from the right ventricle through the ductus.

Prostaglandins may cause pyrexia, jitteriness and apnoea requiring ventilation. Great care should be taken to avoid flushing the intravenous infusion, thereby giving a bolus of prostaglandin. Prolonged use may result in periostitis.

Congestive heart failure

Acute left ventricular failure rapidly progresses to congestive heart failure and occasionally to cardiovascular collapse. Table 17.6 lists causes of congestive cardiac failure in the neonatal period, according to whether they are structural or non-structural.

Clinical features
Congestive heart failure may present with feeding or respiratory difficulties, excessive sweating or

Table 17.6 Causes of congestive heart failure presenting in the newborn period (the commoner ones are discussed in the text)

Structural lesions (the most common in order of frequency)
Patent ductus arteriosus (PDA)
Hypoplastic left heart syndrome (e.g. aortic valve stenosis)
Coarctation of the aorta (includes interrupted aortic arch)
Ventricular septal defect (VSD)
Endocardial cushion defects
Persistent truncus arteriosus
Total anomalous pulmonary venous drainage (non-obstructive)
Aortic stenosis

Non-structural lesions
Transient myocardial ischaemia (association with prenatal asphyxia or severe respiratory distress)
Viral myocarditis (especially Coxsackie, echovirus, rubella, CMV)
Endocardial fibroelastosis
Polycythaemia
Hydrops fetalis
Fluid overload
Hypertrophic subaortic stenosis (especially in infant of diabetic mother)
Hypoglycaemia, hypocalcaemia
Arrhythmias

---

failure to thrive. The cardinal signs of congestive heart failure in the newborn are tachypnoea (respiratory rate greater than 60/min) with mild chest retractions, tachycardia (heart rate greater than 180/min), hepatomegaly (liver more than 3 cm below costal margin), a vigorous precordium and cardiomegaly (often only detected on chest X-ray).

Other signs, such as oedema or excessive weight gain, triple or gallop rhythm, crepitations on chest auscultation, sweating, peripheral cyanosis and cardiovascular collapse, are variable. The position, quality and radiation of any murmurs may be useful in identifying the cardiac lesion.

Hypoplastic left heart

In this condition, affecting 1 in 5500 births, there is failure of development of the left atrium and ventricle and the aortic and mitral valves are usually atretic. The ascending aorta is hypoplastic and blood reaches the systemic circulation retrogradely through the ductus arteriosus. The infant usually develops severe cardiac failure in the first week of life when the ductus closes. The pulses are weak and there is often cyanosis with pallor. There is marked hepatomegaly.

Clinical presentation

Typically this is by prenatal diagnosis after which an expectant neonatal team manages a metabolically stable infant with PGE_1. Alternatively, the infant may present with mild congestive heart failure or a profound circulatory collapse with multiorgan failure after the ductus arteriosus closes.

Investigations

Chest X-ray shows a large heart with plethoric lung fields. The ECG shows little left ventricular activity and RVH. The diagnosis can be made by echocardiography.

Treatment

Infants with a prenatal diagnosis should have the findings confirmed by expert echocardiography shortly after birth. With these infants and those presenting with mild heart failure, many centres offer palliative surgery to establish a viable, haemodynamically stable heart, and this may require a series of operations in the first 2 years of life. In some centres cardiac transplantation is offered following palliative management if the brain and other organs are intact. Before surgical management is considered parents must be fully counselled regarding the mortality risks associated with stage 1 reconstruction (Norwood procedure), especially with associated risks such as LBW or other cardiac lesions, followed by two further cardiac operations and very likely a heart transplant and some degree of cognitive impairment.

Coarctation of the aorta (COA)

Coarctation of the aorta affects 1 in 2500 births. It is an anatomical narrowing of the descending aorta, most commonly at the site of the ductus arteriosus, and is normally associated with bicuspid aortic valve (in 80%) and VSD (in 40%).

If outflow obstruction is severe, then cardiac failure occurs in infancy. Blood enters the aorta retrogradely through the ductus arteriosus, but if the latter closes then the infant rapidly deteriorates, presenting with breathlessness and in cardiac failure. The femoral pulses are weak and the blood pressure considerably higher in the arms than in the legs. About half of patients with COA have a VSD or aortic stenosis, and a murmur is usually audible.

Investigations

Radiographs show a large heart with pulmonary plethora. ECG reveals severe RVH with little evidence of left ventricular activity. Echocardiography may confirm the diagnosis, but requires special training. Cardiac catheterization is necessary to show the extent of the coarctation, as well as the presence of hypoplasia of the ascending aorta.

Treatment

PGE_1 may be life-saving in maintaining ductal flow. Dopamine infusion (5 µg/kg/min) will improve compromised renal blood flow. Surgery is urgent, and angioplasty of the aorta may be remarkably successful. Inotropic support with digoxin and frusemide is best started early and continued postoperatively.

Ventricular septal defect

VSD occurs as an isolated lesion in 1 in 280 live births, and accounts for 40% of all cardiac abnormalities. Lesions may vary in size, but only large defects cause symptoms in infancy. Cardiac failure due to VSD occurs very rarely in the neonate because of a relatively high pulmonary vascular resistance. Usually the only sign is a cardiac murmur in the first weeks of life. The natural history is for small VSDs to undergo spontaneous closure in 50% and for some moderate VSDs to decrease in size.

Investigations

If there is a significant left-to-right shunt, the heart is enlarged on X-ray and pulmonary plethora may be seen. The ECG shows RVH and LVH. A large VSD will be seen on echocardiography and an assessment of flow through the defect may be made at that time.

Treatment

Digoxin (see below) and diuretics are useful in cardiac failure. Banding of the pulmonary artery will protect the pulmonary circulation in the presence of a large left-to-right shunt. In some cases primary closure may be performed rather than banding. Later surgery to patch the defect will always be necessary after banding of the pulmonary artery, and also in large septal defects. Only 1 in 1000 require surgery.

Aortic stenosis

Aortic stenosis affects 1 in 4500 births, but rarely presents in the neonatal period unless it is very severe, when it is likely to be associated with a hypoplastic left ventricle. The prognosis is poor, although PGE_1 and balloon septostomy or urgent balloon valvulotomy may help to stabilize the patient. Critical aortic stenosis has a gradient between the right ventricle and ascending aorta of ≥ 60 mmHg and usually there is severe obstruction *in utero* with marked left ventricular hypertrophy and endocardial fibroelastosis. The presentation of

severe myocardial dysfunction is of congestive heart failure (CHF) and shock.

Management of congestive heart failure (CHF)

General management

Supportive treatment consists of oxygen therapy, elevation of the head of the cot, the provision of a thermoneutral environment, correction of metabolic acidosis with sodium bicarbonate, administration of glucose or calcium when indicated, and tube feeding.

Blood transfusion

An increase in oxygen to the tissues can best be obtained by ensuring an adequate haemoglobin concentration. Anaemia should be treated with blood transfusion of packed cells, and the haemoglobin should be maintained at 12–14 g/dL.

Digitalization

This is a time-honoured method of treating cardiac failure by improving myocardial contraction. Often the newborn myocardium has little inotropic reserve and digoxin is not as effective as in older children. Its main value is in the treatment of cardiac failure due to a large VSD and for supraventricular tachycardia (see p. 190). Digitalis toxicity frequently occurs in the preterm infant, especially with ischaemic and viral myocarditis. The signs are vomiting, lack of interest in feeding and cardiac dysrhythmias.

Digitalizing dose.   In order to avoid the risk of digoxin toxicity, it is preferable to start the baby on maintenance therapy rather than giving a loading dose. Maintenance doses (Table 17.7) take a week

Table 17.7 Dosage regimen for digoxin in the neonate

	Loading dose (µg/kg)	Maintenance dose (µg/kg)
Preterm infants (<1500 g)	20*	2.5
Preterm (1500–2500 g)	20*	5.0
Full-term infants	30	7.5

* Avoid if possible, see text.

to reach steady state. Avoid giving digoxin intramuscularly.

Diuretics

Frusemide in a dose of 1 mg/kg is the usual diuretic used in acute heart failure. Maintenance diuretic therapy consists of frusemide 2 mg/kg/day and spironolactone 2 mg/kg/day, with electrolyte monitoring. Spironolactone may interact with digoxin, leading to toxicity.

Fluid restriction to 100–120 mL/kg/day will act as an adjunct to other therapies.

Captopril, an angiotensin-converting enzyme inhibitor, may be of value in patients who continue to show signs of cardiac failure after maximum diuretic therapy. Captopril causes a fall in blood pressure (p. 178), which must be carefully monitored.

Murmur heard on routine examination

Heart disease may present with a cardiac murmur heard on routine examination in an apparently healthy infant. In such cases evidence of other cardiac disease should be excluded, including a check on the blood pressure in the arms and legs. A chest X-ray and ECG (or echocardiography if available) should be done in all cases other than the softest murmurs. It is necessary to give a full explanation and adequate reassurance to the parents. Most murmurs detected in the neonatal period will disappear in infancy, but arrangements for follow-up must be made.

Circulatory maladaptation at birth

Patent ductus arteriosus (PDA)

Normally the ductus arteriosus is functionally closed by 10–15 h after birth and is anatomically closed by 5–7 days of age. In preterm infants who sustained birth asphyxia or hypoxia after birth, patency of the ductus arteriosus is common. It is rare in term infants unless they are born at high altitude or have rubella embryopathy. A relatively high proportion of very low birthweight (VLBW) infants requiring intermittent positive-pressure ventilation (IPPV) develop delayed closure of the ductus. High fluid volumes are a major factor in its development,

and congestive cardiac failure is seen in about half of these cases.

Clinical features

Preterm infants with respiratory distress develop clinical features of a PDA within the first week or two of life, unlike term infants, who present at 4–6 weeks when the pulmonary vascular resistance has decreased to adult levels.

The classic signs are bounding (collapsing) pulses, a hyperdynamic precordium, a loud second heart sound, and initially a systolic murmur at the upper left sternal edge, with the diastolic component developing later. The absence of a murmur in a clinically significant ductus arteriosus is well recognized (the silent duct), but the peripheral pulses are always abnormal.

Once cardiac decompensation occurs congestive heart failure develops, with tachycardia, tachypnoea, cardiomegaly, hepatomegaly, gallop rhythm and crepitations. Preterm infants with a PDA often develop increasing apnoea, and ventilator and oxygen dependence, and may be predisposed to NEC.

Investigations

Chest X-ray may show an enlarged heart and pulmonary oedema may be present with large left to right shunts. The diagnosis is confirmed by echocardiography which can demonstrate ductal patency and size. Doppler assessment of flow through the ductus may also be helpful in quantifying the shunt, as well as left atrial/aortic ratio.

Treatment

Careful fluid management with avoidance of fluid overload is essential in preventing this condition. Once the infant shows evidence of a haemodynamically significant shunt (collapsing pulses, abnormal echocardiographic findings), fluid restriction should be instituted. Frusemide and top-up blood transfusion, if the patient is anaemic, may be beneficial.

Medical treatment with indometacin is often successful, and is most likely to close the ductus if administered in the first 2 weeks of life and if the gestational age is between 30 and 34 weeks.

Indometacin (indomethacin). PGE$_1$ relaxes the ductus arteriosus, whereas prostaglandin synthetase inhibitors such as indometacin reverse this effect. Unfortunately, indometacin has an effect on all vascular beds, reducing renal blood flow and gut perfusion. The standard dose is 0.1 mg/kg/day for 6 days. A high closure rate has been claimed with early intravenous indometacin.

Contraindications to indometacin include NEC, thrombocytopenia (<100 000 mm^{-3}), creatinine >200 µmol/L, and severe unconjugated hyperbilirubinaemia (>200 µmol/L).

Ibuprofen. This drug has been shown to be as effective as indometacin in closing the ductus, but is associated with fewer complications for the renal vascular bed. Unfortunately ibuprofen is considerably more expensive than indometacin and its benefits may not be justified in cost terms.

If medical closure fails and the infant remains ventilator dependent owing to the large left-to-right shunt, then surgical ligation is necessary.

Persistent pulmonary hypertension of the newborn

The normal changes in the circulation occurring at birth are described in Chapter 2. Conditions that interfere with normal oxygenation or lung expansion after birth may delay the physiological drop in pulmonary vascular resistance, resulting in persistent pulmonary hypertension of the newborn (PPHN). Failure of the pulmonary vascular resistance to fall, with persistence of the intracardiac shunts, leads to severe hypoxia and cyanosis (p. 8).

The tone of pulmonary arterioles is in balance, depending on the opposing influence of vasoconstrictors (e.g. leukotrienes, endothelin-1) and vasodilators (inhaled nitric oxide (iNO), prostacyclins). It is now recognized that iNO has the major influence on pulmonary vasodilatation after birth.

Aetiology

PPHN can have various causes, broadly categorized as primary or secondary:

1 Primary (or idiopathic) PPHN accounts for 20% of all cases and is due to a primary abnormality of the pulmonary arterioles, which have thick walls with a narrowed lumen.

2 Secondary to acute neonatal lung disease such as diaphragmatic hernia, pneumonia, meconium aspiration syndrome and rarely transient tachypnoea of the newborn (TTN) and RDS or chronic neonatal lung disease.

3 Secondary to maladaptation at birth:

(a) hypoxia with metabolic acidosis (e.g. birth asphyxia, RDS, pneumothorax) is a major cause;

(b) hypothermia;

(c) metabolic – hypoglycaemia, hypocalcaemia;

(d) polycythaemia with hyperviscosity;

(e) fetal exposure to prostaglandin synthetase inhibitors, e.g. aspirin, indometacin. Under these circumstances the ductus arteriosus may close *in utero*, leading to persistent pulmonary hypertension, but in practice this is very rare.

Clinical features

The clinical features depend to some extent on the underlying cause, but affected babies usually present shortly after birth with cyanosis and respiratory distress (tachypnoea, grunting and sternal and intercostal recession). In some cases cyanosis may be delayed by several hours, and may initially be intermittent, with wide fluctuations in P_aO_2 from normal to severe hypoxia because of arteriolar lability.

Arterial blood gases show hypoxaemia, acidaemia and variable hypercarbia. These infants resemble those with cyanotic CHD. Untreated their hypoxaemia may become extreme, despite assisted ventilation with high inspiratory pressures. In the survivors the respiratory distress decreases after some days.

It has been suggested that the following conditions should be satisfied before a diagnosis of PPHN can be made:

1 sustained systemic or suprasystemic pulmonary artery pressure;

2 profound hypoxaemia with or without acidosis, while breathing 100% oxygen;

3 normal cardiac anatomy on echocardiographic examination;

4 evidence of right-to-left shunting or bidirectional flow of blood through either the ductus arteriosus or the foramen ovale.

Management

Management should be directed towards the underlying cause of the PPHN if this can be recognized, as well as methods directed towards pulmonary vasodilatation.

General principles.

1 Correct any hypothermia, hypocalcaemia, hypomagnesaemia and hypoglycaemia.
2 Correct metabolic acidosis with sodium bicarbonate or trishydroxyaminomethane (THAM).
3 Treat polycythaemia (packed cell volume (PCV) >65%) with a partial exchange transfusion.
4 Correct systemic hypotension with volume expanders, isoprenaline or dopamine.

Specific management.

1 Provide sufficient oxygen to maintain P_aO_2 in the range 9–13 kPa (70–100 mmHg). Clinicians frequently target higher P_aO_2 levels of >13 kPa [100 mmHg] but there is no evidence for this practice.
2 Ventilatory support should be used to treat hypoxia if the P_aO_2 is <7 kPa (50 mmHg) in 100% oxygen. Both respiratory and metabolic alkalosis lower pulmonary vascular resistance in animal models .However,these therapies are controversial in neonates because low P_aCO_2 levels are associated with neurodevelopment, sernsorineural hearing loss and volutrauma to lungs. Metabolic alkalosis is not well studied in neonates.
3 Ensure an adequate systemic blood pressure. Shunting will be reduced by increasing the differential pressure between the systemic and pulmonary circulations. Inotrope infusion (dopamine and/or dobutamine) is given to increase the systemic blood pressure by at least 20%.
4 Pulmonary vasodilators. There is now a range of vasodilating agents available, which are discussed below.
5 Extracorporeal membrane oxygenation (ECMO). This therapy is aimed at supporting the cardiorespiratory system until pulmonary hypertension settles. It is therefore only indicated for potentially recoverable conditions and is not recommended in diaphragmatic hernia with severe pulmonary hypertension due to lung hypoplasia. A recent British randomized study has shown clearly that the outcome in term babies with severe respiratory failure is twice as good with ECMO than with conventional ventilatory techniques.

Pulmonary vasodilators

The pulmonary artery pressure in PPHN is always higher than the systemic pressure, and right-to-left shunting occurs through the ductus arteriosus and/or the foramen ovale. For therapy to be successful, this shunt must be reduced by selectively reducing the pulmonary vascular resistance while maintaining systemic vascular resistance.

Inhaled nitric oxide (iNO). This is a specific pulmonary vasodilator and has replaced other non-selective agents as the first-line pulmonary vasodilator. iNO is effective in the management of PPHN when given in low concentrations through the ventilator circuit. The therapeutic dose is 5–40 ppm (parts per million), and careful monitoring of inhaled concentration is necessary, as methaemoglobinaemia may occur with higher concentrations. Exhaled gases should be scavenged so that they do not contaminate the air within the nursery.

Prostacyclin. This acts as a vasodilator, but has a very short half-life. There is some evidence that it stimulates endothelial NO release. It is given by continuous intravenous infusion (5–20 mg/kg/min). Like tolazoline it is not a selective pulmonary vasodilator, and systemic hypotension should be anticipated.

Magnesium sulphate. This also acts as a non-specific vasodilator. The recommended dose of $MgSO_4 7H_2O$ is 250 mg/kg as a loading dose over 20 min, followed by 20–50 mg/kg/h.

Dysrhythmias

The newborn infant is subject to disorders of cardiac rate and rhythm, some of which may be detectable before birth with antepartum monitoring. Many are transient, especially following birth asphyxia and birth trauma.

The most important dysrhythmias in the newborn are:
1 supraventricular tachycardia;
2 congenital atrioventricular block;
3 ventricular tachycardia and fibrillation.

Supraventricular tachycardia (SVT)

This is the commonest form of tachycardia and is increasingly recognized *in utero* as a result of cardiotocography monitoring and real-time ultrasound examinations. Prolonged fetal supraventricular tachycardia leads to congestive cardiac failure and hydrops fetalis. If it is considered necessary to treat the fetus medically, the mother may be given an antiarrhythmic drug such as amiodarone or flecanide, which is often effective. Digitalizing the mother is more commenly recommended.

In the newborn SVT may be idiopathic or due to irritation of the sinoatrial node by inadvertent catheterization of the right atrium during umbilical catheterization. Heart failure may develop after a few hours, and treatment includes one of the following:

1 Vagal stimulation by eyeball pressure or an ice pack applied to the face may occasionally be enough to cause reversion to sinus rhythm.

2 Adenosine (150–300 µg/kg by rapid i.v. injection) is the drug of choice in treating neonatal SVT.

3 Once sinus rhythm is restored, maintenance treatment may be necessary with flecanide or amiodorone. These drugs should only be given under paediatric cardiology supervision.

4 DC cardioversion (10 J).

Verapamil is now contraindicated in infancy.

An interval ECG may demonstrate the Wolff–Parkinson–White syndrome (short P–R interval and a wide QRS complex).

Congenital heart block

In 50% of cases this is due to a major congenital cardiac anomaly, such as transposition of the great vessels or Ebstein's anomaly. Some cases are associated with maternal systemic lupus erythematosus, which may be subclinical. Heart block is only likely to cause clinical problems in the newborn period if it is complete (third degree) and associated with profound bradycardia.

Treatment is initially with an infusion of isoprenaline to increase the heart rate. A number of cases are transient and recover fully, but in some infants an electronic pacemaker may be necessary.

Ventricular tachycardia and fibrillation

If these occur they must be rapidly recognized and efficiently treated to avoid cerebral ischaemia. The commonest cause of ventricular tachycardia is hyperkalaemia (p. 167). This occurs spontaneously in some critically ill VLBW infants and may develop if the potassium exceeds 7.5 mmol/L. Treatment of the tachycardia includes

1 calcium gluconate (10%): 1–2 mL i.v. under ECG control;

2 correction of acidosis with sodium bicarbonate infusion;

3 lidocaine (lignocaine) 2 mg/kg by bolus i.v. injection followed by 4 mg/kg by slow i.v. infusion for 1 h;

4 cardioversion (5–10 J).

Usually calcium gluconate is successful in reverting the ventricular tachycardia to sinus rhythm. The treatment of the hyperkalaemia is discussed on p. 167.

Ventricular fibrillation should be treated with external cardiac massage and electrical cardioversion.

PRINCIPLES OF MANAGEMENT

- Seventy percent of major congenital heart lesions are diagnosed antenatally.

- Echocardiography conducted by an experienced cardiologist usually provides a full and accurate diagnosis of neonatal congenital heart disease.

- Palliative care for cyanotic congenital heart disease is achieved with PGE_1 infusion to keep ductus arteriosus patent and improve pulmonary blood flow.

- PGE_1 infusion may be life saving for left heart obstructive lesions by providing systemic blood flow from the right ventricle through the ductus arteriosus.

- Congestive heart failure needs early recognition, supportive care, management of the specific lesion and, rarely, digitalization.

- Inhaled nitric oxide is a specific pulmonary vasodilator and has replaced other non-selective agents as the first-line pulmonary vasodilator for persistent pulmonary hypertension.

References

Adelman RD. The hypertensive neonate. *Clin Perinatol* 1988;**15**:567–585.

Brennan P, Young I. Congenital heart malformation; aetiology and associations. *Semin Neonatol* 2001;**6**:17–25.

Evans N, Archer N. Perinatal cardiology. *Semin Neonatol* 2002;**1**:6.

Moss AJ, Adams FH (eds.). *Heart Disease in Infants, Children and Adolescents*. Baltimore: Williams and Wilkins, 1968.

Scott O. Advances in paediatric cardiology. In: Hull D (ed.) *Recent Advances in Paediatrics* 6, pp. 71–95, Edinburgh: Churchill Livingstone, 1981.

Further reading

Field DJ. Persistent pulmonary hypertension of the newborn. *Semin Neonatol* 1997;**2**:1–79.

Wren C. Cardiac arrhythmias in the fetus and newborn. *Semin Fetal Neonat Med* 2006;**11**:182–90.

CHAPTER 18

18 Haematological disorders

The blood volume and red cell mass at birth and in the neonatal period depend on the volume of the placental transfusion and subsequent readjustments of blood volume.

Placental transfusion

This occurs within 3 min of delivery and contributes 25% of the total neonatal blood volume. This amount will be increased in the following situations:
1 elevated maternal blood pressure;
2 use of oxytocic drugs;
3 late clamping or milking of the cord;
4 infant held in a low, dependent position.

The amount will be reduced by early cord clamping, or holding the infant above the level of the attached placenta.

The average blood volume of a newborn infant is 85–90 mL/kg, but ranges from 75 to 100 mL/kg. The practice of delay in clamping the umbilical cord or milking the cord from the placenta to the baby may result in symptomatic pulmonary plethora as well as hyperbilirubinaemia because of inadvertently high red cell mass.

Readjustment of blood volume

Within the first 3–4 h after birth there is haemoconcentration to compensate for rapid expansion of intravascular volume.

Anaemia

Anaemia is usually defined by a haemoglobin or haematocrit level that is 2.5 SD below the mean for age. The causes of neonatal anaemia are shown in Table 18.1 and will be discussed under the following headings:
1 physiological anaemia;
2 haemorrhage;
3 haemolysis;
4 hypoplasia or aplasia (diminished production).

Physiological anaemia

The full-term infant is born with a haemoglobin concentration in the range 15–23.5 g/dL, whereas in the premature infant the haemoglobin level is slightly lower. Initially there is a slight increase due to haemoconcentration, but then haemoglobin gradually drops and remains low for most of the first year of life (Fig. 18.1). This is known as physiological anaemia.

In term infants the lowest haemoglobin level occurs between 6 and 10 weeks, when it falls to 10–11 g/dL. In premature infants the anaemia occurs earlier and lasts longer, with a nadir of 7–8 g/dL (Fig. 18.1).

Anaemia of prematurity

In the preterm infant physiological anaemia occurs earlier, is more severe and prolonged than in the term infant, and is termed anaemia of prematurity. It is caused by a number of factors.

Table 18.1 Causes of neonatal anaemia

Physiological anaemia
Anaemia of prematurity
Haemorrhage
   Antepartum haemorrhage
   Fetomaternal transfusion
   Twin-to-twin transfusion
   Neonatal internal haemorrhage
Haemolysis (see Table 18.2)
Aplasia: Blackfan–Diamond syndrome

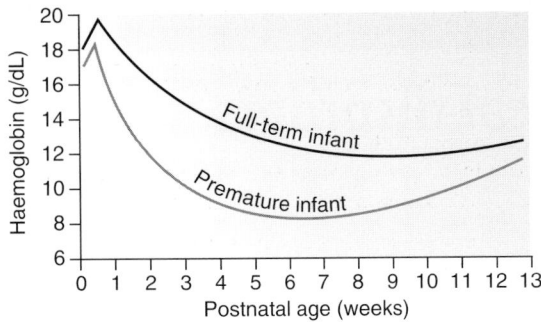

Figure 18.1 Physiological anaemia. The two graphs show the normal fall in haemoglobin with postnatal age in mature and premature infants.

Lack of erythropoietin. At birth the infant moves from a relatively hypoxic fetal state to become relatively hyperoxic. This suppresses erythropoietin secretion for the first 7–8 weeks of life. In addition the bone marrow is probably more resistant to the stimulatory effect of erythropoietin. This phase is terminated when reticulocytes are seen in the peripheral blood film.

Venesection. The preterm infant is subjected daily to repeated blood sampling for laboratory investigation.

Haemodilution. There is an increase in plasma volume over the first months of life and, together with poor red cell production, the haemoglobin falls. This is referred to as 'early anaemia'.

Iron deficiency. The full-term infant is born with sufficient iron stores for the first 4 months of life, but in preterm infants these stores are exhausted more quickly because of the infant's rapid growth rate. An infant of 1.5 kg at birth has half the iron stores of a 3.0 kg neonate. Iron deficiency causes the 'late anaemia' that accounts for low haemoglobin levels after 4 months of age, when hypochromic red cells are seen on a blood film.

Haemolysis. Haemolysis may occur in preterm infants as a result of vitamin E deficiency. Administration of vitamin E (25 mg/day) may reduce the extent of late anaemia of prematurity.

Treatment

A daily dose of 1–2 mg/kg/day of elemental iron (equivalent to 30–60 mg of ferrous salt) is associated with a good response in most cases, but routine iron supplementation from an early age to 'prevent' anaemia is controversial and not practised universally.

Transfusion (10 mL/kg) may be necessary in premature infants if the haemoglobin falls below 7–8 g/dL and the infant is symptomatic. Symptoms include breathlessness with feeds, tachycardia, apnoea and bradycardia or failure to gain weight. Blood transfusion will suppress erythropoietin activity, and if the infant shows a reticulocyte count of more than 5% then transfusion may be delayed, depending on the infant's condition. Premature infants receiving intensive care do end up receiving repeated blood transfusions. In such situations, exposure to multiple blood donors can be avoided by using the same batch blood from a single donor and stored in mini packs. Donor blood should be screened for blood-borne viruses.

The following formula may be used to calculate the volume of blood to be transfused for an anaemic infant (Hct, haematocrit):

$$\text{Donor blood required (mL)} = \frac{(\text{desired Hct} - \text{actual Hct}) \times \text{body weight (kg)} \times 90}{\text{donor Hct}} \qquad (18.1)$$

The administration of subcutaneous recombinant human erythropoietin to preterm infants has been shown to stimulate red blood cell production, thereby avoiding the need for frequent blood transfusions. But this treatment has not been shown to be cost-effective and is not widely used.

Haemorrhage

This may be due to
1 Haemorrhage before and during delivery from
   (a) placenta – placenta praevia, placental abruption, incision into the placenta during caesarean section;

(b) cord–rupture or torn vessels on insertion into the placenta;

(c) fetal–fetomaternal or twin-to-twin transfusion;

2 Neonatal haemorrhage:

(a) trauma–bleeding may occur into brain, lung, peritoneum or bowel;

(b) haemorrhagic disease of the newborn (see p. 203).

Investigations

These will depend on the likely diagnosis, but include

1 haemoglobin and haematocrit;

2 blood group (mother and baby);

3 cross-matched blood (against mother's and baby's blood);

4 Kleihauer's test (to assess the presence of fetal cells in maternal blood, indicating fetomaternal transfusion);

5 coagulation studies (indicated if a bleeding diathesis is suspected);

6 investigations to determine site of bleeding, e.g. lumbar puncture, ultrasound of head or abdomen, testing stools for blood.

Treatment

The clinical examination for hypovolaemia and shock includes assessment of colour, blood pressure, heart rate, tissue perfusion and urine output.

Severe haemorrhage may be a neonatal emergency and may require an immediate blood transfusion to prevent irreversible shock. If blood is not immediately available, i.v. normal saline, plasma or plasma substitute (purified protein fraction 20 mL/kg) may be given via a peripheral vessel. Umbilical transfusion via the umbilical vein may be life-saving in the shocked patient. In an emergency, group O rhesus-negative blood may be used, but formal cross-matching should be done whenever possible. Remember babies rarely die of anaemia, and hypovolaemia is much more damaging. Restoration of a circulating blood volume with fluid (crystalloid or colloid) is life saving before administering blood.

Haemolysis

The causes of neonatal haemolysis are shown in Table 18.2. Unconjugated hyperbilirubinaemia and

Table 18.2 Causes of immune and non-immune neonatal haemolysis

Immune haemolysis (positive Coombs' test)
Rhesus incompatibility
ABO incompatibility
Minor blood group incompatibility (e.g. Kell, Duffy, Kidd)
Maternal autoimmune diseases (e.g. SLE)
Non-immune haemolysis (negative Coombs' test)
Congenital infection
DIC
G6PD deficiency
Pyruvate kinase deficiency
Hereditary spherocytosis
α-Thalassaemia
Infantile pyknocytosis
Vitamin E deficiency

reticulocytosis are usually associated with haemolysis, the causes of which can be divided into immune and non-immune.

Rhesus haemolytic disease

This occurs because the mother's immune system has been sensitized by rhesus-positive cells from her fetus. Sensitization may be due to

1 fetomaternal transfusion;

2 rhesus-incompatible transfusions.

The rhesus factor is complex, comprising CDE/cde antigens. The commonest antigen is D, and this accounts for 95% of cases. Approximately 83% of the population are D positive, that is, rhesus positive (Rh +ve). If sensitization occurs, maternal immunoglobulin G (IgG) crosses the placenta to cause haemolysis of 'foreign' fetal erythrocytes. IgG remains present in the neonatal circulation for up to 3 months and neonatal haemolysis may continue to occur for some weeks after birth.

Prevention

Rh IgG prophylaxis (anti-D gammaglobulin) is indicated in the management of all non-immunized pregnant women who are Rh negative. Current recommendations include the routine administration of IgG at 28 weeks' gestation to all pregnant women who are RhD negative, and within 72 h of delivery to all rhesus-negative women who give birth to rhesus-positive infants. If antibodies are already present anti-D is not given. The standard dose of 300 µg is sufficient for protection for up to 30 mL of fetal blood. This provides satisfactory prophylaxis for 99% of all term deliveries. Women should have a Kleihauer test following the administration of anti-D gammaglobulin to test whether the dose was adequate to neutralize all rhesus-positive red blood cells.

Anti-D gammaglobulin should also be given to at-risk rhesus-negative women after abortions and after amniocentesis if the Kleihauer test shows a fetomaternal transfusion.

Anti-D gammaglobulin is ineffective against non-D rhesus antigen (usually C, E). If a large transfusion of fetal blood occurs, the standard dose of 300 µg/kg may be insufficient. In women at high risk, a Kleihauer–Berke smear test can be performed to quantitate for the fetal blood present. For every 30 mls of fetal blood detected, an additional 300 µg of IgG can be administered.

Management during pregnancy

Routine testing. Rhesus-negative women should be screened for rhesus antibodies at their first antenatal visit, and at 28, 32 and 36 weeks' gestation. If antibodies are detected at any of these times, more frequent testing will be necessary.

Antibodies present. If antibodies are present, then depending on the level and/or whether the titre is rising, an amniocentesis should be performed.

This should also be done if there is a history of a previously affected infant who required exchange transfusion, or if there has been a previous stillbirth because of rhesus disease. Amniocentesis is commonly done at 30–32 weeks but may be performed earlier, depending on the level of antibodies, and particularly on the history of previous pregnancies. Amniocentesis is carried out under ultrasound control so that the placenta can be localized and avoided. A Kleihauer test is done before and after amniocentesis, and a lecithin/sphingomyelin (L/S) ratio will be done on the amniotic fluid obtained. The timing of delivery will depend on the antibody levels, amniocentesis result and previous history of affected infants.

Assessment of bilirubin in liquor amnii. Fetal rhesus disease is now a relatively rare condition, and affected pregnancies should be managed in recognized regional centres experienced in treating these women and their babies. Traditionally the amount of bilirubin in the amniotic fluid was assessed by a spectrophotometric technique at a wavelength of 450 nm, which is the region of maximal absorption of bilirubin. The optical density difference between the patient's amniotic fluid and normal amniotic fluid at a specific gestational age is plotted on either the Liley (Liley 1961) or the Queenan (Queenan *et al.* 1993) chart. Figure 18.2 superimposes Queenan and Liley charts (Scott & Chan 1998).

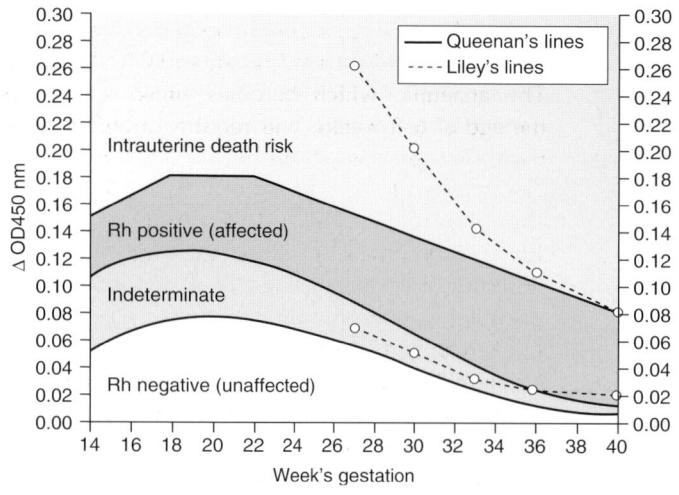

Figure 18.2 Superimposed 'Queenan' and 'Liley' charts of the deviation of optical density at a wavelength of 450 nm in amniotic fluid (OD450) vs. gestation. Note that 'Liley's' lines only started at 27 weeks. These lines are not linear on this graph because the scale for OD450 is not logarithmic on 'Queenan's' chart. Also note that the division lines for 'Queenan's' chart are lower at all gestations compared to 'Liley's'. (Reproduced from Scott & Chan 1998 with permission of John Wiley & Sons Ltd.)

The Liley chart provides guidelines for the severity of rhesus isoimmunization, treatment and expected cord blood haemoglobin. It allows the obstetrician to plan when to deliver the infant. This chart, which starts at 27 weeks' gestation, has been largely superseded by the Queenan chart, which commences at 14 weeks' gestation. Maternal fetal medicine specialists often also use fetal Doppler blood flow assessment, liver length and assessment of fluid in visceral cavities to estimate the timing of fetal blood transfusion. If the fetus is severely affected and is too immature to deliver, then *in utero* blood transfusion is necessary by percutaneous injection directly into the fetal umbilical cord under ultrasound control. This may need to be performed weekly in severe cases until the baby is mature enough for delivery.

Ultrasound. High-resolution ultrasound is an essential adjunct to the assessment of isoimmunized pregnancies. It allows early detection of hydrops, assessment of fetal behaviour (biophysical profile, which provides important evidence of fetal wellbeing), and interventions such as fetal blood samplings and transfusion. Ultrasound is used to assess the amniotic fluid index, hepatomegaly, subcutaneous oedema, ascites and increases in middle cerebral artery blood flow.

Management of the rhesus-immunized infant

The baby should be assessed for maturity, pallor, jaundice, hepatosplenomegaly, oedema, ascites, ecchymoses, heart failure and respiratory distress. The placenta is examined for the presence of oedema, weighed and sent to the pathology department for confirmation of the diagnosis.

Investigations at birth. Cord blood is taken for grouping, direct Coombs' test, haemoglobin and platelet count and total bilirubin estimation. The Coombs' test is always positive in rhesus incompatibility, unless an intrauterine transfusion with rhesus-negative blood has recently been performed. The more positive the Coombs' test, the more severely affected the infant is likely to be.

Indications for immediate exchange transfusion. The principal indications for exchange transfusion are:
● Cord haemoglobin <8 g/dL
● Hydrops fetalis

Indications for early exchange transfusion.
1 Cord bilirubin >85 µmol/L (5 mg/100 mL).
2 Cord haemoglobin 8–12 g/dL.
3 Rapidly rising serum bilirubin that crosses the level for exchange transfusion on the charts shown on p. 136.
4 A very strongly positive Coombs' test.

Interval exchange transfusion. This is done to prevent the serum unconjugated bilirubin reaching a potentially dangerous level (250 µmol/L in preterm, 340 µmol/L in term infants). This is usually carried out as an adjunct to phototherapy, and guideline graphs are useful (see p. 136).

Exchange transfusion. This is performed with less than 5-day-old warmed (37°C) whole blood. The infant is given a double-volume exchange (180 mL/kg). The blood should be rhesus negative and ABO compatible with the mother's blood. The method for exchange transfusion is described on p. 137.

Complications of rhesus incompatibility

The complications include
1 Kernicterus and bilirubin encephalopathy (see p. 138).
2 Hyaline membrane disease.
3 Beta-cell hyperplasia of the pancreas, resulting in hypoglycaemia.
4 Hypoalbuminaemia and lung oedema.
5 Thrombocytopenia and disseminated intravascular coagulopathy.
6 Inspissated bile syndrome.
7 Complications of exchange transfusion (see p. 139).
8 Anaemia. This results from ongoing haemolysis. The anaemia, which becomes most severe by the age of 6–8 weeks, will require careful assessment by determining haemoglobin levels and reticulocyte counts. Treatment includes folic acid administration and 'top-up' transfusions. Iron therapy is not necessary unless the infant is born prematurely.

ABO incompatibility

Haemolytic disease caused by ABO incompatibility is now the commonest cause of isoimmune haemolytic anaemia, but is generally less severe than that caused by rhesus incompatibility.

The naturally occurring anti-A or anti-B antibody is of the IgM type, which does not cross the placenta. Approximately 10% of women carry 'immune' anti-A or anti-B antibodies of the IgG class. It is in the pregnancies of these women that ABO incompatibility occurs, as the IgG crosses the placenta to haemolyse fetal red cells. Women with blood group O are most likely to have anti-A and anti-B IgG agglutinins, and it is this maternal blood group that accounts for the vast majority of ABO incompatibility. The mechanisms of development of this antibody are disputed. ABO incompatibility may occur in the first pregnancy, and subsequent pregnancies may be relatively unaffected.

ABO incompatibility generally occurs with the blood group combinations listed in Table 18.3.

Clinical features

The usual presentation is with jaundice on the first day or two of life but without hepatosplenomegaly. Kernicterus is an unusual complication, and hydrops fetalis has only occasionally been reported. Unlike rhesus disease, late anaemia is seldom a problem but folic acid is recommended because of ongoing haemolysis.

Investigations

ABO incompatibility is usually suspected in the presence of maternal blood group O and when the infant is either blood group A or, less commonly, group B.

1 The direct Coombs' test on the infant's blood is usually negative or only weakly positive, but the indirect Coombs' test may be positive.

2 A blood smear from the infant may show features of haemolysis, often with microspherocytes. Spherocytes are rarely seen in rhesus disease.

3 If the mother's serum causes haemolysis of adult A or B cells, this strongly suggests that she carries

α or β haemolysins. Maternal blood should be examined for haemolysins.

4 Immune anti-A or anti-B may be eluted from fetal red blood cells or cord blood.

Treatment

This is as for rhesus haemolytic disease, but intrauterine fetal transfusion is much less likely to be required.

Minor blood group incompatibilities

Rarely blood group incompatibilities are caused by Duffy, Kell, Kidd and C and E antibodies. They usually present with mild jaundice, but hydrops fetalis has been reported.

Glucose-6-phosphate dehydrogenase (G6PD) deficiency

This disease is inherited in an X-linked recessive manner and is due to a deficiency of the G6PD enzyme within the red blood cells, thereby rendering the cells more susceptible to haemolysis. More than 100 million people throughout the world, mainly Chinese, southern Mediterranean, black American or black African, have this abnormality. It usually occurs in males, although the heterozygote female may manifest mild features of the disease (an example of the Lyon hypothesis; see p. 153). There are many variants of this condition, some requiring an oxidizing agent to trigger haemolysis and others that cause haemolysis spontaneously. Some infants with the enzyme deficiency develop jaundice in the newborn period without exposure to oxidant drugs, but in other variants of the condition oxidant drugs are required to trigger haemolysis. In later years otherwise healthy children may become acutely ill with anaemia when exposed to drugs.

Table 18.4 lists the more commonly used drugs that may cause haemolysis in susceptible neonates. Some drugs excreted in breast milk are liable to haemolyse red cells in G6PD-deficient infants, including nitrofurantoin, sulfonamides and sulfasalazine. In addition, respiratory viruses, viral hepatitis and fava beans cause haemolysis in susceptible infants. Naphthalene in mothballs is a potent inducer of haemolysis in susceptible infants. Routine administration of 1 mg vitamin K_1 to G6PD-deficient infants is safe.

Table 18.3 Blood group combinations causing ABO incompatibility

Mother	Infant	Frequency
O	A or B	Common
A	B or AB	Rare
B	A or AB	Rare

Table 18.4 Drugs that may cause haemolysis in infants with G6PD deficiency

Antimalarials (primaquine, quinine)
Nitrofurantoin
Sulfonamides
Phenacetin
Acetylsalicylic acid
Nalidixic acid
Methylene blue
Naphthalene
Vitamin K (large doses)
Chloramphenicol

Clinical features

Haemolysis may occur spontaneously or after exposure to infection or drugs. Jaundice and pallor may be the only clinical signs. It may be severe and require exchange transfusion. Hepatosplenomegaly is uncommon.

Investigations

Anaemia with spherocytosis, reticulocytes and crenated red cells is seen. Heinz bodies are another feature of the haemolytic anaemia. A screening test for G6PD deficiency is available and is reliable in infants of Chinese and Mediterranean extraction. In black infants, once haemolysis has occurred, a population of young red cells may remain with normal enzyme activity, and this makes the screening test unreliable. Black infants and those positive on the screening test should have the enzyme level directly assayed.

Treatment

Infants born into families known to have G6PD deficiency should not be exposed to agents likely to cause haemolysis. Spontaneous haemolysis may occur, and the treatment is as for any cause of unconjugated hyperbilirubinaemia. Anaemia may require transfusion.

Pyruvate kinase deficiency

This is an autosomal recessive condition affecting glucose metabolism within the red cell membrane. Spontaneous haemolysis occurs in the neonatal period with anaemia and jaundice. Splenomegaly is always present. Diagnosis is made by enzyme assay.

Hereditary spherocytosis (HS)

This is an autosomal dominant condition that may cause early neonatal haemolysis. The blood film shows spherocytes with little splenomegaly initially. ABO incompatibility may present in a similar way, and a family history of HS is an important diagnostic point. The spherocytes show an increased osmotic fragility, although this may not be apparent in the first few months of life. Severe haemolysis with very high levels of hyperbilirubinaemia may occur suddenly.

α-Thalassaemia

Classic β-thalassaemia major does not affect neonates because the majority of the haemoglobin is in the fetal (HbF) form. α-Thalassaemia is a rare and severe condition that causes hydrops and severe anaemia. The α chain is manifested by a double allele, so that four different types of α-thalassaemia may be recognized:

Hb Barts (hydrops fetalis) is homozygous for both alleles and is denoted -/-.

HbH disease is both homozygous and heterozygous for alleles α-/--.

α-Thalassaemia minor may be α-/α-; or --/αα-, and α-thalassaemia trait αα/α-.

Infantile pyknocytosis

This is a rare cause of neonatal haemolysis and is diagnosed by finding large numbers of small distorted 'pyknocytes' in the peripheral blood film. The greater the numbers of pyknocytes, the greater the tendency to haemolysis. This condition may be due to vitamin E deficiency and is self-limiting.

Hydrops fetalis

This term is used to describe an infant who shows severe and generalized oedema and fluid in at least two visceral cavities (pleural effusions, ascites, pericardial effusions).

Causes

The many causes of hydrops fetalis can be broadly categorized as immune and non-immune.

Immune. The principal immune cause is severe haemolytic disease of the newborn (rhesus, ABO, minor blood groups).

Non-immune. Non-immune causes fall into various subcategories, as follows:

1 Severe chronic anaemia *in utero*:
- fetomaternal haemorrhage;
- homozygous α-thalassaemia;
- chronic fetomaternal transfusion or twin-to-twin transfusion.

2 Cardiac failure:
- severe congenital heart disease;
- premature closure of foramen ovale;
- large atrioventricular (A-V) malformation (haemangioma);
- fetal supraventricular tachycardia.

3 Hypoproteinaemia:
- renal disease:
  –congenital nephrosis
  –renal vein thrombosis
  –congenital hepatitis

4 Infections (intrauterine):
- syphilis;
- toxoplasmosis;
- cytomegalovirus;
- parvovirus B19 (this usually causes hydrops secondary to severe anaemia).

5 Miscellaneous:
- maternal diabetes mellitus;
- parabiotic syndrome (multiple pregnancy);
- sublethal umbilical or chorionic vein thrombosis;
- fetal neuroblastomatosis;
- Chagas' disease;
- choriocarcinoma *in situ*.

6 Congenital malformations:
- cystic adenomatoid malformation of the lung;
- obstructive uropathy;
- achondroplasia;
- pulmonary lymphangiectasia;
- Gaucher's disease.

7 Genetic abnormality:
- trisomy 21, 18 and 13;
- Turner syndrome (45XO);
- triploidy;
- Noonan syndrome.

8 Idiopathic. This may account for up to 50% of cases where after extensive investigations no obvious cause is found.

Management
Investigations are done to determine the cause of the hydrops fetalis and include:
1 Coombs' test and full blood count;
2 haemoglobin electrophoresis;
3 Kleihauer test;
4 TORCH (toxoplasmosis, other, rubella, cytomegalovirus, herpes simplex type II)/syphilis investigations;
5 placental examination;
6 chest X-ray;
7 detailed ultrasound examination;
8 echocardiography;
9 total serum proteins and serum albumin;
10 chromosomal analysis;
11 dysmorphology evaluation;
12 autopsy.

Treatment
This will include paracentesis of the abdomen and chest, transfusion, intubation and positive-pressure ventilation, plus diuretic and intravenous albumin therapy. Despite intensive treatment, prognosis for non-immune hydrops remains poor, particularly if there are structural defects or its cause is not known, compared with cases caused by isoimmunization.

Aplasia

Impaired erythrocyte production is an unusual cause of anaemia in the newborn. The most common cause is the Diamond–Blackfan syndrome, also known as congenital hypoplastic anaemia.

Polycythaemia

Polycythaemia in the newborn is common and is defined as a venous haematocrit of 65% or more (approximating to a haemoglobin of 22 g/dL), during the first week of life. Polycythaemia does not mean the blood is hyperviscous. Blood viscosity depends largely on packed cell volume (haematocrit), but the deformability of red blood cells and the plasma viscosity may also be significant factors. The relationship between viscosity and haematocrit is linear below a haematocrit of 60–65%, but increases exponentially above this level. Viscosity is much greater in small vessels than in large ones.

Polycythaemia should only be diagnosed on a free-flowing venous specimen and not from a heel-prick sample.

The causes of polycythaemia are listed in Table 18.5.

Clinical features
The infant looks plethoric, and polycythaemia may cause problems in a number of organ systems owing to diminished blood flow through small vessels. The clinical signs associated with polycythaemia/hyperviscosity are illustrated in Fig. 18.3.

$$\text{Volume (MI) to be exchanged} = \frac{(\text{actual Hct} - \text{desired Hct}) \times \text{body weight (Kg)} \times 90}{\text{actual Hct}} \tag{18.2}$$

Table 18.5 Causes of neonatal polycythaemia

Chronic intrauterine hypoxia:
  SGA infants
  Post-maturity
Excessive transfusion of blood
  Placental transfusion due to delayed clamping
  Twin-to-twin transfusion
  Maternofetal transfusion
Infants of diabetic mothers
Down syndrome
Neonatal thyrotoxicosis
Congenital adrenal hyperplasia
Beckwith–Wiedemann syndrome

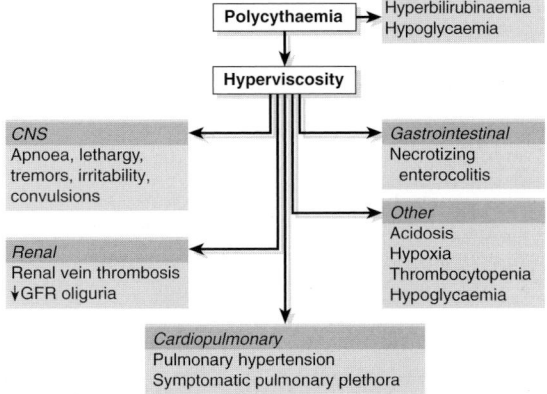

Figure 18.3 The interrelationship between polycythaemia and hyperviscosity and their contribution towards clinical signs. CNS, central nervous system; GFR, glomerular filtration rate.

Management
Infants at risk of polycythaemia should have a haematocrit measured on free-flowing venous blood. Babies without symptoms of polycythaemia but a venous haematocrit greater than 70% should have a dilutional exchange transfusion. Those with a venous packed cell volume (PCV) of 65–70% may require dilutional exchange if symptoms are present.

A dilutional exchange is performed with plasma and is aimed at reducing the haematocrit (Hct) to about 50% by the following formula:

where 90 refers to the blood volume (MI) per kg.

Bleeding and coagulation disorders

These may be due to thrombocytopenia, clotting factor deficiency, abnormal capillaries or a combination of these. Coagulation is a complicated process and is relatively less efficient in the newborn (particularly premature infants) than in older children.

When the vascular endothelium is damaged specific factors are released that cause platelet aggregation, upon which thrombus is deposited. This induces fibrin formation, which further induces platelets to be deposited, leading to the creation of a platelet–fibrin syncytium that prevents further bleeding. Thrombin is formed from prothrombin by the action of factor X. Factor X may be activated by either the intrinsic or the extrinsic pathway to precipitate a cascade of clotting factors, culminating in the production of fibrin. Plasminogens act to remove fibrin (fibrinolysis), and in the healthy state this system is balanced with the clotting mechanism by a series of inhibitors.

Clinical features
Bleeding may be overt, from venepuncture sites or the umbilical stump. Bruising (ecchymoses), purpura or petechial haemorrhages may be present at birth or develop in the neonatal period.

A careful maternal history should be taken, including a family history of bleeding, drugs (warfarin, aspirin), idiopathic thrombocytopenic purpura (ITP) and recent viral illness

Neonatal examination includes

1 site of bleeding: examination will determine the origin of bleeding, such as the gastrointestinal tract, umbilicus or circumcision;

2 purpura suggesting thrombocytopenia;

3 hepatosplenomegaly: infection (TORCH, bacterial);

4 congenital anomaly, e.g. giant haemangioma, thrombocytopenia with absent radii (TAR) syndrome.

Investigations

Platelet count

A platelet count less than 100 000/mm³ is usually classified as thrombocytopenia. A useful guide to severity is

50–100 000: mild thrombocytopenia (bleeding with surgery);

25–50 000: moderate thrombocytopenia (bleeding with minor trauma);

<25 000: severe thrombocytopenia (spontaneous bleeding is likely).

Infants with long-standing thrombocytopenia may have no spontaneous bruising even with platelet concentrations as low as 10 000/mm³.

Coagulation profile

Bleeding time. This measures the time to stop bleeding after a standard small wound, as from an Autolet device. The upper limit of normal for this test in the neonate is 3.5 min. Prolonged bleeding time is seen in thrombocytopenia, von Willebrand's disease and disseminated intravascular coagulation (DIC).

Prothrombin time (PT). This assesses the extrinsic clotting pathway (factors II, V, VII and X). This is not markedly affected by heparin.

Partial thromboplastin time (PTT). This assesses the intrinsic clotting pathway (most factors except VII and XII) but is prolonged by heparin contamination. It is the most sensitive test for coagulation disturbances.

Thrombin clotting time. This assesses fibrinogen activity and requires calcium for activation.

Fibrinogen degradation products (FDPs). Fibrin is deposited during coagulation and is simultaneously degraded by plasminogens to FDPs. The presence of increased levels of FDPs or elevated D-dimer indicates that fibrinolysis is occurring, usually following thrombosis.

Clotting factor analysis. Specific factors can be assayed individually, but interpretation may be difficult because of uncertainty as to the normal range in very immature infants.

The normal ranges for some of these tests are shown in Table 18.6.

Thrombocytopenia

Petechiae and ecchymoses, which may be present at birth or appear after birth, are the characteristic lesions produced by platelet deficiencies. Whereas bleeding may occur from any site, intracranial haemorrhage is the most devastating complication. Table 18.7 lists the causes of neonatal thrombocytopenia.

Alloimmune thrombocytopenia

This is analogous to rhesus isoimmunization but is a much rarer condition. A transfusion of fetal A1 antigen-positive platelets into the maternal circulation may produce maternal IgG antibodies if the mother is platelet A1 antigen negative. The mother has normal numbers of platelets. Thrombocytopenia in the neonate may be severe, but is transient. The disease presents with intracranial haemorrhage (often fetal) in 20%. *In utero* treatment consists of

Table 18.6 Normal results for some of the more commonly used tests of coagulation

Test	Preterm (30–36 weeks)	Term
PT (s) (I, II, V, VII, X)	13–23	13–17
Thrombotest (TT;%) (II, VII, IX, X)	15–50	15–60
PTT (s) (I, II, V, VII, IX, X, XI, XII)	35–100	35–70
Thrombin time (s)	12–24	12–18
Reptilase time (s)	18–30	18–24
Fibrinogen concentration (g/L)	1.2–3.8	1.5–3.5

Table 18.7 Causes of neonatal thrombocytopenia

Infection:
    Any bacterial infection
    TORCH infections
Isoimmune
Maternal disease:
    Severe toxaemia of pregnancy
    Idiopathic thrombocytopenic purpura
    Systemic lupus erythematosus
    Drug induced (hydralazine, thiazides)
Neonatal drug exposure:
    Thiazide diuretics
    Quinine
    Sulphonamides
Disseminated intravascular coagulation
Thrombocytopenia with absent radii (TAR syndrome)
Giant haemangioma (Kasabach–Merritt syndrome)
Fanconi's anaemia
Leukaemia
Pancytopenias

fetal platelet transfusion and regular gammaglobulin therapy. Neonatal treatment is valuable, using platelet transfusions, gammaglobulin and steroids.

Maternal idiopathic thrombocytopenia

Transplacental maternal antibodies cause thrombocytopenia in the neonate and the mother will usually have thrombocytopenia. The lower the concentration of maternal platelets, the more severely affected the infant may be. Prenatal administration of corticosteroids or high-dose intravenous IgG has been advocated to reduce the incidence and severity of neonatal thrombocytopenia, but the response to these treatments is uncertain and unpredictable. The use of IgG infusion in the thrombocytopenic neonate may rapidly cause the platelet count to increase.

It has been suggested that delivery by caesarean section should be undertaken in severely thrombocytopenic fetuses to avoid trauma, but recent evidence suggests that intracerebral bleeds may occur before the onset of labour.

Prednisolone (4 mg/kg/day) may be given to the severely affected neonate, but the condition is transient, lasting at most 12 weeks. Treatment of severe thrombocytopenia includes fresh whole blood or platelet transfusion (10 mL/kg). Serious neonatal haemorrhage does not occur if the platelet count is above 50 000/mm³.

Haemorrhagic disease of the newborn

Classic haemorrhagic disease of the newborn is caused by a deficiency of the vitamin K-dependent clotting factors, and its decline in incidence is due to the routine administration of vitamin K_1 (1 mg i.m. or by mouth) at birth. Vitamin K is produced by the bacterial flora of the gastrointestinal tract, but as the newborn infant has a sterile bowel at birth there is little production from this source in the first weeks of life.

Clinical features
Spontaneous bleeding can occur from any site but is usually gastrointestinal (producing haematemesis or melaena), umbilical or associated with circumcision. It occurs late in the first week of life, especially in the breastfed infant owing to the low vitamin K levels in human milk.

Gastrointestinal bleeding in the infant must be differentiated from swallowed maternal blood from antepartum haemorrhage, episiotomy or cracked nipples.

The Apt test, which depends on the resistance of haemoglobin F (fetal red cells) to denaturation by sodium hydroxide, will distinguish the infant's blood (predominantly fetal) from maternal blood (adult blood). Most centres will now perform Hb electrophoresis to identify if it is predominantly fetal or adult haemoglobin to identify the source of bleeding.

Investigations
The diagnosis is confirmed by a prolonged PT but a normal PTT.

Treatment
Vitamin K_1 1 mg i.m. or i.v. is given after blood has been obtained for investigations. Whole-blood transfusion (30 mL/kg) will be indicated for hypovolaemic shock.

Vitamin K prophylaxis
Routine administration of intramuscular vitamin K to all newborn babies will prevent bleeding from vitamin K deficiency. Concerns about the safety of

intramuscular vitamin K, in particular the risk of cancer, were raised in the early 1990s and although there are few data to support this, a small risk of leukaemia cannot be excluded. In order to avoid the potential risk of intramuscular injection a number of countries have recommended oral administration of vitamin K in all healthy full-term infants. Unfortunately, it appears that the protection this policy provides for the development of late-onset haemorrhagic disease of the newborn is not ideal, and approximately 2/100 000 cases of late-onset bleeding have been reported.

There is no doubt that the only certain way to prevent serious late-onset vitamin K deficiency bleeding is to give intramuscular vitamin K. If this is not acceptable to the parents, then oral administration can be used, but in exclusively breastfed babies, who constitute the highest-risk group for this condition, three doses are necessary to give full protection. Konakion MM paediatric drops are licensed in the UK for use in healthy neonates of 36 weeks' gestation and older. The recommended dosage regimen is 2 mg orally shortly after birth, a further 2 mg at 4–7 days and, if the baby is exclusively breastfed, a third dose of 2 mg should be given at 1 month of age. Failure to give a complete dosage regimen appears to be the reason for the re-emergence of serious late-onset vitamin K deficiency haemorrhage. In rare situations where haemorrhagic tendency still persists after administration of vitamin K, one should exclude the possibility of cystic fibrosis and α_1-antitrypsin deficiency.

Disseminated intravascular coagulation (DIC)

DIC is an acquired coagulation disorder characterized by the intravascular consumption of platelets and clotting factors II, V, VIII and fibrinogen. Widespread intravascular coagulation results from the deposition of thrombi in small vessels and the consumption of clotting factors, with consequent haemorrhage. DIC is recognized as a complication of an increasing variety of neonatal conditions, including

1 septicaemia;
2 severe shock;
3 severe perinatal asphyxia;
4 hyaline membrane disease in very low birthweight (VLBW) infants;

5 severe rhesus disease;
6 TORCH infections;
7 hypothermia;
8 maternal DIC with a transplacental effect – this occurs secondary to antepartum haemorrhage, a dead twin fetus or amniotic fluid embolism.

Investigations
1 Blood film shows haemolysis with fragmented and distorted red cells.
2 Thrombocytopenia.
3 Prolonged PT, PTT and thrombin time.
4 Low fibrinogen.
5 Increased FDPs.
Not all these features are necessary to make the diagnosis, but the presence of three or more makes DIC very likely.

Treatment
This is a complex disorder and haematological consultation will often be necessary. Treatment consists of:
● Treating the underlying disease process.
● Treatment of the haematological abnormality, including exchange transfusion with fresh whole blood and/or replacement of clotting factors with fresh frozen plasma, platelet concentrates and cryoprecipitate. Heparinization is unlikely to be of any benefit.

Inherited disorders of coagulation

Coagulation factors are not transferred from the maternal circulation to the fetus. Severe forms of haemophilia A (factor VIII deficiency) and Christmas disease (factor IX deficiency) account for the majority of haemorrhagic problems of the newborn caused by congenital coagulation abnormalities. Bleeding in these X-linked recessive diseases occurs when male infants are subjected to surgical procedures such as circumcision, or from either birth trauma or routine sampling of capillary blood. The diagnosis is confirmed by a prolonged PTT, normal PT and decreased factor VIII assay. Factor XI deficiency (haemophilia C) is inherited as an autosomal recessive disease and is not usually diagnosed in the neonatal period. Excessive bleeding typically occurs in the post-traumatic or postoperative settings such as after circumcision. Factor XI deficiency has been described as a common finding in Noonan syndrome.

von Willebrand disease does not usually present in the neonatal period. However, because von Willebrand factor (vWF) serves as a carrier for factor VIII, those who are symptomatic in early infancy often have signs and symptoms associated with low factor VIII. Laboratory testing requires determination of vWF antigen and vWF activity and a platelet function test in addition to ascertaining factor VIII activity.

Management

A specific diagnosis may be difficult to make at birth because in the healthy infant many of the clotting factor assays are low. Treatment consists of transfusion with fresh blood, and sometimes cryoprecipitate when a specific diagnosis can be made.

Congenital deficiency of anticoagulant proteins

The anticoagulant proteins, protein C, protein S, antithrombin III and heparin cofactor II, are all inherited in an autosomal dominant manner. Homozygous protein C or protein S deficiency causes serious thrombotic events in the postnatal period. The parents, who usually are asymptomatic, are heterozygous for deficiency of the suspected protein. Factor V Leiden, a mutation in coagulation factor V that renders it resistant to cleavage by activated protein C, is now the most common abnormality found in patients with excessive venous thrombosis. Such patients require anticoagulation with heparin and warfarin.

References

Liley AW. Liquor amnii analysis in management of pregnancy complicated by rhesus sensitization. *Am J Obstet Gynecol* 1961;**82**:1359.

Queenan JT, Tomai TP, Ural SH, King JC. Deviation in amniotic fluid optical density at a wavelength of 450 nm in Rh-immunised pregnancies from 14 to 40 weeks gestation: a proposal for clinical management. *Am J Obstet Gynecol* 1993;**168**:1370–1376.

Scott F, Chan FY. Assessment of the clinical usefulness of the 'Queenan' chart versus the 'Liley' chart in predicting severity of Rhesus isoimmunization. *Prenatal Diag* 1998;**18**:1143–1148.

Further reading

Arceci R, Hann I, Smith O. *Pediatric Hematology*. Oxford: Blackwell Publishing, 2006.

Lanzkowsky P. *Manual of Pediatric Hematology and Oncology*, 3rd edn. New York: Academic Press, 2000.

19 Neurological disorders

Brain development

There is a continuum of brain development from the time of conception right through gestation and until the end of the first decade of life. The pattern of brain growth and development is illustrated in Fig. 19.1.

Neuronogenesis　The first neural tissue appears at about 18 days with the neural crest, from which the neural tube develops. There is a phase of rapid neuronogenesis occurring from 4 to about 18 weeks of gestation.

Differentiation　The primitive neural cells differentiate into the different populations of cells, both neurons and glia, that make up the mature brain. This process occurs mainly from weeks 4 to 18.

Proliferation　There is a vast increase in the number of neuronal cells up to about 18 weeks of gestational life, most of which die as part of the neuronal regression process (see below).

Neuronal migration　Neurons are produced deep in the brain and migrate to the cortex and other sites.

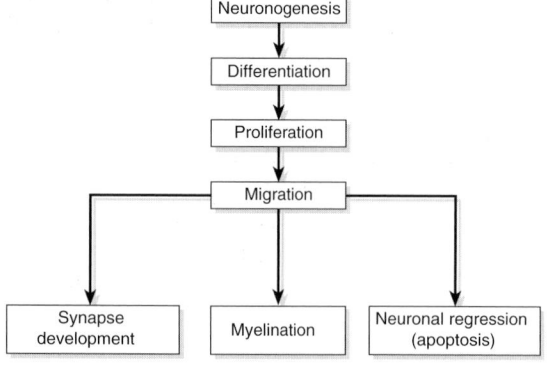

Figure 19.1 The sequence of brain development.

Final migration of neurons has been achieved by 25 weeks of gestation.

Neuronal regression　The process of apoptosis ensures that only neurons that have achieved a functional capacity within the nervous system survive. Most neurons, during the course of migration, do not acquire this function and regress as part of normal brain development.

Synapse development　Full function in the brain depends on the dendrites of each neuron developing and making many connections (on average each neuron is in contact with 10 000 other neurons). These connections are called synapses. Establishing new synaptic contacts is part of the process of development and learning.

Myelination　Glial cells are associated with the process of myelination and there is rapid growth of these cells from 24 weeks as they migrate to their final sites. Myelination is not complete until about 12 years.

Factors adversely influencing brain growth and development may operate at different times. Community-based studies of disabled children, relating the timing of the brain insult to either prenatal, perinatal or postnatal events, show that prenatal insults account for more disability than perinatal and postnatal causes together. The approximate proportions for neurological handicap in a community are shown in Table 19.1. Table 19.2 lists the relatively common insults that may cause prenatal, perinatal or postnatally acquired disability.

The brain is not a homogeneous organ. Specific areas of the brain grow at different times and rates. Thus, growth restriction at any one time (e.g. due to malnutrition) distorts the general growth of the brain and may selectively affect a particular area.

Unlike general body growth, the brain has only one opportunity to develop properly and thus interference with growth at a particular time in development may be irreversible.

Malformations of the central nervous system

Abnormalities of the brain can be classified as malformations (a developmental defect in which the brain was never normal) and deformations, where an external insult has affected normal brain development causing an abnormality in subsequent structure.

The incidence of major central nervous system (CNS) abnormalities in the UK has fallen more than tenfold in the last 30 years and in 2005 was less than 0.5/1000 live births. In Australia the incidence is approximately 1.2/1000.

Malformations of the CNS apparent at birth result from abnormalities in CNS development. These can be divided into two groups:
1 disorders of dorsal induction;
2 disorders of ventral induction.

Dorsal induction refers to the formation and migration of the neural tube, with subsequent development of the anterior tube into the primitive brain structures. These processes occur during the third and fourth weeks of gestation. Disorders occurring at this time include anencephaly, encephalocoele, myelomeningocoele and meningocoele. These are collectively known as neural tube defects, and the incidence of babies born with these disorders has fallen markedly over the last 10 years.

Ventral induction refers to development at the ventral end of the neural tube, and particularly cleavage into bilateral hemispheres and ventricles, with thalamic and hypothalamic growth. These processes occur mainly in the fifth and sixth weeks of gestation. The commonest disorder occurring at this time is holoprosencephaly, which may be associated with abnormalities in facial development.

Neural tube disorders

Aetiology
Neural tube disorders in general, and spina bifida in particular, have become much less common than they were previously. There are two main reasons for this: periconceptual folate supplementation and antenatal fetal screening. In some women the risk of a baby with neural tube disorders (NTDs) is increased. This includes families with a history of an affected child, or where the mother herself has the condition. A number of anticonvulsant drugs administered to the mother (particularly sodium valproate) are associated with a considerably increased risk.

It is now known that folic acid is an important substrate for normal early neural tube development, and periconceptual supplementation of at-risk women with folic acid reduces the incidence of this condition by approximately 75%. As it is not possible to know which women are at increased risk until their first baby is born with spina bifida, it

Table 19.1 Estimated timing of events which cause neurological handicap in a community

Prenatal	70–75%
Perinatal	20%
(Premature	60%)
(Full-term	40%)
Postnatal	5–10%

Table 19.2 Causes of neurological disability related to the timing of onset of the insult

Prenatal	Perinatal	Postnatal
Down syndrome	Birth asphyxia	Hypothyroidism
Neural tube defects	Intracranial haemorrhage	Meningitis
Other chromosomal disorders	Periventricular leukomalacia	Inborn errors of metabolism
Viral infection	Ototoxic drugs	Trauma
Intrauterine growth restriction	Kernicterus	
Toxins and drugs	Hypoglycaemia	

is now recommended that all women intending to become pregnant take regular folate for 3 months prior to conception.

The second factor in the falling incidence of NTDs is early fetal ultrasound to detect congenital spine or brain abnormalities. In many developed countries virtually all pregnant women are screened at about 18 weeks of gestation. The detection of a seriously abnormal fetus offers the opportunity for the parents to consider terminating the pregnancy.

Anencephaly

In this condition the forebrain is absent (Fig. 19.2); it occurs as the result of an insult before 24 days' gestation. With routine fetal scanning and termination of pregnancy this condition is now rarely seen at birth. Anencephaly is incompatible with life and results in stillbirth or neonatal death.

Encephalocoele

In this condition there has been failure of midline closure of the skull, usually with herniation of the brain. Up to 80% of cases occur in the occipital region (Fig. 19.3). This lesion occurs about 28 days after conception. The prognosis depends on the amount of brain in the sac. If the infant is microcephalic with a large encephalocoele, the prognosis is very poor. Neurosurgery is necessary to close the defect.

Spina bifida

This is a developmental failure of fusion of the vertebral column, often with an external protrusion of the meninges and cord. A meningeal sac of cerebrospinal fluid (CSF) with normal underlying spinal cord is referred to as a meningocoele, and if there is

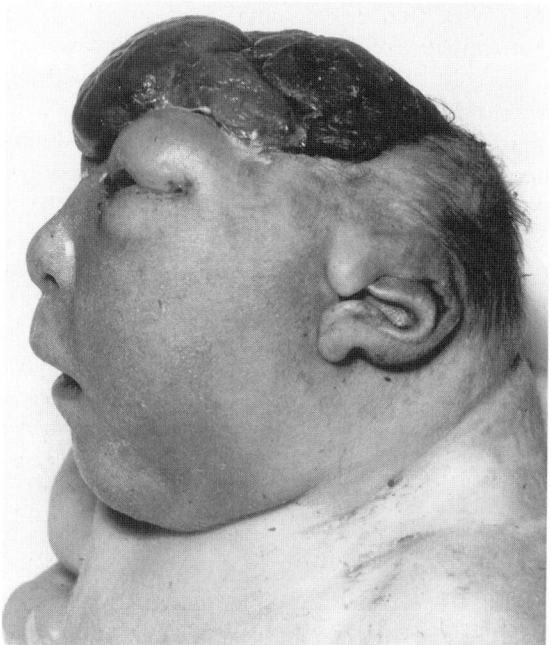

Figure 19.2 Anencephaly.

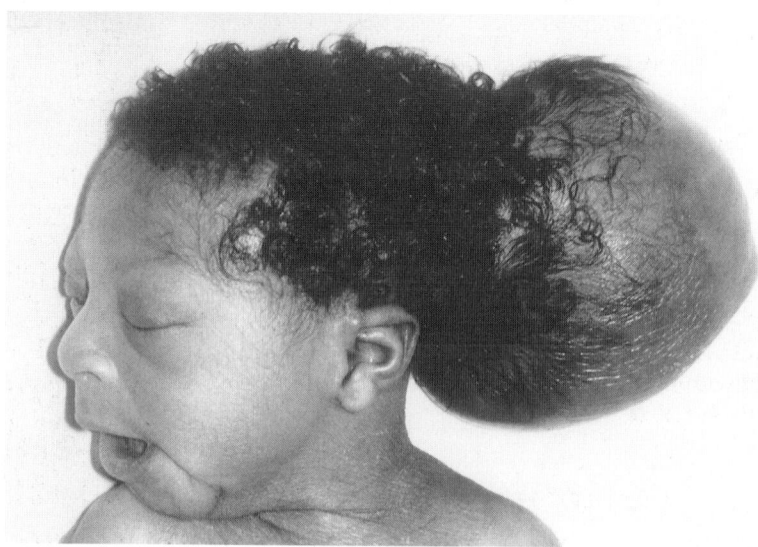

Figure 19.3 Occipital encephalocoele. This infant was operated on. Although he has severe visual impairment, at 2 years he was otherwise normal.

associated abnormality of the cord it is a meningo-myelocoele. The abnormalities produced may be classified according to their severity.

Spina bifida occulta

In this condition the vertebrae are bifid but there is no meningocoele or myelomeningocoele sac (Fig. 19.4). This abnormality is seen in 10% of the population and is usually of no clinical significance. In a small proportion the spinal cord may be tethered and with growth becomes stretched, causing irreversible neurological signs in the lower limbs and bladder. This condition should be suspected if there are lesions over the midline of the lower back. Such lesions include:

- a deep sinus;
- a naevus;
- a tuft of hair;
- a soft fatty swelling referred to as a lipomyelomeningocoele – this is particularly likely to be associated with later neurological signs.

All newborn infants with any of these clinical features should be investigated with real-time ultrasound and, if spinal cord tethering is suspected, referred to a neurosurgeon. The prognosis is much better with early repair prior to the onset of neurological symptoms.

Spina bifida cystica

This includes meningocoeles and myelomeningocoeles (Fig. 19.4). The incidence of this lesion in live-born infants is now about 1/1000 births, but is considerably higher in some parts of the world.

Meningocoeles These account for 20% of spina bifida cystica lesions. In this condition there is no herniation of nervous tissue, and consequently no neurological deficit. There is a risk of meningitis if the sac leaks CSF.

Meningomyelocoeles (Fig. 19.5) These account for 80% of spina bifida cystica lesions. They are associated with herniation of nervous tissue and permanent neurological deficit.

Clinical features

The antenatal features and diagnosis may be similar to those seen with anencephaly, as the spinal

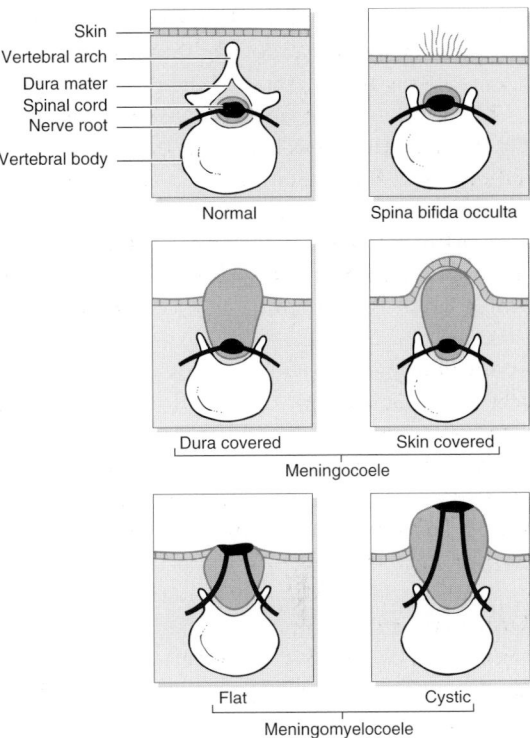

Figure 19.4 The varieties of spina bifida.

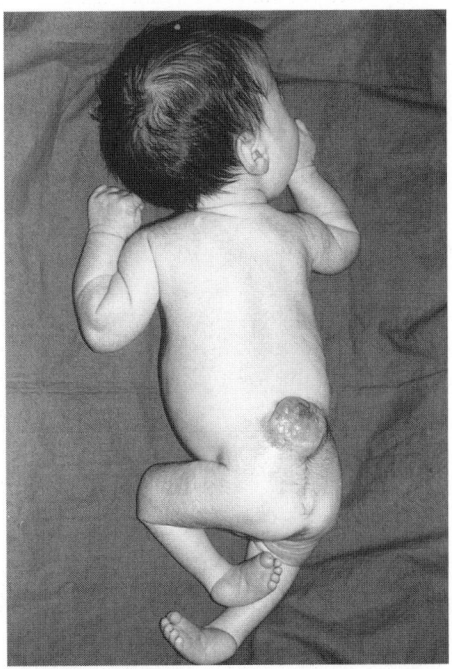

Figure 19.5 Lumbosacral meningomyelocoele.

abnormality is obvious at birth; clinical examination should assess the following features:

1 *Site of lesion.* About 70% are lumbosacral.

2 *Covering of sac.* Usually meninges, but occasionally the sac is ruptured, leading to CSF leakage and consequent risk of meningitis.

3 *Clinical assessment*:

(a) motor loss – this is generally lower motor neuron in type and the extent depends on the site of the lesion;

(b) sensory loss – this depends on the position of the lesion, and the level is often asymmetrical;

(c) neurogenic bladder – the patient usually dribbles urine constantly and has a distended expressible bladder;

(d) patulous anal tone.

4 *Hydrocephalus.* Ninety percent of infants with meningomyelocoeles have an associated abnormality of the brain and skull base, referred to as the Arnold–Chiari type II malformation. This includes prolapse of the medulla, cerebellum and fourth ventricle through an abnormal foramen magnum into the cervical canal. Not all infants develop hydrocephalus, but most have ventricular dilatation on ultrasound scans. Progressive enlargement of the head may occur with advancing age;

5 *Orthopaedic abnormalities.* These are common and include talipes, dislocated hips, kyphosis, scoliosis and contractures of the lower limbs.

6 *Miscellaneous abnormalities.* These include renal, cardiac and visceral defects and chromosome disorders.

Investigations

The neural arches of the vertebrae are poorly mineralized at birth, and spinal radiography is of little value except for the assessment of scoliosis. Ultrasound examination of the spine in the newborn period allows visualization of the spinal cord: if it does not move with respiration, this suggests that there may be tethering.

Management

With antenatal diagnosis at 17–19 weeks' gestation in the majority of cases a paradigm shift in decision-making has occurred from the neonatal period to this gestational stage. A careful assessment of the newborn infant by appropriate specialists is necessary

before a definite treatment plan can be formulated. Treatment is always discussed with the parents, whose wishes should be considered. Many centres use Lorber's (1971) criteria for conservative treatment. Lorber followed a large number of babies with meningomyelocoele during the period when all babies were energetically treated, and identified the following bad prognostic criteria:

1 total paralysis of the legs;

2 thoracolumbar or thoracolumbosacral lesions;

3 severe kyphoscoliosis;

4 hydrocephalus at birth;

5 other major congenital malformations, e.g. Down syndrome, congenital heart lesion.

If one or more of these features are present at birth, he recommended conservative management. This consists of nursing care only, but does not rule out subsequent reappraisal of the need for neurosurgery.

If active treatment is indicated, the following approach would be adopted:

1 *Early neurosurgery.* Closure of the sac within 24 h of birth, with ongoing assessment for hydrocephalus and insertion of a ventriculoperitoneal shunt, if indicated.

2 *Orthopaedic assessment and treatment* as necessary.

3 *General surgical treatment.* Urinary incontinence is a major problem, and girls usually require an ileal conduit, whereas boys may be managed at least initially with a penile collecting system or intermittent catheterization. The aim of treating faecal incontinence is to produce a firm stool to prevent soiling and faecal impaction.

4 *Supportive care.* Pressure sores need to be prevented by careful positioning and skin care. Psychological and social problems are common and parents need careful support and counselling. Schooling and employment also present difficult problems.

5 *Genetic counselling.* This will be necessary for future pregnancies.

Screening for neural tube defects

There are two main aspects of screening for NTDs:

1 α-*Fetoprotein* (*AFP*). Blood is taken from the mother at 14–18 weeks' gestation and the level of AFP is measured. AFP in the first trimester normally increases with gestational age, and an accurate assessment of the duration of pregnancy is essential in assessing the significance of the AFP level. Those women with high serum levels should have repeat samples taken 1 week later. Only 10% of pregnancies complicated by a high serum AFP level are associated with NTDs. Multiple pregnancies, exomphalos and other abnormalities may cause high levels. AFP is raised in 90% of cases of anencephaly, and in most cases of open myelomeningocoele. A skin-covered lesion will not have raised levels.

2 *Ultrasound screening.* Various abnormalities are assessed, including careful examination of the lower spine for a skin defect and examination of the skull base for the 'banana' sign (a feature of the Arnold–Chiari malformation) or a 'lemon' sign involving the frontal bones.

Disorders of ventral induction

Holoprosencephaly

This is a rare condition where there is a failure of midline fusion of the CNS, resulting in a single cerebral vesicle. There may also be midline defects of the eyes, lips and palate. Chromosome analysis should be carried out, as half of these lesions are associated with abnormal chromosomal patterns, most often trisomy 13 or 18. The prognosis for normal development is hopeless.

Holoprosencephaly may present as complete alobar forms or as partial forms, referred to as lobar or semilobar, and the diagnosis is made on ultrasound or computed tomography (CT) examination. The appearances of agenesis of the corpus callosum and septo-optic dysplasia may be confused with holoprosencephaly if care is not taken. If septo-optic dysplasia is suspected assessment of the baby's vision and hypothalamic/pituitary function should be made.

Microcephaly

Microcephaly occurs as the result of a variety of brain insults. It is defined as an occipitofrontal head circumference more than two standard deviations below the mean for the infant's gestational age. The child may show microcephaly in proportion to his or her weight and length (generalized growth restriction), or more ominously have a small head but a normally grown body. Microcephaly may be primary or secondary. Secondary microcephaly implies normal growth up to a point when a major insult has occurred, after which brain growth fails. Table 19.3 lists various causes of microcephaly.

The underlying cause should be diagnosed and treated wherever possible. The prognosis is usually poor and treatment is supportive.

Craniostenosis (craniosynostosis)

In this condition the skull sutures fuse prematurely, with resultant cranial distortions (Fig. 19.6). The

Table 19.3 Causes of primary and secondary microcephaly

Primary	Secondary
Familial	Intrauterine growth retardation
Autosomal recessive	Meningitis
X-linked recessive	Hypoglycaemia
Chromosomal	Asphyxia
Trisomy 13	Periventricular leukomalacia
Trisomy 18	
TORCH infections	
Maternal phenylketonuria	
Lissencephaly	
Fetal alcohol syndrome	

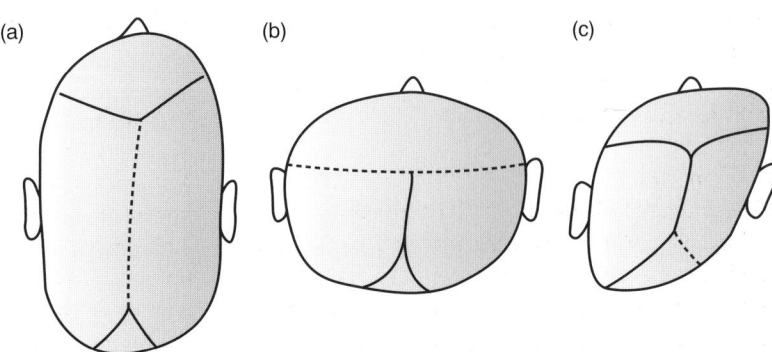

(a) (b) (c)

Figure 19.6 Premature suture closure leading to craniostenosis. (a) Scaphocephaly (sagittal suture); (b) turricephaly (coronal suture); and (c) plagiocephaly (single lambdoid suture).

most common form of craniostenosis is premature closure of the sagittal suture, giving a scaphocephalic head shape. Premature closure of the coronal suture leads to a turricephalic head, and closure of one lambdoid suture results in plagiocephaly (parallelogram-shaped head). Plagiocephaly also results from the baby lying on one side of the head with resultant distortion in shape. Autosomal dominantly inherited craniofacial deformities include:

1 Apert syndrome (acrocephalosyndactyly);
2 Crouzon syndrome (craniofacial dysostosis);
3 Carpenter syndrome (acrocephalopolysyndactyly).

Management
Skull X-rays are necessary to confirm the clinical suspicion. Surgery is indicated for cosmetic reasons or, rarely, if premature fusion of the sutures causes raised intracranial pressure.

Hydrocephalus

Hydrocephalus is caused by an imbalance between the production and the absorption of CSF, with resultant dilatation of the cerebral ventricles. Later a rapid increase in head size can occur as a result of progressive ventricular dilatation. The term 'hydrocephalus' has often been used inappropriately to describe an excessively large head without ventricular enlargement. The term megalencephaly is more appropriate under these circumstances. Babies can have considerable ventriculomegaly but, at least in the early stages, have normal head size.

Classification

Non-obstructive hydrocephalus
In this extremely rare type there is no interference with CSF flow. The excessive production of CSF is usually due to a papilloma of the choroid plexus.

Obstructive hydrocephalus (see Fig. 19.7 for site of obstruction)
Obstructive hydrocephalus can be divided into non-communicating and communicating.

Non-communicating. There is little or no communication between the ventricles and the subarachnoid space. There are three common sites of obstruction:
1 Aqueduct of Sylvius (due to stenosis or atresia).

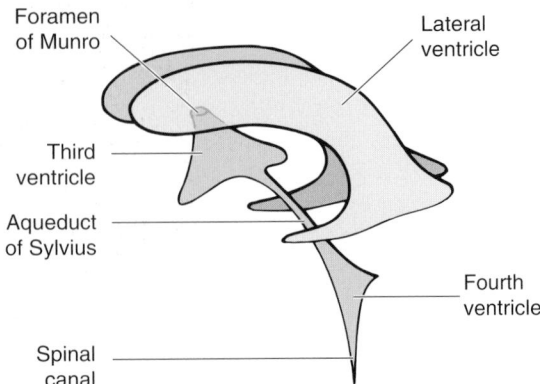

Figure 19.7 Diagram to show intracerebral drainage of cerebrospinal fluid. (Reproduced from Levene 1987, with permission of Churchill Livingstone.)

2 Occlusion of the foramina of Luschka and Magendie as a result of basal adhesions. This is the commonest site of blockage and is usually due to intraventricular haemorrhage.
3 Arnold–Chiari type II malformation secondary to spina bifida cystica.

Communicating. CSF can escape from the intracranial system via the foramina of Luschka and Magendie, but cannot be absorbed at the arachnoid granulations situated over the surface of the brain. This is usually due to arachnoiditis following either meningitis or intracranial haemorrhage (ICH). Ventricular dilatation occurring following intraventricular haemorrhage (IVH) is due to non-communicating causes in only 15%; in 85% of cases it is communicating.

Clinical features

Hydrocephalus due to congenital abnormalities may be present at birth or diagnosed *in utero* by ultrasound examination. Follow-up studies have shown that about 50% of babies born with apparently isolated fetal ventriculomegaly (no other congenital malformation detected) are normal. The prognosis is poor if the ventriculomegaly is associated with spina bifida.

Ventricular dilatation occurring after IVH can be detected by cranial ultrasound examinations (Fig. 19.8). Ventriculomegaly may be quite advanced before abnormal head growth is noted. A 'sunset'

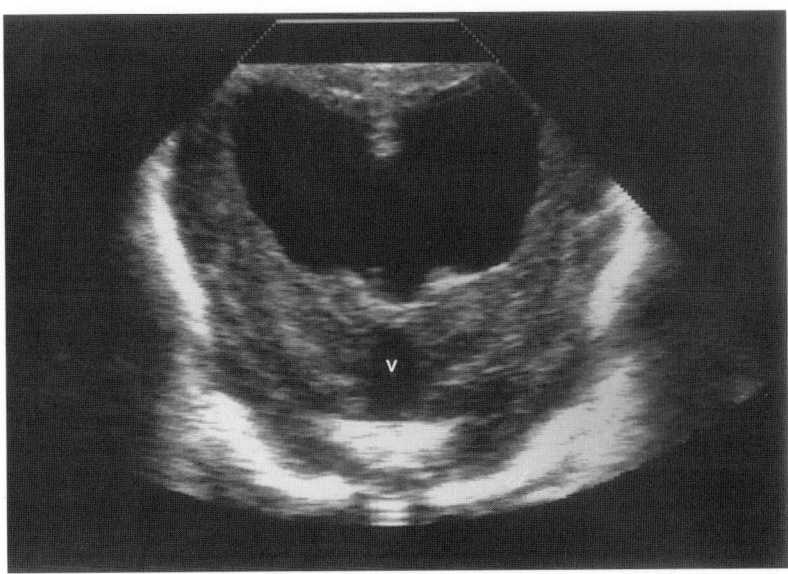

Figure 19.8 Coronal ultrasound scan showing massive dilatation of both lateral and third ventricles (v).

appearance of the eyes is a late sign in neonatal hydrocephalus and may be seen in infants without dilated ventricles.

Investigations

It is recommended that all infants with IVH have weekly ultrasound scans to detect ventricular dilatation. Accurate measurement of the occipito-frontal circumference at weekly intervals is essential in all infants, especially those with intracranial pathology.

Management

This depends on the underlying cause and the degree of ventriculomegaly.

Congenital hydrocephalus

If treatment of the general condition (e.g. spina bifida) is thought to be appropriate, then ventriculoperitoneal shunting is the treatment of choice. If the infant is unfit for surgery, then temporizing management is necessary by intermittent or continuous drainage of CSF from the ventricles.

Posthaemorrhagic ventricular dilatation

The management of posthaemorrhagic ventricular dilatation (PHVD) remains controversial. There is no convincing evidence that infants who develop ventricular dilatation following ICH are at markedly greater risk of adverse neurodevelopmental outcome than those with haemorrhage of the same size but without ventriculomegaly. It is the extent of the haemorrhage that carries the major adverse risk, rather than posthaemorrhagic hydrocephalus per se.

Research into the management of posthaemorrhagic hydrocephalus has not suggested that early or aggressive therapy is advantageous to the baby. The European multicentre study (Ventriculomegaly Study Group 1990) on the management of PHVD showed that early treatment (lumbar puncture taps) to prevent further ventriculomegaly gave no benefit in terms of reducing subsequent disability, compared with conservative treatment started when the head circumference exceeded the 97th centile. The use of acetazolamide and furosemide (frusemide) treatment in established posthaemorrhagic hydrocephalus is associated with a worse prognosis than babies not treated with these drugs. In the last five years, evaluation of the direct instillation of thrombolytic agents into the ventricles of babies with early posthaemorrhagic hydrocephalus has not been promising for the safe treatment of this condition.

The important factors in the management of PHVD are probably the extent of the initial haemorrhage and the intraventricular pressure.

A management protocol is as follows:

1 Twice weekly ultrasound measurement of ventricular size.

2 If there is progressive ventricular dilatation, then careful measurement of occipitofrontal head circumference should be performed on alternate days.

3 Measurement of CSF pressure if:

(a) there is a progressive increase in ventricular size on ultrasound to a point 4 mm above the normal ventricular index (Fig. 19.9);

(b) there is a progressive increase in occipitofrontal head circumference above the 97th centile;

(c) there are symptoms of raised intracranial pressure (apnoea, poor feeding, irritability, etc.).

CSF pressure can most safely be measured by lumbar puncture. Pressure is measured either by a fluid manometer and measuring the height of a column of CSF in cmH_2O, or by a non-fluid displacement technique by attaching a pressure transducer to the hub of the needle. Two important criteria must be applied to these measurements:

1 There is free flow of CSF. If less than 5 mL of fluid is obtained, it suggests that the obstruction is non-communicating and that the pressure can only be measured by ventricular tap.

2 The infant is lying quietly when the pressure measurement is made. If the infant is agitated or crying, the measurement is unreliable. Sometimes it will be necessary to sedate the infant to obtain accurate measurements.

In infants with non-communicating ventricular dilatation, or those who are very unstable and in whom the handling involved in lumbar puncture is unacceptable, ventricular tap is the alternative (see p. 312).

If the pressure is elevated (>10 cm H_2O, >7.5 mmHg), then further treatment is warranted. If the CSF protein is <1 g/L, then a ventriculoperitoneal shunt should be inserted. If the protein is >1 g/L, a ventricular reservoir or access device will be necessary to prevent the maintenance of raised intracranial pressure. This can later be converted to a shunt. Drug treatment for posthaemorrhagic hydrocephalus should be avoided.

Prognosis

Complications of surgery include shunt obstruction, ventriculitis and the need for shunt revision. The long-term outlook depends on the cause and severity of the hydrocephalus and any subsequent complications.

Hydranencephaly

In this condition there has been almost total loss of all cerebral substance owing to an early massive insult *in utero* such as a vascular insult, infection or trauma after the 12th week of pregnancy. There is usually sparing of the cerebellum and basal ganglia. The skull is entirely filled with fluid and at birth the head may be normal or enlarged. There is no treatment and the prognosis is hopeless.

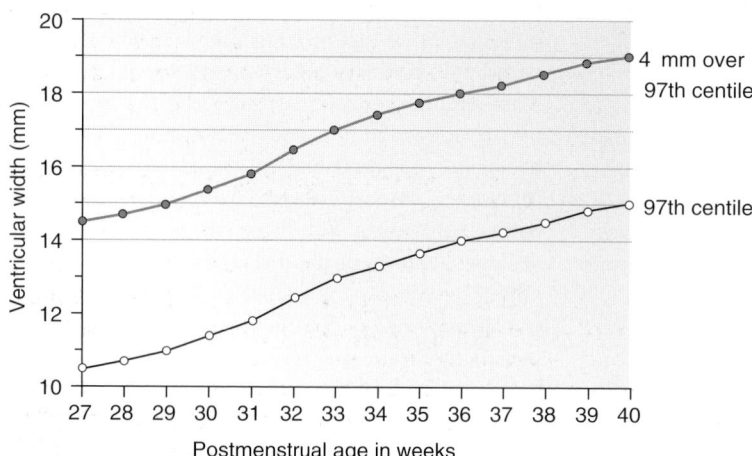

Figure 19.9 Indication for significant ventriculomegaly. The lower line is the 97th centile for normal ventricular size. The upper line defines ventricular dilatation severe enough to require treatment.

Porencephaly

Porencephaly is the name given to cystic cavities in one or both cerebral hemispheres, which may or may not communicate with the lateral ventricles. They can be congenital or acquired following meningitis, ICH or cerebral atrophy. The commonest cause is following an intraparenchymal haemorrhage (see p. 216).

Diagnosis is made by ultrasound or magnetic resonance imaging (MRI) examination. Rarely 'expanding porencephaly syndrome' is seen, in which the porencephalic cavity progressively enlarges. This may require ventriculoperitoneal shunting.

Lissencephaly

This is an abnormality of neuronal migration and may be due to an intrauterine viral infection, or vascular or asphyxial insult that occurs in the first half of pregnancy. The brain appears smooth and is often accompanied by microcephaly. Lissencephaly is usually associated with dysmorphic features and neonatal convulsions that are very difficult to control. It may also be due to a genetic disorder, including Miller–Dieker syndrome and Walker–Warburg syndrome.

Intracranial haemorrhage (ICH)

ICH in the newborn is a common finding at autopsy, and 70% of infants who die have evidence of some degree of ICH. Subdural haemorrhage, which 50 years ago was the most common type of ICH, is now rare, and intraventricular haemorrhage (IVH) has replaced it as the commonest ICH seen in the newborn infant. There are five important types of neonatal ICH:

1 subarachnoid;
2 subdural;
3 intraventricular;
4 intracerebral;
5 intracerebellar.

Subarachnoid haemorrhage (SAH)

Blood in the subarachnoid space is most commonly secondary to IVH, which tracks through the ventricular system.

Primary subarachnoid haemorrhage (SAH) is a common, and usually benign, condition and is seen in both premature and full-term infants. It occurs as a response to hypoxia or trauma, and is usually seen as a discrete area over the convexity of the brain.

Clinical features

SAH is usually asymptomatic, but when symptoms do occur seizures and apnoea are most commonly seen in full-term infants on the second day of life. Between seizures the infant is usually neurologically normal.

Diagnosis

Ultrasound is very unreliable in detecting SAH, and CT or magnetic resonance imaging (MRI) are much more sensitive for this diagnosis. The CSF is usually heavily bloodstained and does not clear in successive tubes.

Prognosis

A good prognosis can be given if there are minimal neurological signs in the neonatal period and if the predisposing traumatic or hypoxic injury is mild.

In approximately 90% of cases infants with seizures as the primary manifestation of the haemorrhage are normal on follow-up. Rarely the patient dies or is left with serious neurological sequelae, such as hydrocephalus, which presents weeks to months after the initial insult.

Treatment

There is no specific treatment. Bleeding disorders should be excluded and, if present, treated appropriately (see Chapter 18). Shunting for posthaemorrhagic hydrocephalus may rarely be required.

Subdural haemorrhage

Subdural haematoma was formerly relatively common but now rarely causes encephalopathy owing to a reduced incidence of birth trauma associated with a reduction in the use of high and mid-cavity forceps deliveries, fewer prolonged labours and a concurrent increase in caesarean section births. It is classically due to rapid changes in head shape during labour and delivery. More frequent use of brain imaging has shown that clinically insignificant, relatively small subdural haemorrhages are a common feature of babies born by vacuum extraction.

Pathogenesis

There are three basic origins of subdural haemorrhage:

1 tentorial laceration with rupture of the straight sinus, resulting in an infratentorial haematoma;

2 falx cerebri laceration and rupture of the inferior sagittal sinus, giving rise to a haematoma of the longitudinal cerebral fissure;

3 rupture of superficial cerebral veins with a subdural haematoma over the temporal lobe – usually unilateral and accompanied by subarachnoid blood.

Predisposing factors

Several predisposing factors have been established:

1 Rigid birth canal – primipara, elderly multipara, small pelvis.

2 Infant with large head.

3 Labour – precipitous, prolonged.

4 Presentation – breech, foot, face, brow.

5 Delivery – difficult forceps, difficult rotation.

6 Vacuum extraction.

Clinical features

Subdural haematomas may present as a recognizable symptom complex including tense fontanelle, hypotonia, lethargy and facial palsy. If the haemorrhage involves the posterior fossa, then apnoea, irregular sighing respiration, fixed bradycardia, opisthotonus and skew deviation of the eyes may occur. If there is only a minor haemorrhage, the baby may be asymptomatic. Signs of hydrocephalus may develop. Asymptomatic subdural haemorrhage is increasingly recognized by increased use of MR imaging.

Investigations

Subdural haemorrhage over the brain convexity or associated with tentorial tears may be seen on ultrasound, particularly if large. A midline shift may be the only clue to a convexity subdural collection. A CT/MRI scan is more sensitive for diagnosis than ultrasound.

Treatment

In convexity subdural haemorrhage, subdural taps through the anterior fontanelle under strict aseptic conditions are necessary. Repeated taps may be required (see p. 312). Neurosurgical evacuation of thrombus is rarely required.

Intraventricular haemorrhage (IVH)

IVH is a description of blood within the ventricular system and may be due to:

1 germinal matrix haemorrhage; or

2 choroid plexus haemorrhage – this is usually a relatively benign condition occurring in an asphyxiated full-term infant.

IVH is usually assumed to have arisen from the rupture of capillaries within the germinal matrix of the caudate nucleus. The condition occurs in premature infants and its incidence is approximately 33% in infants of birthweight 1500 g or below. In some infants the bleeding may be massive, with involvement of the cerebral parenchyma (Fig. 19.10). The initial bleeding occurs into the germinal matrix (also called the subependymal plate), which lies over the head of the caudate nucleus. The germinal matrix is present between 24 and 34 weeks

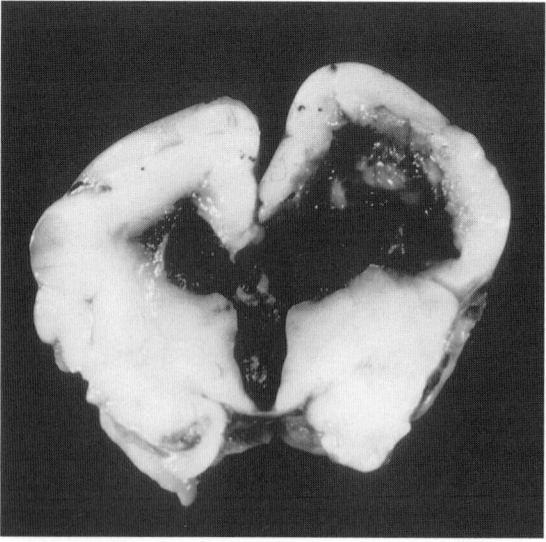

Figure 19.10 Bilateral intraventricular haemorrhage with massive parenchymal extension into the right hemisphere.

of gestation and rapidly involutes after this time. Rupture into the ventricles (hence the term IVH) occurs in 80% of cases of germinal matrix haemorrhage. Rarely IVH is seen in full-term infants. Changes in cerebral blood flow probably precipitate the bleeding, and infants with respiratory distress syndrome (RDS) are most likely to have an unstable cerebral circulation. The following are the most important clinical features associated with IVH:

1 prematurity;
2 RDS;
3 intermittent positive-pressure ventilation;
4 hypercapnia;
5 metabolic acidosis;
6 birth outside a perinatal centre;
7 coagulation disorder.

Clincial features

1 *Minimal signs.* Approximately 60% of infants with IVH have no major clinical symptoms. Neurological examination (see p. 31) reveals subtle changes in tone, including a tight popliteal angle, and roving eye movements (slow nystagmus) for some weeks after the haemorrhage has occurred.

2 *Intermittent deterioration* over a period of days, with increasing signs of apnoea, bradycardia, metabolic acidosis and seizures.

3 *Massive collapse* with neurological signs (seizures, coma), shock and anaemia. This is a rare clinical presentation and is more likely to occur as the result of other neonatal complications, including infection and respiratory complications.

Diagnosis

Real-time ultrasound is the method of choice. There is no generally agreed method for grading the severity of IVH. The two most commonly used schemes are outlined below:

Grade 1 – subependymal and/or minimal IVH (Fig. 19.11);

Grade 2 – intraventricular clot within the lateral ventricle;

Grade 3 – intraparenchymal involvement. This is usually unilateral and occurs as a result of venous infarction. In this case the intraventricular clot reduces venous drainage in the periventricular white matter of one hemisphere, causing stasis

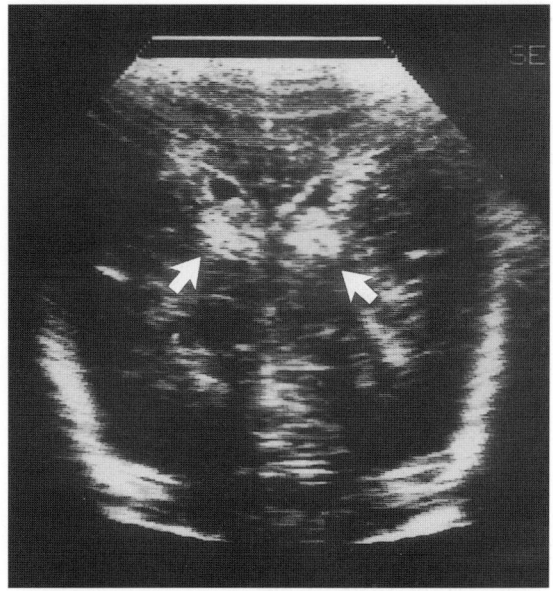

Figure 19.11 Coronal ultrasound scan showing bilateral haemorrhage in the region of the germinal matrix (arrowed).

with infarction (periventricular haemorrhagic infarction). If the parenchymal 'haemorrhage' is bilateral, then it is more likely to be due to bleeding into a primary ischaemic area of the brain, and this is referred to as *periventricular leukomalacia (PVL)* (see below).

The second scheme is called the Papile classification:

Grade 1 – subependymal germinal matrix haemorrhage;

Grade 2 – IVH with no ventricular dilatation;

Grade 3 – IVH with ventricle distended by blood;

Grade 4 – intraparenchymal haemorrhage.

Complications

There are two main complications of IVH:

1 PHVD – this occurs in approximately 25% of infants with IVH (see 'Hydrocephalus' above).

2 Porencephaly (see p. 215).

Treatment

There is no specific treatment once IVH has occurred. Careful attention to respiratory management, coagulation disturbances and blood pressure is important in ill infants in an attempt to reduce the likelihood of IVH.

Prevention

A variety of drugs have been evaluated to assess their effectiveness in preventing IVH when given shortly after birth. Only two, indometacin (indomethacin) and etamsylate (ethamsylate), have been shown on the basis of randomized controlled trials to reduce the incidence and severity of IVH. There is no convincing evidence that these drugs reduce adverse outcome in survivors. In our view the currently available evidence suggests that no drug should be routinely administered to very premature babies to reduce the incidence of IVH.

Intracerebral haemorrhage

In 80% of cases this is due to venous infarction secondary to IVH or to rebleeding into periventricular ischaemic areas of the brain. Other causes of primary intracerebral haemorrhage include:
1 coagulation disturbances;
2 cerebral artery occlusion;
3 TORCH (toxoplasmosis, other, rubella, cytomegalovirus, herpes simplex type II) infection;
4 thalamic haemorrhage;
5 arteriovenous malformation (very rare);
6 tumour (very rare).

Diagnosis is made by ultrasound examination or CT/MRI.

Intracerebellar haemorrhage

This type of haemorrhage occurs in about 5% of preterm infants. It may be due to hypoxic insults, a traumatic breech delivery or head compression. No treatment is available and cerebellar hypoplasia may develop in surviving infants.

Periventricular leukomalacia (PVL)

Periventricular leukomalacia literally means softening of the white matter around the ventricles, and if severe is a major risk factor for the subsequent development of cerebral palsy. It is due to damage to the developing oligodendroglial cells inhabiting the periventricular white matter during the vulnerable period between 26 and 34 weeks of gestation.

Causes

It used to be thought that cerebral underperfusion of the periventricular white matter, as occurs in neonatal hypotension, is the cause of PVL because of the potential vascular watershed at an immature gestation, but more modern studies have shown this proposal to be unlikely. A number of associated factors are correlated with the development of PVL and these include:
1 Twin-to-twin transfusion syndrome (p. 268).
2 Maternal chorioamnionitis. It is now recognized that infection of the fetal membranes or the fetoplacental unit releases inflammatory proteins called cytokines, which are neurotoxic to the immature brain. There is currently no known way of protecting the fetal/neonatal brain from the effects of cytokine release.
3 Severe fetal asphyxia (e.g. massive placental abruption, cord prolapse).
4 Complications of severe neonatal lung disease such as tension pneumothorax.
5 Hypocarbia. Studies have shown a consistent association between severe and probably prolonged hypocarbia (low P_{CO_2} <3 kPa) and the development of PVL. It is important to avoid hypocarbia by appropriate blood gas monitoring with changes to mechanical ventilator settings. Marked fluctuations in P_{CO_2} are most likely during transport and following surfactant instillation.
6 Necrotizing enterocolitis (this may be due to cytokine release).
7 Postnatal dexamethasone administration for chronic lung disease if given in the first 96 hours of life (Halliday *et al.* 2003).

Diagnosis

Diagnosis is made by real-time ultrasound, which initially shows areas of echodensity in the white matter; these may resolve spontaneously or progress to cystic degeneration after 10–21 days. Multiple cavities or cavities in the occipital region are known to carry a high risk of less severe cerebral palsy, and small or single cavities predispose the baby to a greater risk of adverse outcome. The prognosis for babies who show persistent echodensity ('flare') is uncertain. More subtle white matter damage may be detected on MRI, and this may not be evident on ultrasound, but the clinical significance of these lesions is probably negligible.

Neonatal convulsions

The terms 'convulsion', 'fit' and 'seizure' are used interchangeably to describe clinically evident, episodic events occurring in the neonatal period and arising from a brain disorder. The incidence of neonatal seizures is 5–8/1000 live-born infants. It may be difficult to decide whether movements made by the sick neonate are abnormal or not. In addition, jitteriness must be distinguished from the infant having convulsions. Table 19.4 lists important differences between these two conditions:

1 *Irritability*. This is due to CNS depression and the infant behaves in an abnormal manner, lying quietly until disturbed, when he or she cries excessively. The cry may be high pitched, the baby is difficult to console and takes longer to settle than normal.

2 *Jitteriness*. The jittery infant shows exaggerated responses to stimuli, with an exaggerated startle to noise or handling, and has exaggerated fine tremulous movements.

The essential difference between irritability and jitteriness is that the former is non-stimulus sensitive, whereas the latter occurs in response to minor stimulation.

Seizure type

The five basic descriptive types of convulsions in the newborn are subtle, tonic, multifocal clonic, focal clonic and myoclonic. The preterm infant with a less well-organized immature CNS is more likely to show subtle convulsions.

Subtle

These may be difficult to distinguish from jitteriness. There are a number of recognized types:

1 horizontal deviation of the eyes with or without jerking;

2 chewing or sucking movements;

3 bicycling movements;

Table 19.4 Important features in distinguishing the jittery infant from one who is having convulsions

	Jitteriness	Convulsions
Stimulus provoked	Yes	No
Predominant movement	Rapid, oscillatory	Clonic, tonic
Movements cease when limb is held	Yes	No
Conscious state	Awake or asleep	Altered
Eye deviation	No	Yes

4 rhythmic or dancing movements of the eyes;

5 apnoea, which may be the only feature of seizures.

Tonic

Tonic convulsions are characterized by extensor spasms of the trunk and limbs with opisthotonic posturing. They may occur predominantly in preterm infants.

Multifocal clonic

These involve a non-ordered progression of clonic movements of the limbs. They occur predominantly in term infants.

Focal clonic

Well-localized clonic jerking of a limb or jaw is seen with the focal clonic type. They are sometimes associated with a convexity haemorrhage (e.g. subdural).

Myoclonic jerks

Occasional myoclonic jerks may be normal in the newborn but multiple myoclonic jerks are usually pathological. They may be difficult to distinguish from jitteriness.

Electroconvulsive dissociation (ECD)

With the introduction of more clinical cotside continuous monitoring of brain electrical function, referred to as 'cerebral function monitoring' (CFM) or 'amplitude integrated EEG' (aEEG), it has become apparent that the correlation between abnormal clinical movements and electrical abnormalities is often poor. This is referred to as electroconvulsive dissociation. ECD becomes more apparent after

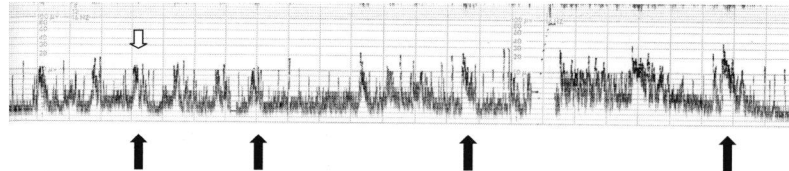

Figure 19.12 Trace from a cerebral function monitor. There are frequent electroconvulsive seizures (one indicated by white arrow). The clinically evident seizures are marked with black arrows showing electroconvulsive dissociation.

treatment with antiepileptic drugs (see below). CFM or aEEG is increasingly used in neonatal units to determine whether apparently abnormal movements are due to cortical seizure activity. Figure 19.12 shows an example of ECD. Whether all electroconvulsive seizures require drug treatment is controversial and is discussed below.

Aetiology

The major causes of neonatal convulsions depend on the time of onset and whether the infant is term or preterm. Table 19.5 lists the more common causes of neonatal seizures and indicates their time of onset.

Perinatal asphyxia

This accounts for 50% of cases and is the commonest cause of neonatal seizures. Such seizures usually present on the first day of life as subtle in type, progressing to multifocal clonic and tonic seizures. They usually improve and cease within 4–5 days. Status epilepticus may occur with severe hypoxic ischaemic encephalopathy. This condition is discussed fully in Chapter 3.

Intracranial haemorrhage

All types of ICH may present with fits. The infant who convulses as a result of SAH usually appears to be neurologically normal between fits. Seizures secondary to cerebral contusion, especially a convexity subdural or subarachnoid collection, may exhibit predominantly focal features. All full-term infants with convulsions should have an ultrasound scan to exclude this as the cause.

Infections

Intracranial bacterial and non-bacterial infections account for a significant number of neonatal

Table 19.5 Causes of neonatal convulsions indicating whether they occur early or late. The overall frequency of convulsions is indicated by the number of '+' signs shown

	Time of onset and relative frequency	
	0–2 days	2–10 days
Asphyxia	+++	−
Intracranial haemorrhage	++	+
Hypocalcaemia	++	+
Hypoglycaemia	++	+
Infection	+	++
Developmental abnormalities	+	+
Drug withdrawal	+	
Inborn errors of metabolism	+	+
Pyridoxine deficiency	++	
Fifth-day fits	−	++

convulsions. The most common infecting organisms are the Gram-negative bacilli, group B β-haemolytic streptococcus and the TORCH group.

Drug withdrawal (narcotics and barbiturates)

Over 65% of the babies of opioid-dependent women will show withdrawal symptoms in the first 3–5 days after birth. Symptoms of the neonatal abstinence syndrome include irritability, hypertonia, tremors and hyperactivity in over 70% of affected infants. Convulsions occur in less than 10% of cases. Other common symptoms include yawning, snuffliness, sweating, sneezing, diarrhoea, vomiting and poor feeding.

Management of the drug-addicted infant is discussed in Chapter 14 (p. 146).

Crack cocaine is becoming a commonly abused drug in pregnancy. It may cause fetal cerebral artery infarction, with resultant neonatal convulsions.

Metabolic

Derangements of electrolytes such as hypocalcaemia, hypomagnesaemia, hyponatraemia and hypernatraemia as well as hypoglycaemia and hyperbilirubinaemia may cause convulsions.

Inborn errors of metabolism

These are individually very rare and include maplesyrup urine disease, urea cycle defects, organic acidaemias and galactosaemia. They often present once the baby is on full milk feeds and there may be a family history. Screening investigations when inborn errors of metabolism are suspected include urinary amino acids and organic acids, serum lactate and ammonia.

Pyridoxine deficiency

This is very rare but must be considered where there is a history of very early convulsions and where the convulsions are resistant to standard anticonvulsant medication.

Fifth-day fits

This is almost certainly not a single entity, but rather a group of benign conditions with unrecognized causes. The baby develops seizures on the fourth or fifth day of life, and these are self-limiting. Between seizures the infant appears to be entirely normal. The diagnosis is made by excluding other causes for the convulsions.

Diagnosis

Newborn infants with convulsions need a diagnostic evaluation, consisting of a careful history and examination and laboratory investigations. It is unusual not to find a cause for the convulsions as idiopathic epilepsy rarely, if ever, commences in the newborn period.

An approach to diagnosis is:
1 *History*. Family history of neonatal convulsions, maternal drug ingestion, antenatal and intrapartum infections, perinatal asphyxia, birth trauma.

2 *Examination*. Developmental anomalies, signs of sepsis.
3 *Metabolic*. Test for hypoglycaemia. Blood is obtained for assay of calcium, magnesium, phosphate and sodium.
4 *Lumbar puncture*. Meningitis, haemorrhage.
5 *Septic work-up and TORCH serology*. Meningitis, encephalitis.
6 *Ultrasound scan of the brain*. Intracranial haemorrhage, developmental anomalies of the brain.

Additional investigations include:
1 urinary and serum amino acids;
2 urine for organic acids;
3 serum lactate;
4 serum ammonia;
5 galactose-1-phosphate uridyl transferase activity.

Treatment

Specific treatment

The underlying cause of the convulsion is treated if possible.

Hypoglycaemia If the infant is hypoglycaemic (see p. 158), 25% dextrose (2 mL/kg) should be given intravenously followed by an infusion of 10% dextrose.

Hypocalcaemia If serum calcium is less than 1.5 mmol/L, the baby is given 200 mg/kg of 10% calcium gluconate intravenously with electrocardiogram (ECG) monitoring. If convulsions are recalcitrant to calcium and the serum magnesium level is low, 50–100 mg/kg of 50% magnesium sulphate heptahydrate should be administered by slow intravenous infusion under ECG control.

Asphyxia This is discussed fully in Chapter 3.

Infection The management of meningitis is discussed in Chapter 7.

Inborn errors of metabolism Exchange transfusion may be helpful in some cases, and megavitamin therapy is also recommended (Wraith 2001).

Anticonvulsant drug treatment

Before considering drug treatment it is necessary to ask whether convulsions are just a marker of existing brain damage or whether the seizures in their own right cause additional neuronal injury. Recent animal studies support the notion that short but frequent seizures do cause both additional structural and functional brain damage. This swings the pendulum towards more aggressive management with antiepileptic drugs (see Levene 2002 for review).

In neonatal practice, treatment of neonatal convulsions is often unsuccessful in abolishing all seizure activity apparent either clinically or on EEG monitoring. A randomized controlled trial showed that EEG seizures were abolished in less than 50% of babies given either phenytoin or phenobarbitone separately, and when both drugs were used together seizures were stopped in only 59% of cases. Infants with the least severe electrical seizures were the ones who responded to treatment best (Painter *et al.* 1999).

In practice, frequent or prolonged seizures should be aggressively treated but drug treatment in babies with severe seizure activity is often only partially successful. It is also known that high-dose antiepileptic drugs in the newborn are toxic and may also cause neuronal injury or apoptosis. A sensible approach to management is required with no more than three drugs being used at any one time.

First-line anticonvulsant therapy is with intravenous phenobarbitone (20 mg/kg) loading dose with a further 10 mg/kg for persistent seizures. If the baby continues to have seizures then phenytoin (20 mg/kg) should be given by slow intravenous infusion. Third-line anticonvulsant management is with midazolam infusion (150–200 µg/kg i.v. followed by continuous infusion of 1–5 µg/kg/min). Lidocaine by continuous infusion is becoming more widely used for resistant seizures but must not be used if phenytoin has been given previously because of the possibility of cardiotoxic effects.

Stopping anticonvulsant drugs
Only about 10% of babies with neonatal seizures will have convulsions in the first year of life after discharge from the hospital. It is therefore advisable to stop all anticonvulsant medication in the newborn, provided the baby is showing no abnormal neurological signs.

Prognosis

The prognosis for infants who have had neonatal convulsions depends on the underlying cause. A summary of the outcome following neonatal convulsions is given in Table 19.6.

Neonatal hypotonia ('floppy infant')

There are a large number of causes of neonatal hypotonia (see Mercuri *et al.* 2001 for review). Hypotonia is a very significant symptom and should never be ignored. Generalized floppiness may be due to abnormalities in a variety of anatomical sites:
1 brain (asphyxia);
2 spinal cord (trauma);
3 anterior horn cell (spinal muscular atrophy);
4 nerve root (brachial plexus injury) – this causes hypotonia only of the affected limb;
5 peripheral nerve (trauma);
6 neuromuscular junction (myasthenia gravis);
7 muscle (congenital dystrophy).

Clinical features

These infants are lethargic, show little movement and lie in the classic 'frog' posture with the hips abducted and external rotation of the limbs (Fig. 19.13). This posture must be differentiated from the normal posture of a preterm infant.

Table 19.6 The chance of normal outcome depending on the cause of the neonatal seizure

Cause of seizures	Chance of normal development (%)
Hypoxic-ischaemic encephalopathy	50
Subarachnoid haemorrhage	90
Other intracranial haemorrhage	50
Hypoglycaemia	50
Hypocalcaemia	90
Bacterial meningitis	20–50
Developmental abnormality	0
Fifth-day fits	100
Idiopathic	75

There are two main groups of infants in this category:

1 *Non-paralytic:* weak infant with hypotonia and normal muscles, e.g. cerebral hypoxia. (This form may progress to cerebral palsy with increased tone.)

2 *Paralytic:* weak infant with hypotonia and muscular disease, e.g. spinal muscle atrophy (Werdnig–Hoffmann disease).

The two groups can be distinguished by the ability of the infant to move his or her limbs against gravity, either spontaneously or following a stimulus. The paralytic infant is unable to maintain the posture of an elevated limb, and has a poverty of spontaneous movement. Table 19.7 lists causes of paralytic and non-paralytic hypotonia.

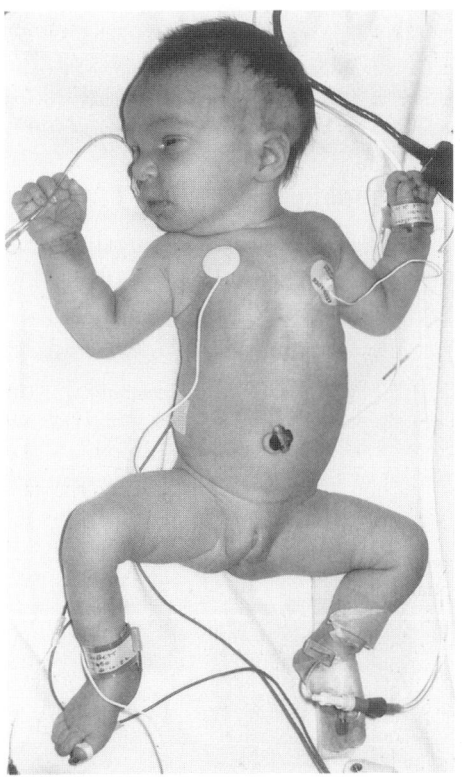

Figure 19.13 An infant with severe hypotonia showing the characteristic 'frog' posture.

Spinal muscular atrophy (Werdnig–Hoffmann disease)

This is caused by an abnormality of the anterior horn cells in the spinal cord and is an autosomal recessive disorder. The infant presents with profound weakness and hypotonia, although the face is usually striking by its expressiveness because the facial muscles are not involved. Congenital contractures are sometimes present. Diagnosis is made by muscle biopsy. There is no treatment and the infant dies before the first birthday.

Myasthenia gravis

Ninety percent of cases of myasthenia gravis occur as a result of maternal disease but are transient and last 6–12 weeks, with complete recovery. Rarely a congenital form occurs without maternal disease. Infants show intermittent hypotonia responsive to Tensilon or neostigmine (0.5 mg/kg).

Congenital muscular dystrophy

A condition of unknown cause but inherited as an autosomal recessive disorder, this may present in the newborn period with generalized hypotonia; the infant is often born with severe contractures. The prognosis may be reasonably good, as improvement in the weakness may occur. Diagnosis is by muscle biopsy.

Table 19.7 Causes of hypotonia in the newborn

Paralytic	Non-paralytic
Spinal muscular atrophy (Werdnig–Hoffmann)	Birth asphyxia
Congenital muscular dystrophy	Down syndrome
Congenital myopathy	Prader–Willi syndrome
Congenital myotonic dystrophy	Skeletal and connective tissue disorders
Myasthenia gravis	Drugs
	Benign congenital hypotonia

Congenital myotonic dystrophy

This a genetic disorder due to chromosomal triplet repeat expansion (p. 150), but the mother is the affected parent in 90% of cases of neonatal disease. The mothers of all floppy infants should be screened for clinical evidence of myotonia or weakness (inability to close the eyelids tightly and bury her eyelashes).

Benign congenital hypotonia

This is a diagnosis of exclusion and cannot be made in the neonatal period. Prader–Willi syndrome needs to be excluded.

Investigations

In all infants with significant weakness or hypotonia the following investigations should be performed:

1 Creatinine phosphokinase (CPK). This is often high in the first week of life in normal children. Only in blood taken after 2 weeks of life are high levels of CPK of clinical significance.
2 Electromyography.
3 Motor nerve conduction velocities.
4 Muscle biopsy, only if the pathology department has adequate facilities for sophisticated histochemical staining techniques.

Prognosis

This depends on the underlying cause of the hypotonia. In many cases the prognosis is poor and for this reason establishing a reliable histological diagnosis is very important.

References

Halliday HL, Ehrenkrantz RA, Doyle LW. Early postnatal (<96 hours) corticosteroids for preventing chronic lung disease in preterm infants (review). *Cochrane Database of Systematic Reviews* 2003, Issue 1: Art No CD001146.

International PHVD Drug Trial Group. International randomised controlled trial of acetazolamide and furosemide in posthaemorrhagic ventricular dilatation in infancy. *Lancet* 1998;**352**:433–440.

Kaiser A, Whitelaw A. Cerebrospinal fluid pressure in infants with post-haemorrhagic ventricular dilatation. *Arch Dis Child* 1985;**46**:783–787.

Levene M. The clinical conundrum of neonatal seizures. *Arch/Dis Child Fetal Ed.* 2002;**86**:F75–77.

Lorber J. Results of treatment of myelomeningocoele. *Dev Med Child Neurol* 1971;**13**:279–289.

Mercuri E, Heckmatt J, Dubowitz V. Neuromuscular disorders. In: *Fetal and Neonatal Neurology and Neurosurgery* (senior eds MI Levene, FA Chervenak, M Whittle), pp. 709–726. Edinburgh: Churchill Livingstone, 2001.

Painter MJ, Scher MS, Stein AD *et al.* Phenobarbital compared with phenytoin for the treatment of neonatal seizures. *N Engl J Med* 1999;**341**:485–489.

Ventriculomegaly Study Group. Randomised trial of early tapping in neonatal posthaemorrhagic ventricular dilatation. *Arch Dis Child* 1990;**65**:3–10.

Further reading

Levene MI, Chervenak FA, Whittle M. *Fetal and Neonatal Neurology and Neurosurgery*, 4th edn. Edinburgh: Churchill Livingstone, 2008.

Volpe JJ. *Neurology of the Newborn*, 4th edn. Philadelphia: W.B. Saunders, 2001.

Wraith JW. Inborn errors of metabolism, postnatal diagnosis and management. In: *Fetal and Neonatal Neurology and Neurosurgery* 4th edn. (eds) MI Levene, F Chervenak London: Churchill Livingstone, 2008.

20 The special senses: hearing and vision

Profound hearing and visual impairments are major causes of severe disability arising from the neonatal period. Assessment of both hearing and vision in infants is usually possible before the child leaves the neonatal unit, and early diagnosis is essential for optimal management of any deficiencies.

Hearing impairment

The importance of early diagnosis in hearing-impaired children is obvious, as appropriate sound amplification and the provision of specialized educational facilities will enable the deaf child to realize his or her maximal potential. Speech in deaf children is much better if hearing aids are fitted in the first 6 months of life.

Hearing impairment takes one of the following forms:

1 *Conductive*. This involves abnormalities of the external auditory meatus, the tympanic membrane or the ossicles within the middle ear. This can rarely be congenital if the meatus has not yet canalized, but much more commonly it is due to infection or serous exudate within the middle ear.

2 *Sensorineural*. Abnormalities or damage to the cochlea or brainstem nuclei cause 'nerve' deafness. These conditions are considered below.

3 *Mixed*. Not uncommonly children with sensorineural deafness may also develop infection, which may further impair hearing as a result of conductive loss.

Screening

Since 2006 all babies born in the UK have been screened as newborns to assess their hearing. Two methods for screening are used: the otoacoustic emissions (OAE) and auditory brainstem response (ABR) tests. All newborns will have OAE testing and some high-risk ones will go on to have an automated ABR test. Most Australian states have introduced Newborn Hearing Screening programs with ABR and/or OAE.

● *Otoacoustic emissions (OAEs)*. This technology detects the physiological response from the outer hair cells within the cochlea, which are present in 98% of normally hearing babies. As sensorineural hearing impairment is due to abnormal function of the outer hair cells this is a very sensitive and accurate test for hearing impairment. An automated OAE test is used for routine screening of all newborn infants in UK.

● *Auditory brainstem responses (ABRs)*. This technique measures evoked electrical signals detected by surface electrodes from within the hearing pathways of the brain in response to sounds at predetermined frequencies and loudness. ABR tests the whole auditory pathway rather than just the cochlea and is more valuable in screening high-risk babies, particularly those who have been subject to neonatal intensive care, as they are at more risk of developing retrocochlear hearing impairment (auditory neuropathy).

It is important to be able to refer babies with abnormal responses to neonatal hearing tests for rapid assessment and treatment with hearing aids if deafness is confirmed. Part of the screening protocol requires appropriate response, follow-up and treatment.

Incidence

Deafness remains a common cause of disability, with approximately 2–3/1000 children requiring hearing aids and a considerably larger number having a permanent mild bilateral impairment or significant unilateral deafness.

The prevalence of severe congenital or early hearing impairment is 1.5–2/1000 live births, and in 90% this is due to sensorineural causes. Deafness is, however, much more common in infants who have received intensive care, and studies of this high-risk group report an incidence of moderate or severe hearing impairment of the order of 30/1000, a marked increase compared to the general population.

Although conductive deafness is an uncommon cause of permanent hearing loss, it is a common condition. In a study of infants receiving intensive care, up to 25% were found to have evidence of otitis media while on the neonatal unit (Berman *et al.* 1978). In many of these infants there were clear signs of systemic sepsis, but middle ear disease was never considered as the cause. Babies intubated and receiving ventilatory support are most at risk of otitis media. If this condition is recognized and adequately treated, it is unlikely to lead to long-term hearing impairment.

Aetiology

There are a large number of causes of sensorineural hearing loss affecting the newborn. Many high-risk babies can be recognized on history taking and physical examination (Table 20.1). The most important are detailed below.

Table 20.1 Indications for routine auditory assessment

Family history of hearing impairment
Congenital perinatal infection, particularly rubella, CMV, syphilis
Anatomical malformations:
   Cleft palate
   Ear anomalies
   Syndromes (e.g. Down, Treacher–Collins)
Hyperbilirubinaemia:
   >340 μmol/L for full-term infants
   >240 μmol/L for infants <1500 g
Bacterial meningitis
Severe perinatal asphyxia
High aminoglycoside serum levels

Genetic causes

With the reduction in incidence of rubella embryopathy, inherited causes now account for 50% of all cases of severe sensorineural hearing impairment. Eighty percent are due to single gene autosomal recessive disorders and 15% to autosomal dominant disorders. Deafness due to chromosomal abnormalities or syndromic causes is rare. Genetic disorders often present late and are frequently progressive. The age of onset of hearing loss is not useful in distinguishing environmental from genetic loss.

Syndromic causes

The main syndromes causing hearing impairment are:

1 Branchio-oto-renal syndrome. Although this is a rare dominant disorder (1:40 000) it is the commonest syndromic cause of deafness. There are branchial clefts, ear abnormalities and renal anomalies.
2 Pendred syndrome (autosomal recessive): goitre and profound deafness.
3 Waardenburg syndrome (autosomal dominant): white forelock, different-coloured eyes and deafness.
4 Usher syndrome (autosomal recessive): retinitis pigmentosa leading to blindness and deafness.

Congenital infection

A variety of prenatally acquired viruses can cause permanent deafness.

Rubella

The full-blown syndrome (now very rarely seen) includes microcephaly and cataracts in addition to deafness, but hearing impairment may be the only abnormality. Active infection may continue well after birth, and deafness that is inapparent in the newborn period may develop later in childhood.

Cytomegalovirus

In infants with evidence of cytomegalovirus (CMV) infection at birth, 30% will have hearing impairment, and in those with asymptomatic infection almost 20% will subsequently develop hearing loss. As hearing loss is usually progressive, repeat screening might be indicated, and targeted testing at 9–12 months is recommended.

Meningitis

Deafness is an important complication of neonatal meningitis, and the organisms *E. coli*, group B β-haemolytic streptococcus and *Listeria* are particularly liable to cause deafness. The infection causes direct inflammatory involvement of inner ear structures leading to permanent hearing loss. It has been suggested that dexamethasone may reduce the chances of deafness in neonatal meningitis, but as this has not been consistently shown it cannot be recommended as part of meningitis treatment.

Bilirubin toxicity

Sensorineural deafness is part of the clinical spectrum of kernicterus, which includes mental retardation, choreoathetosis and failure of upward gaze. It is due to the penetration of unconjugated bilirubin into the brain, with staining and damage to the basal ganglia and deposition of bilirubin in the cochlear nuclei. Deafness may be the only neurological manifestation. Neonates whose cochlear nuclei are damaged by hyperibirubinaemia may pass an OAE screening test, but will be picked up on an abnormal ABR. The sicker the infant, the more likely he or she is to develop kernicterus. This is presumably because penetration of unconjugated bilirubin into the brain is more likely to occur in sick immature infants. There is evidence (although not conclusive) that it is the free (non-protein-bound) bilirubin that causes the neural toxicity. It has been suggested that damage to the blood–brain barrier allows the entry of bilirubin into the brain, thereby predisposing the infant to deafness.

Unfortunately, there are no adequate guidelines as to what levels of bilirubin are dangerous. It is clear that the sick premature infant is more liable to this complication, and treatment should be commenced earlier in this group than in more mature babies. de Vries *et al.* (1985) suggested that sensorineural hearing loss only occurred in very low birthweight (VLBW) infants whose total serum bilirubin exceeded 240 µmol/L (14 mg/dL). The recommended charts for the treatment of hyperbilirubinaemia are shown on p. 136.

Drugs

Aminoglycoside antibiotics (gentamicin, amikacin, netilmicin, tobramycin and kanamycin) are potentially ototoxic but the risk of deafness in neonates treated with these drugs is probably overestimated. Provided that the appropriate dosages and intervals between doses are used together with measurements of trough and peak drug levels, these drugs are unlikely to contribute significantly to the numbers of deaf neonates. Peak serum levels (1 h after drug administration) and trough levels (immediately before the next dose) are used to calculate the drug regimen. High peak levels indicate too high a dosage, and high troughs indicate that the interval between dosages should be lengthened. Recent studies have suggested that combined use of aminoglycosides and furosemide (frusemide) increases the risk of sensorineural hearing loss in LBW infants.

Incubator noise

It has been suggested that noisy incubators are an important cause of neonatal deafness, but there are few data to support this in the present era of relatively quiet incubators. Unnecessary environmental noise should always be avoided in the neonatal nursery.

Hypoxia

It is extremely difficult to evaluate the importance of hypoxia as an independent variable in causing neonatal deafness. Hypoxia usually indicates that an infant is sick, and there is little evidence that auditory pathways are more sensitive than other areas of the brain to hypoxia.

Management

Now that routine neonatal screening for deafness is widely used and high-risk babies are screened by ABR, more rapid diagnosis of deafness is made with more effective intervention. Fitting of hearing aids from a young age is important, and a cochlear implant later in childhood has been shown to be effective for certain children.

Visual impairment

Visual impairment as a result of prematurity is relatively common, although usually not severe; however, approximately 2% of babies born extremely preterm are registered blind. The most important cause of blindness is retinopathy of prematurity (ROP), but in term infants severe asphyxia may cause cortical visual impairment as well as other disabilities.

In a follow-up study of visual problems at 10–12 years of age in a group of babies weighing ≤1701 g at birth a significant reduction in visual acuity and contrast sensitivity was found compared with children born at full term even when ROP was not present (O'Connor *et al.* 2004). Amblyopia was particularly common in the preterm group as a result of stasbismus.

Retinopathy of prematurity (ROP)

ROP, formerly known as retrolental fibroplasia, is a relatively common condition affecting the most immature infants. Studies in the 1950s proved a direct association between oxygen dosage and the development of retinal abnormalities, and the controlled use of oxygen reduced the incidence of this condition in mature neonates. More recently, it has been noted that the relationship between oxygen and ROP is more complex than was originally thought, particularly in preterm babies.

The key to the pathophysiology of ROP is abnormality in the expression of the vascular endothelial growth factor (VEGF), which is normally stimulated by relative hypoxia as occurs in the fetus. Hyperoxia after birth causes VEGF to be downregulated with consequent vaso-obliteration and cessation in the growth of new blood vessels within the retina. This in turn leads to hypoxia of the non-perfused retina with secondary local upregulation of VEGF leading to neovascularization and in some cases the development of retinal fibrosis and detachment.

Classification

The diagnosis of ROP is made clinically by means of indirect ophthalmoscopy after prior pupillary dilatation with 0.5% cyclopentalate eyedrops. The examination is performed by a paediatric ophthalmologist, as considerable expertise is required. The description of ROP given here follows the recommendations of the international classification of the staging of ROP (Anon. 1984).

Severity

Stage 1 (demarcation line). A thin white line of demarcation in the periphery of the retina separating the avascular retina anteriorly from the vascularized retina posteriorly.

Stage 2 (ridge). The line is more extensive and forms a ridge.

Stage 3 (proliferation). Ridge with vascular proliferation immediately posterior to it.

Stage 4. Retinal detachment – subtotal.

Stage 5. Retinal detachment – total.

Mild ROP never progresses beyond stage 2 and does not require treatment. Stage 3 or worse is severe.

Location by zone

The location of ROP is described by the zone involved (Fig. 20.1). The zones are centred on the optic disc.

Zone 1. Extends from the optic disc to twice the disc–foveal distance.

Zone 2. From the periphery of the nasal retina in a circle around the anatomical equator.

Zone 3. This is anterior to zone 2 and is present temporally, inferiorly and superiorly, but not in the nasal retina.

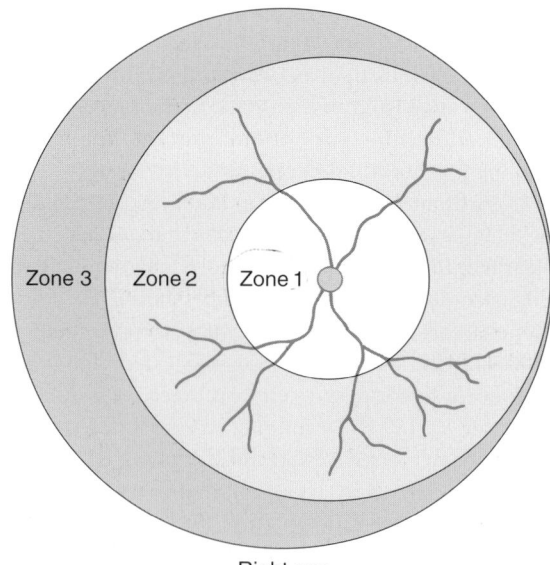

Right eye

Figure 20.1 The three zones shown on the right retinal field.

Extent
The extent is recorded in 'clock hours' 1–12 around the retinal circumference.

'Plus' disease
'Plus' is added to any stage of ROP if the following signs of activity are seen:
1 tortuosity and engorgement of retinal vessels;
2 vascular engorgement and rigidity of the iris;
3 vitreous haze;
4 pupil rigidity.

Threshold disease
A further concept is 'threshold' disease. This refers to the presence of a combination of five continuous clock hours or eight cumulative hours of stage 3 ROP in zones 1 and 2 together with 'plus' disease.

More recently it has been recognized that the most immature infants may develop a more virulent form of ROP referred to as 'pre-plus disease' and aggressive posterior ROP. These babies may need treatment earlier than more mature infants (see below).

Incidence

ROP is common in very premature infants; the incidence is 65–70% in babies of birthweight <1251 g, but only about 5% of these require treatment and 1–2% are blind as a result of severe ROP. In Western countries ROP accounts for only 6% of children with severe visual impairment, usually in the most immature infants. By contrast, in developing countries ROP is the cause of visual impairment in about 40% of children, and often affects larger babies of 1.5–2.0 kg. More severe forms of ROP (stage 3 or worse) occur in about 50% of babies <750 g, 30% of babies 750–999 g and in only 18% of babies 1000–1250 g.

Screening
Screening with indirect opthalmoscopy is recommended in all babies weighing <15001 g or <1250 g or <31 weeks' gestation at birth. In the event of sight-threatening disease (prethreshold, threshold plus disease or stage 3) developing, it will only occur at or after the baby is 31 weeks of postmenstrual age (PMA = gestational age + postnatal age) and after

4 weeks from birth. No new sight-threatening ROP occurs after 46 weeks PMA. Therefore in order to detect all cases of acute ROP in a timely manner so that appropriate treatment may be started, babies should be screened for signs of potentially severe disease starting at 31 weeks PMA and thereafter weekly. If significant disease is not present by 45 weeks PMA, screening can be stopped.

Prevention

The Po_2 of at-risk infants should be maintained at 6–8 kPa (45–60 mmHg). There has been much speculation as to appropriate levels for setting saturation monitor alarms to prevent ROP. Tin *et al.* (2001) showed that infants who were given controlled oxygen to maintain their oxygen saturation in the 70–90% range had four times less ROP than those nursed in saturation levels of 88–98%.

Treatment of acute ROP

The Multicentre Trial of Cryotherapy for ROP (Cryotherapy for ROP Cooperative Group 1988) has shown that cryotherapy saves vision in infants with severe disease. Now laser therapy has become more widely used to than cryotheropy treat ROP. Treatment should be confined to centres with special expertise in its use. More recently early laser treatment of pre-threshold ROP in very immature babies has been shown significantly to reduce visual impairment (Anon. 2003).

Cerebral visual impairment

This refers to an abnormality of the brain that renders the child functionally blind or with a major visual disability where the child finds it difficult to make visual sense of the world. These children often have major disability acquired in the perinatal period including cerebral palsy.

Causes of cerebral visual impairment include:
- brain malformations;
- periventricular leukomalacia (PVL) (p. 218);
- hypoxic-ischaemic brain injury (p. 21);
- hydrocephalus (p. 212);
- meningitis and encephalitis (p. 72).

Cataracts

Cataracts account for blindness in 20% of children with severe visual handicap. The causes of cataracts seen in the neonatal period include:

1 congenital rubella syndrome (see p. 64);
2 other prenatal infections (CMV and *Toxoplasma*) less commonly;
3 prematurity: cataracts may be due to trauma rather than prematurity per se, and are usually transient requiring no treatment;
4 galactosaemia (see p. 174);
5 hypocalcaemia;
6 Lowe syndrome (oculocerebrorenal syndrome): an X-linked condition;
7 Down syndrome: 5–10% of these children have cataracts at birth;
8 inherited: usually as an autosomal dominant condition;
9 idiopathic: accounts for up to 50% of cases.

Diagnosis

Cataracts should always be sought at the routine neonatal examination. Normally, on shining a light directly into the infant's eye, a red reflex is seen. If a white reflection is seen, then this is suggestive of a cataract, although retinoblastoma will give a similar appearance. If there is any doubt, careful ophthalmic examination should be performed under anaesthetic by an experienced person.

Treatment

Urgent referral to an ophthalmologist is essential. Unless most of the pupil is occluded by the cataract, it can be left and observed. If surgical treatment is necessary, the lens is removed and contact lenses are placed.

Glaucoma (buphthalmos)

Congenital glaucoma occurs in 1/10 000 births and is usually bilateral. It may be a familial condition.

The eye appears large (buphthalmos) in only one-quarter of infants with congenital glaucoma. The commonest presentation is the observation of a cloudy cornea. The treatment is surgical.

References

Anonymous. An international classification of retinopathy of prematurity. *Brit J Ophthalmol* 1984;**68**:690–697.

Anonymous. Revised indications for the treatment of retinopathy of prematurity. *Arch Ophthalmol* 2003;**121**:1684–1696.

Berman SA, Balkany T, Simmons M. Otitis media in the neonatal intensive care unit. *Pediatrics* 1978;**62**:198–203.

Cryotherapy for ROP Cooperative Group. Multicentre trial of cryotherapy for retinopathy of prematurity results. *Arch Ophthalmol* 1988;**106**:471–479.

Davis A, Bamford J, Wilson I *et al.* A critical review of the role of neonatal hearing screening in the detection of congenital hearing impairment. *Health Technol Asses* 1997;**1**:10.

Joint Working Party on Retinopathy of Prematurity. *Guidelines for Screening and Treatment.* London: The Royal College of Ophthalmologists and the British Association of Perinatal Medicine, 1995.

O'Connor AR, Stephenson TJ, Johnson A *et al.* Visual function in low birthweight children. *Brit J Ophthalmol* 2004;**88**:1149–1153.

Tin W, Milligan DWA, Pennefather P, *et al.* Pulse oximetry, severe retinopathy and outcome at one year in babies of less than 28 weeks gestation. *Arch Dis Child Fetal Neonatal Ed* 2001;**84**:F106–F110.

de Vries LS, Lary S, Dubowitz LMS. Relationship of serum bilirubin levels to ototoxicity and deafness in high risk low birth weight infants. *Pediatrics* 1985;**76**:351–354.

Further reading

Fielder A, Newton V (eds) Special senses: Vision and hearing. *Semin Neonatol* 2001;**6**:451–551.

21 Congenital postural deformities and abnormalities of the extremities

It is convenient to discuss congenital postural deformities and abnormalities of the extremities together. In some cases there may be an obvious cause for the deformity, such as posture in the uterus, but in others there may be a mixed aetiology, including chromosomal abnormalities and genetic factors. Sometimes no obvious cause can be found. It is not unusual for an infant to show several postural abnormalities, for example facial asymmetry, talipes and congenital dislocation of the hip. For predisposing factors, see Chapter 14.

Abnormalities of the extremities

Malformations of digits

Malformations of the digits are common and frequently inherited as autosomal dominant disorders. They are usually symmetrical. The principal types are:
- *Syndactyly:* fusion of the fingers or toes.
- *Polydactyly:* extra digit.
- *Ectrodactyly:* 'lobster claw' deformity.

Limb malformations

These may be symmetrical but occasionally they affect only one joint. The main types are:
- *Amelia:* absence of a limb or limbs.
- *Ectromelia:* gross hypoplasia or aplasia of one or more limbs.
- *Phocomelia:* partial deficiency of the proximal segment with preservation of distal parts ('seal-like' limbs).
- *Hemimelia (reduction malformation):* rudimentary formation of the distal part of a limb with normal development of the proximal part.

- *Amputations in utero:* thought to be due to amniotic bands.

Management
Orthopaedic or plastic surgery will be necessary to achieve maximal function and acceptable cosmetic appearance.

Abnormalities of the lower limbs

Lower limb abnormalities are common and may vary from a mild postural problem to more marked intrauterine compression leading to talipes calcaneovalgus or equinovarus. The latter conditions can be severe and there may be associated muscle wasting; they are illustrated in Fig. 21.1.

Talipes equinovarus (clubfoot) occurs in 1/1000 births and is ten times more common than severe calcaneovalgus. Minor degrees of postural

(a)   (b)

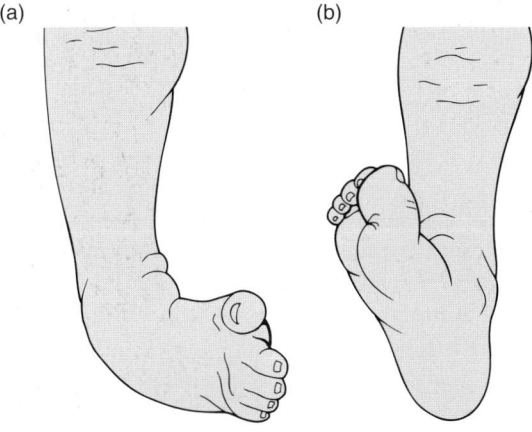

Figure 21.1 Talipes: talipes equinovarus (a) and talipes calcaneovalgus (b).

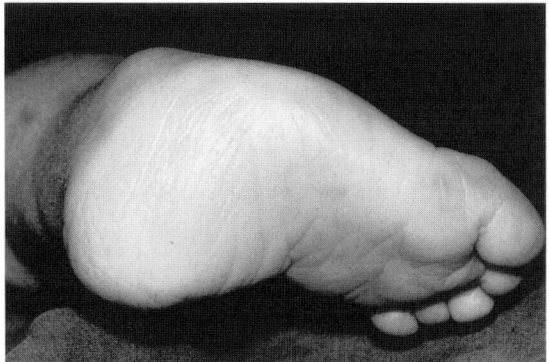

Figure 21.2 Metatarsus varus.

calcaneovalgus deformity are common. When either of these conditions is seen, other associated congenital abnormalities should be sought (e.g. dislocation of the hip and myelomeningocoele).

Metatarsus varus is a common disorder affecting the feet (Fig. 21.2). It may be present as an isolated finding or seen in conjunction with talipes.

Management

If the foot can be passively corrected to the position opposite the deformity, it is considered to be mild. Mild positional deformities will require simple passive exercise treatment by a physiotherapist and the parents. More severe deformities will require explanation, physiotherapy, splinting, and possibly surgical correction under orthopaedic supervision.

The parents of children with metatarsus varus should be strongly reassured that the disorder is usually self-correcting.

Genu recurvatum

This is a rare disorder in which the knees are hyperextensible. In severe cases there may be dislocation of the knee joint, and splinting may be necessary. The cause is multifactorial, with mechanical and genetic elements. Recurvatum at the knee sometimes approaches 90°. A lateral X-ray shows that the tibia is anterior to the femur.

Femoral retroversion

This is a common condition seen at the follow-up examination of infants leaving the neonatal unit.

The child lies or stands with his or her legs externally rotated at 90° ('Charlie Chaplin' gait). There is little or no internal rotation when in extension, but good external rotation. This condition often causes distress to the parents but they should be strongly reassured as it rapidly corrects within a year of the child learning to walk. It is, however, important to exclude congenital dislocation of the hip as the cause of the external rotation.

Developmental dysplasia of the hip (DDH)

Also known as congenital dislocation of the hip (CDH), DDH is an important asymptomatic neonatal congenital condition that should be detectable during the routine screening examination at birth.

Examination

Examination of the hip should start with observation for signs of established dislocation, such as unequal leg length and asymmetry of the thighs. The physical examination should be undertaken in two parts.

Ortolani's (reduction) test

This test assesses whether the hip is already dislocated. With the baby relaxed on a firm surface the hips and knees are flexed to 90°. The examiner grasps the baby's thigh with the middle finger over the greater trochanter and lifts it to bring the femoral head from its dislocated posterior position to opposite the acetabulum. Simultaneously, the thigh is gently abducted, reducing the femoral head over the posterior lip of the acetabulum. In a positive finding the examiner senses reduction by feeling a 'clunk', and there is a movement forwards of the head of the femur (Fig. 21.3).

Barlow's (dislocation) test

This test assesses whether the hip is dislocatable and is really a reversal of Ortolani's test. With one hand fixing the pelvis with the thumb anteriorly over the symphysis pubis and the other fingers posteriorly over the coccygeal region, the other hand grasps the baby's thigh and adducts it gently downwards. Dislocation is palpable as the femoral head slips over the posterior lip of the acetabulum (Fig. 21.4).

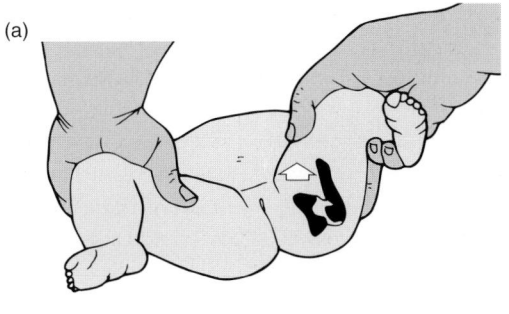

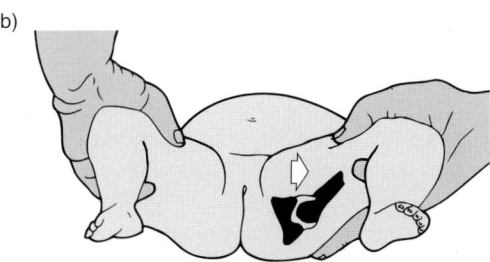

Figure 21.3 Ortolani's test. The hip cannot be abducted because of posterior dislocation of the femoral head. The hip is pulled upwards (a) and the head clunks into the acetabulum, permitting abduction (b).

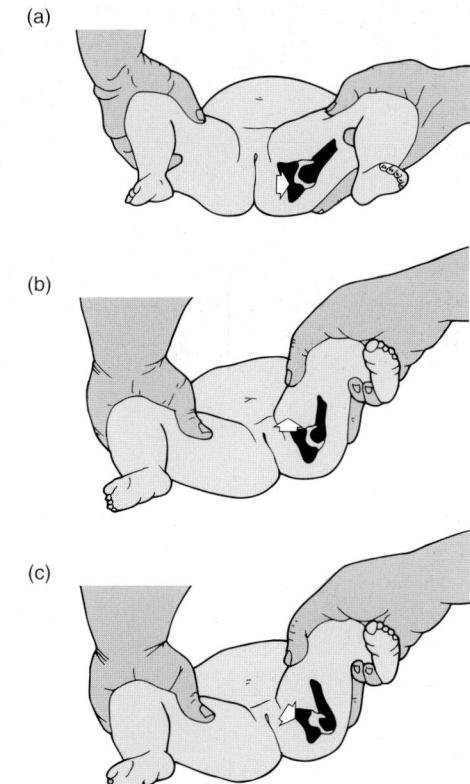

Figure 21.4 Barlow's test. The hip is abducted to establish that it is not dislocated (a). The adducted hip is then pulled upwards (b) and the femoral head pushed downwards and laterally to see whether it is dislocatable (c).

It is known that infants may have normal hips at birth that can dislocate some time later. For this reason, the hips should be examined at a 6-week assessment. Failure to abduct a hip is a very significant sign. Shortening of the leg, and asymmetrical skin creases in the newborn period, may not be reliable clinical signs of a dislocated hip.

Aetiology

Hip dislocation diagnosed in the neonatal period occurs in 1–2/1000 births. The left hip is dislocated four times more commonly than the right, and this is due to the fetal position causing the left hip to be more adducted than the right. The following associations are described with CDH:

1 *Polygenic or multifactorial condition.* This condition recurs in families at a rate of about 1/30.

2 *Presentation.* Breech/vertex ratio 10:1. The incidence of CDH in singleton breech deliveries is 14%.

3 *Gender.* Female/male ratio 6:1.

4 *Race.* Incidence is increased in some countries (Italy) and reduced in others (China).

5 *Abnormalities producing muscular imbalance around the joint,* e.g. spina bifida, hypertonia, congenital hypotonia, arthrogryposis congenita multiplex.

6 *Syndromes:* e.g. trisomy 13, trisomy 18.

7 Multiple congenital abnormalities.

Terminology

A variety of terms are used to describe abnormal hips. At the newborn examination the hips are carefully examined using both the Ortolani and the Barlow manoeuvres. The hips are then described as follows.

Stable. There is no abnormal movement of the joint.

Clicking. The hips are stable but a click is heard or felt during examination. This is probably normal if there is no excessive movement of the femoral head in the joint. Some paediatricians recommend that the hip should be examined again at 6 weeks of age. Clicking occurs as a result of ligamentous laxity and is found in up to 10% of newborn infants.

Dislocatable joint. The femoral head is in the joint (the hip can be fully abducted), but when Barlow's test is attempted on adduction the hip dislocates posteriorly.

Dislocated joint. The hip is out of joint at birth and cannot be abducted. It is detected on Ortolani's test.

Imaging

Ultrasound is the best method for imaging the hips. There is no place for X-ray examination for the assessment of hip dislocation until ossification occurs in the femoral epiphysis at about 3–4 months of age.

Ultrasound clearly defines the hip anatomy and allows evaluation of the shape of the acetabulum. Routine ultrasound examination of the hips of all babies is not recommended, but ultrasound examination of the hips is indicated in the following cases:
1 clinical instability;
2 family history of unstable hips;
3 breech presentation;
4 associated lower limb abnormality.

Management

There are many ways to treat this condition in the newborn period. The principle is to keep the hip immobilized in an abducted position for 2–3 months to allow the acetabular rim to develop and the hip ligaments to strengthen. Several varieties of splint are used, including the Aberdeen and Von Rosen splints and the Pavlik harness. There is no place for treatment with 'double nappies'. After 3 months the splint may be removed and, if the hip is clinically stable, check X-rays are taken usually at 6 and 12 months of age. Fixed dislocations of the hip, failure to respond to treatment and late-diagnosed dislocated hips will require individual orthopaedic consideration. The success of treatment depends on accurate and early diagnosis of the condition.

Scoliosis

Severe curvature of the spine (scoliosis) is usually due to vertebral defects resulting from either failure of formation (hemivertebrae) or failure of segmentation (unsegmented bars) or mixed. Milder cases may be caused by abnormal posture in the uterus.

Management will depend on the severity and cause, and orthopaedic consultation with regular follow-up is necessary. Congenital genitourinary malformation occurs in 20% of babies with congenital scoliosis and should be ruled out by a renal ultrasound scan.

Mandibular asymmetry, torticollis and plagiocephaly

These deformities may be due to abnormal posture of the fetus in the uterus. They usually correct either spontaneously during the first year of life or with the assistance of physiotherapy. Torticollis may also be associated with a sternomastoid tumour (see Chapter 15).

Arthrogryposis multiplex

This term describes multiple joint deformities involving more than one limb (Fig. 21.5). It is caused by restriction of joint movement *in utero* and there may be a variety of underlying causes:
1 neuromuscular – congenital dystrophy, spinal muscular atrophy;
2 oligohydramnios;
3 bicornuate uterus.

All infants with this disorder require orthopaedic referral and vigorous physiotherapy. An underlying neuromuscular problem should be considered, and creatinine phosphokinase levels measured. Other investigations are described in Chapter 19.

Neonatal dwarfism

Dwarfism may be classified as either primordial or chondrodystrophic.

Primordial

This generic term is used to cover a wide variety of different syndromes associated with dwarfism and having a variety of characteristic features, including mental retardation. These children are severely growth retarded at birth (intrinsic group) but there is no selective shortening of the limbs. Examples of

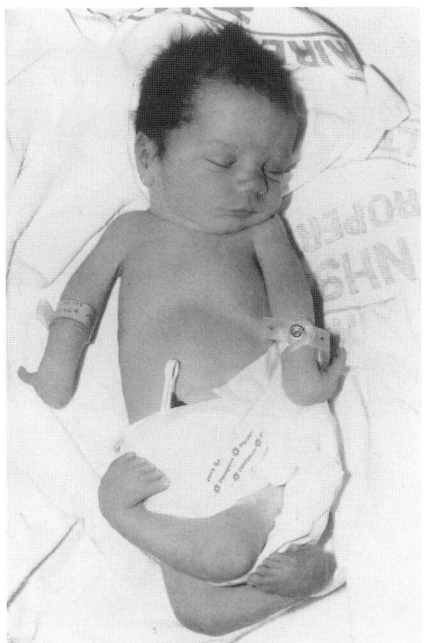

Figure 21.5 Arthrogryposis multiplex.

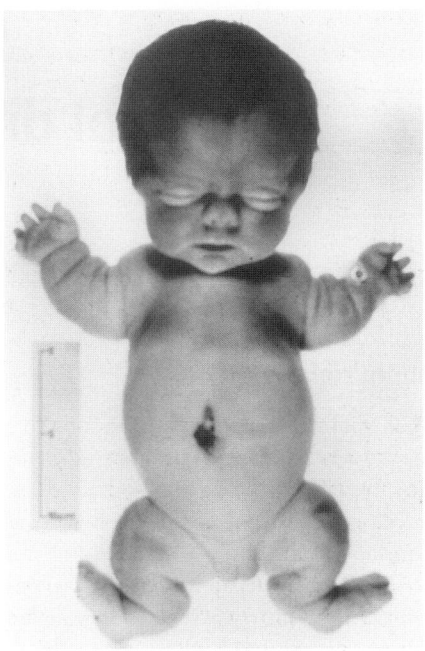

Figure 21.6 Thanatophoric dwarf.

these dwarf syndromes include Russell–Silver, Cornelia de Lange, Conradi, Seckel's bird head, Cockayne, leprechaunism and progeria.

Chondrodystrophic (skeletal dysplasia)

An underlying skeletal dysplasia should be suspected in any baby who is small for gestational age with other congenital abnormalities and who has disproportionate shortening of the limbs and trunk.

Skeletal dysplasias may present simply as short stature or disproportionate body habitus, but a variety of other anomalies, such as hydrocephalus, craniostenosis, cleft lip and palate, polydactyly, syndactyly, dislocated hips and dysmorphic facial features, may coexist.

There are many classifications of the more than 100 distinct syndromes. The most commonly recognized syndromes in the newborn are:

1 achondroplasia;
2 osteogenesis imperfecta: types I–V;
3 asphyxiating thoracic dystrophy;
4 thanatophoric dwarf (Fig. 21.6);
5 osteopetrosis (marble bone disease);
6 diastrophic dwarf;
7 Ellis–van Creveld syndrome.

Achondroplasia. This is the most common skeletal dysplasia that produces shortening of the limbs. The proximal segment of the limbs (i.e. humerus and femur) is more involved than the lower segments (i.e. radius and ulna or tibia and fibula). The head is typically enlarged; there are disproportionately short limbs but the trunk appears normal. It is inherited as an autosomal dominant trait but approximately 80% of cases are new mutations.

Osteogenesis imperfecta. This is an inherited (autosomal recessive) disorder of connective tissue. In its milder form, affected infants have increased susceptibility to fracture and hearing loss in later childhood, but at its most severe it is lethal and perinatal death is the rule. These babies have blue sclera and their bones fracture *in utero*.

Further reading

Jones KL, Smith DW. *Smith's Recognizable Patterns of Human Malformation*, 5th edn. Philadelphia: W.B. Saunders, 1997.

CHAPTER 22

22 Renal disorders in the newborn

Renal physiology

The fetus does not depend on the kidney to excrete waste products, instead relying on the placenta to perform this function. The fetal kidney does, however, produce very dilute urine, and this is the major contribution to the volume of amniotic fluid. An absence of fetal urine as a result of severe renal impairment is usually associated with severe lung hypoplasia (see below).

Renal function in the newborn depends on both gestational and postnatal age. Renal function rapidly matures within the first week after birth.

Glomerular filtration rate

The newborn infant has a very low glomerular filtration rate (GFR) compared to the older child. This is partly related to a relatively fewer number of nephrons. For this reason, the neonate cannot excrete a water load as well as older children. After 34 weeks of gestation and in response to birth there is a marked increase in GFR. The measurement of serum creatinine is the most convenient index of GFR in immature infants, but plasma urea is unreliable as it increases with catabolism even in the presence of normal renal function. The normal limits of creatinine are shown in Table 22.3 (see p. 241).

Tubular function

The concentrating ability of the developing kidney increases throughout gestation and improves rapidly after birth. This is due partly to elongation of the collecting tubes and partly to a hormonal effect (see below).

Tubular function can most easily be assessed by measuring the fractional excretion of sodium (FES):

$$FES = \frac{urine\ Na}{serum\ Na} \times \frac{serum\ creatinine}{urine\ creatinine} \times 100 \quad (22.1)$$

In the newborn FESNa should be <2.5%.

Sodium conservation

The fetus has a very poor ability to conserve (reabsorb) sodium. The stress of birth rapidly matures the ability of the tubules to conserve sodium, and this is related to the renin–aldosterone response. Sodium conservation is closely related to gestational age as well as postnatal age. All babies born <30 weeks of gestation have a negative sodium balance when fed on standard formulas, but this improves with increasing gestational age.

Hormonal function

The kidney is influenced by a variety of hormones.
- *Antidiuretic hormone (ADH)*. This increases water reabsorption from the collecting ducts. It is present from early in fetal life but the fetal kidney is relatively insensitive to it. After birth the collecting ducts become more sensitive and ADH is active in very premature infants, and even the most immature infant is capable of concentrating the urine to a remarkable extent within days of birth.
- *Renin–aldosterone*. Renin levels are higher in newborn infants than in adults and increase in response to sodium loss. However, the adrenal does not respond with high aldosterone levels and consequently sodium retention is poor, but matures in response to birth.

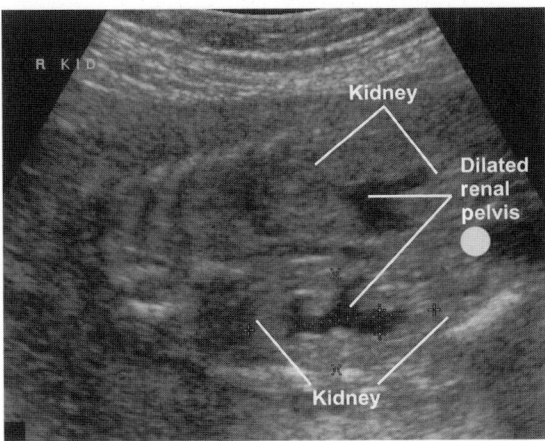

Figure 22.1 Longitudinal ultrasound view of fetal abdomen showing bilateral renal pelvocalyceal dilatation. (Courtesy of Dr R. Cincotta.)

Investigation of renal disease

Ultrasound

This is the mainstay of investigating the structure of the renal tract both before and after birth (Fig. 22.1).

MAG 3 renogram

A MAG 3 (mercapto-acetyltriglycine) renogram is a kinetic scan that involves intravenous injection of a radioactive tracer, which is taken up by the kidney thereby enabling excretion curves to be plotted. Delay in excretion of isotopes from the kidney is suggestive of obstructive uropathy such as PUJ (pelvi-ureteric junction obstruction). It is also possible to estimate differential kidney function using this scan prior to the excretion phase.

DMSA scan

A dimercaptosuccinic acid (DMSA) radionuclide scan is a static scan that delineates renal scarring or dysplasia and allows better estimation of differential renal function. It may show false positive results if done during or soon after an episode of acute urinary tract infection.

Micturating cystourethrogram (MCUG)

This is the investigation of choice for vesico-ureteric reflux. It involves urethral catheterization with the injection of radio-opaque dye into the bladder and observation of whether the dye refluxes into the ureters on micturition. It is a very invasive procedure and the child must be covered with trimethoprim antibiotic for at least 48 hours prior to and after the procedure.

Presentation of renal disease

Genitourinary disease in the newborn may present in a number of different ways. These are discussed separately.
1 Potter's syndrome.
2 Obstructive uropathy.
3 Acute renal failure.
4 Infection.
5 Renal mass.
6 Haematuria.
7 Congenital abnormalities.

Prenatal diagnosis

Most significant structural renal anomalies are detected antenatally as the result of routine fetal anomaly scanning. Some diagnoses are so severe (renal agenesis) that termination of pregnancy may be offered to the parents, but in other cases the neonatal team will be notified prior to delivery of a baby with a renal anomaly and a variety of investigations are pursued after birth.

The most common abnormal feature detected by prenatal scanning is renal pelvis dilatation. This may represent PUJ obstruction or vesico-ureteric reflux but may simply be due to atonic dilatation of the ureter. The size of the pelvic dilatation determines how rapidly after birth the baby is investigated. If the fetal renal pelvis measures 6–10 mm and the fetal ureters appear normal then there is no reason to investigate the baby until one month of age with a postnatal renal ultrasound scan. If the pelvis measures >10 mm or if the ureters are dilated then the baby should have a renal scan immediately after birth and be started on prophylactic antibiotics until the precise cause of the anomaly is fully investigated. Figure 22.3 illustrates an algorithm to investigate prenatally detected renal dilatation.

Potter's syndrome

Potter's syndrome refers to the association of dysmorphic clinical features and bilateral renal agenesis. The incidence of this condition is 1/4000 births, with a male predominance. Failure of renal development is associated with oligohydramnios and retardation of lung development. These infants usually have severe lung hypoplasia, which is incompatible with life. The oligohydramnios also gives rise to characteristic facial features, including a beaked nose, low-set abnormal ears, prominent epicanthic folds and an antimongolian slant to the eyes (Fig. 22.2). The fetal surface of the placenta often shows amnion nodosum, which is small white plaques of fibrinoid necrosis.

Facial features identical to those seen in Potter's syndrome are seen in other causes of oligohydramnios due to urinary outflow obstruction, sometimes referred to as pseudo-Potter's syndrome. In these cases large kidneys are usually palpable.

Infants with Potter's syndrome are severely asphyxiated at birth and, although often resuscitated, die within several hours owing to their lung hypoplasia. Prenatal ultrasound may detect renal agenesis, but large adrenals (common in this condition) may be confused with normal kidneys. The syndrome is usually considered to be sporadic, but may be polygenic with a recurrent risk of unilateral or bilateral renal agenesis of approximately 1%.

Obstructive uropathy

Causes of urinary obstruction are listed in Table 22.1. These usually occur in males, but the commonest cause (pelvi-ureteric junction obstruction) occurs equally in both males and females.

Clinical features

Diagnosis of uropathy is often suspected antenatally as described above. Infants may present with an abdominal mass (bladder and/or kidney) or dribbling urine. If obstruction has been severe, the infant may be born with the facial appearances of Potter's syndrome and lung hypoplasia. Prune-belly syndrome should be obvious from the wrinkled appearance of the abdomen. The penis should be examined carefully for a normal meatus. The spine should be inspected for meningomyelocoele.

A strategy for investigation

A suggested algorithm for investigation of babies with renal dilatation is shown in Fig. 22.3. In cases where more severe disorders are suspected investigations must proceed rapidly and imaging as well as functional assessment may need to be repeated at intervals to observe progression in renal disease. The investigations referred to in Fig. 22.3 are described above. As well as investigating the cause of the uropathy, the neonatologist must also protect the baby's

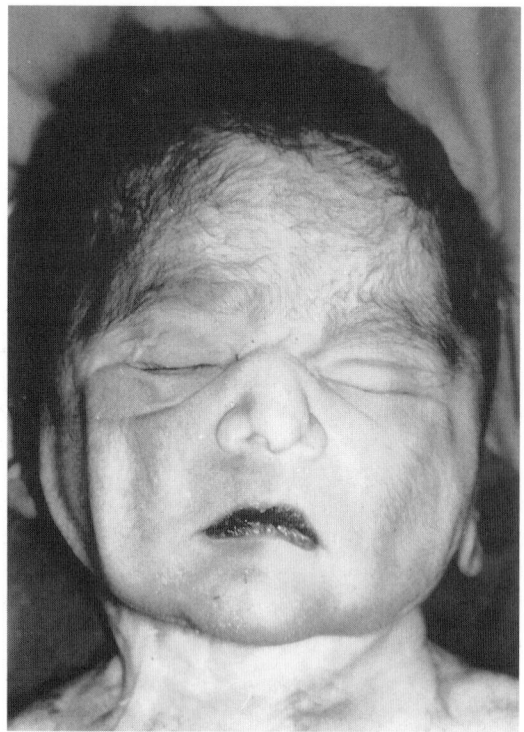

Figure 22.2 *Potter's syndrome.* Note the beaked nose as if the face has been pressed up against a windowpane, and the prominent epicanthic folds.

Table 22.1 Causes of obstructive uropathy in the newborn

Pelvi-ureteric junction obstruction
Posterior urethral valves
Urethral meatal stenosis in males
Neurogenic bladder
Ureterocoele
Prune-belly syndrome

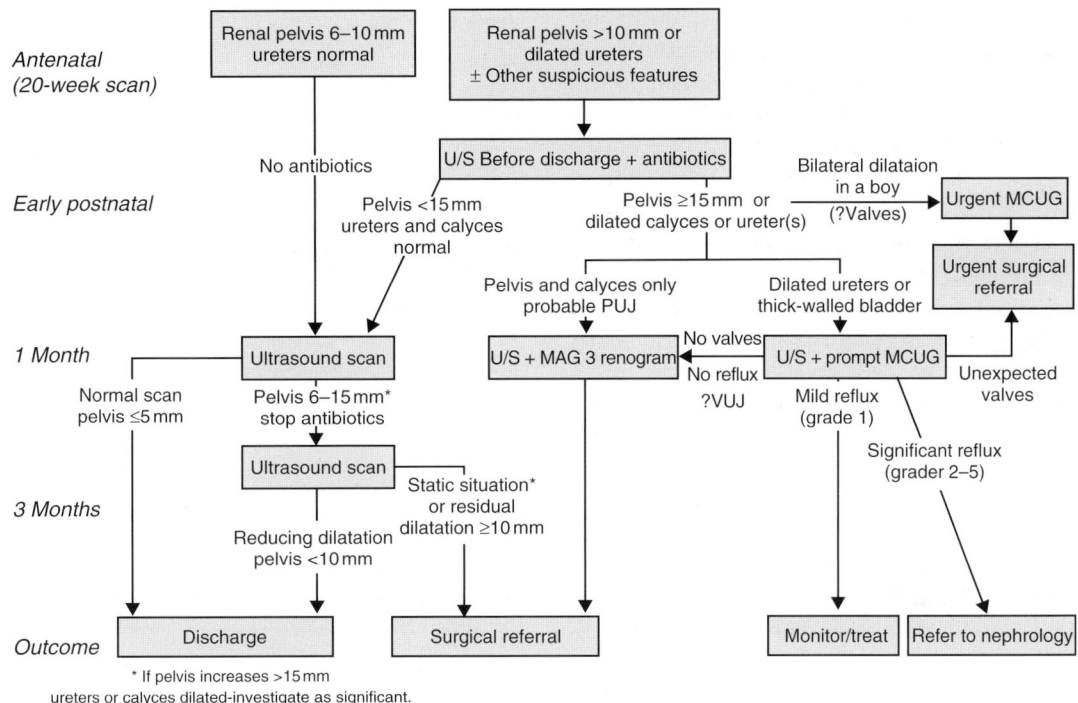

Figure 22.3 Algorithm for investigating a fetus or newborn with renal dilatation.

renal tract from further damage due to infection. The use of prophylactic antibiotics is essential in some cases until definite management is introduced. In complicated cases early referral to a paediatric nephrologist and/or paediatric urologist is necessary.

Prune-belly syndrome (triad syndrome)

This occurs mainly in males. There is an absence of the musculature of the anterior abdominal wall, with bladder neck obstruction in 25%, dilatation of the ureters and undescended testicles. It is probably due to degeneration of the abdominal musculature as a result of a distended bladder.

Treatment is directed towards draining the bladder and preventing infection. Cosmetic surgery for the abdominal wall deficiency may be necessary.

Posterior urethral valves

This condition occurs only in male infants and successful treatment depends on early diagnosis, which

is often made on fetal ultrasound scanning. Urine dribbling from the penis is always an ominous sign and should alert the clinician to the presence of urethral valves. There is proximal obstruction of the urethra, owing to mucosal folds arising from the verumontanum producing a valve-like obstruction. This causes hypertrophy and dilatation of the urethra, bladder, ureters and kidneys.

On examination of the abdomen, a hard muscular bladder is felt arising from the pelvis. In addition, both kidneys are easily palpable.

Ultrasound will confirm the presence of a hypertrophied bladder and establish the degree of upper tract involvement. The bladder should be drained by a urethral or suprapubic catheter. A micturating cystourethrogram will confirm the diagnosis.

Management

If the lesion is mild, surgical resection of valve cusps through a cystoscope is all that is necessary. Antenatal diagnosis and the insertion of a vesico-amniotic catheter into the fetal bladder are indicated in highly selected cases of severe obstruction. If renal impairment has occurred, urinary drainage via bilateral cutaneous ureterostomies or vesicostomy will be necessary before resection of the valves.

Ureterocoele

This is a ballooning of the intravesical portion of the distal ureter into the bladder, which obstructs the drainage of the kidney on that side. Investigation is by ultrasound, cystogram or cystoscopy. The ureterocoele should be excised and the ureter reimplanted to avoid urinary reflux.

Pelvi-ureteric junction obstruction

This is usually unilateral, but in 25% of cases is bilateral. It presents as a unilateral mass in the loin, which may become massive. If the kidney is grossly hydronephrotic with less than 20% function as shown by a functional MAG 3 scan, then nephrectomy is the best treatment. In milder or bilateral cases plastic repair of the pelvi-ureteric junction may be all that is necessary.

Acute renal failure

Acute renal failure may occur as the result of numerous disease processes, many of which are detected on antenatal ultrasound (Fig. 22.1); these can be divided into prerenal, renal and postrenal causes (Table 22.2). Prerenal failure is the commonest variety and usually occurs with severe respiratory disease or as a postoperative complication.

Clinical features

The baby develops oliguria (urine output <1.0 mL/kg/h), a rising serum creatinine and blood urea, and electrolyte disturbances in which potassium and phosphate are increased, and the calcium and magnesium are often decreased. Metabolic acidosis commonly develops. Fluid retention with oedema commonly occurs, and cardiac dysrhythmias may develop as a result of hyperkalaemia.

Oliguria may be difficult to detect early in the infant's life as the passage of urine may have occurred unnoticed or may not have been recorded.

Table 22.2 Causes of renal failure in the neonate

Prerenal	Renal	Postrenal
Dehydration	Cystic disease	Obstructive uropathy (see Table 22.1)
Hypotension due to:	Acute tubular necrosis	
Haemorrhage	Cortical necrosis	
Infection	DIC	
Cardiac dysrhythmia	Infection (pyelonephritis)	
Asphyxia	Haemolysis	
Hypothermia	Venous thrombosis	
	Congenital nephrotic syndrome	
	Drugs (aminoglycosides)	

DIC, disseminated intravascular coagulation.

Over 90% of normal infants pass urine in the first 24 h of life, and 98% have voided by 48 h from birth. If oliguria is suspected, then a urinary catheter will determine whether urine is present in the bladder and allow assessment of the volume. Abdominal ultrasound may also be useful in showing whether there is urine in the bladder.

In oliguric infants there may be difficulty in distinguishing prerenal from renal failure. FESNa may be used in such cases. In prerenal failure the urine is concentrated and the serum and urinary creatinine measurements are high. If doubt still exists, an infusion of blood or plasma (20 mL/kg) with a dose of furosemide (frusemide) (3 mg/kg) should resolve the issue. Postrenal causes of acute renal failure must be excluded (see p. 238).

Pathological examination of the kidneys of infants dying with acute renal failure shows acute tubular necrosis, acute cortical necrosis or bilateral renal vein thrombosis. With renal vein thrombosis, loin masses are generally palpable and the baby has haematuria.

Creatinine

The most important index of renal function in the newborn is serum creatinine. The plasma urea is unreliable as it increases with catabolism even in

Table 22.3 Upper limit for normal serum creatinine levels (μmol/L) in neonates

Gestational age (weeks)	Age of infant (days)				
	2	7	14	21	28
28	220	145	118	104	95
30	192	132	107	95	87
32	175	119	97	86	78
34	158	109	88	78	71
36	143	98	80	71	64
38	130	89	72	64	59
40	118	81	66	57	53

The figure represents the 95th centile of normality for gestational age. (Reproduced from Rudd et al. 1983, with permission)

the presence of normal renal function. The normal limits of creatinine are shown in Table 22.3.

Management

In established renal failure the following management regimen should be carried out under the direction of a nephrologist. The underlying cause should be treated wherever possible.

Fluid restriction

Water intake is necessary to replace insensible water loss as well as the urinary loss. These losses are calculated separately. Insensible loss depends on the infant's birthweight and gestational age. In the first week of life the following approximate figures apply:

<1250 g	60 mL/kg/24 h
1250–1750 g	30 mL/kg/24 h
>1750 g	20 mL/kg/24 h

For all infants over 1 week of age the insensible water loss is approximately 20 mL/kg. The volume of urine voided by the infant every 12 h should be added to the input over the next 12 h. Daily weighing is an accurate way of assessing fluid balance, and no change in weight is to be aimed for.

Protein and potassium restriction

Potassium should not be given unless the infant is hypokalaemic. To avoid endogenous protein breakdown, a high carbohydrate infusion (15% dextrose) should be given. The volume depends on the infant's output (see above).

Correction of electrolyte imbalance

Hyponatraemia is usually due not to sodium depletion but rather to fluid overhydration. Water should be restricted until this is corrected.

Metabolic acidosis

Sodium bicarbonate is carefully administered if the pH falls below 7.25. Care is necessary to avoid hypernatraemia.

Anaemia

Fresh blood (10 mL/kg) is given if the haemoglobin falls below 8 g/dL.

These measures are usually sufficient to maintain homeostasis until renal function recovers.

Constant attention should be paid to life-threatening complications, including:

1 Hyperkalaemia (>7.5 mmol/L). Calcium resonium enemas should be given when hyperkalaemia occurs. An intravenous infusion of salbutamol (4 μg/kg as a single dose over 5 minutes) reduces serum potassium and may need to be given once the serum K+ is >7.5 mmol/L. Insulin and dextrose may also be necessary to drive potassium into the cells.

2 Severe metabolic acidosis (pH<7.20).

3 Fluid overload with severe oedema and congestive cardiac failure.

4 Hypertension, usually due to fluid overload.

5 Severe uraemia with central nervous system (CNS) depression.

Under these circumstances peritoneal dialysis may be indicated (see p. 312).

Infection

The incidence of symptomatic urinary tract infection in the neonatal period is 1%. The symptoms of urinary tract infection in the newborn are generally non-specific, with jaundice, vomiting, failure to thrive, temperature instability, lethargy and poor feeding. Specific symptoms of dysuria, frequency and abdominal discomfort are rarely seen. Urinary tract infections in the newborn are more common in the male and may be bloodborne, ascending or secondary to an abnormality of the urinary tract. In the neonatal period pyelonephritis is usually due to bloodborne infection.

Urinary tract infection should be suspected in infants with non-specific symptoms. A 'clean voided' bag sample of urine is used only as a screen and is never the basis for a definitive diagnosis. If the bag sample suggests a urinary tract infection or if the baby is sick and in need of urgent treatment, either a 'clean catch', suprapubic aspiration or a urinary catheter sample will be necessary. The following interpretations can be made on an adequately collected urine sample.

Microurine. A white cell count of more than 30 000/mL suggests infection and a count of less than 10 000/mL is probably normal. Some normal newborn infants have up to 30 000 white cells/mL, even on a bladder tap aspirate of urine. White cell counts in urine specimens from collecting bags are high and should be interpreted carefully, and only in conjunction with colony counts.

Culture. More than 100 000 organisms/mL indicates a significant infection, less than 10 000/mL or mixed organisms suggests contamination, and counts between 10 000 and 100 000/mL indicate that the urine sample should be repeated. If any growth of organisms is obtained on bladder tap, this is significant. The infecting organisms are usually coliform bacteria or rarely Gram-positive cocci. The presence of budding hyphae in the urine strongly suggests systemic fungal infection (see p. 73).

Treatment

Antibiotics that are excreted in the urine should be started immediately in an infant for whom there is a strong clinical suspicion of urinary tract infection. This is particularly important in pyelonephritis. In the presence of severe or suspected infection, therapy is usually commenced with an intravenous aminoglycoside (e.g. gentamicin) and ampicillin. Once cultures and sensitivities are known, an inappropriate antibiotic may be deleted. Co-trimoxazole (Septrin) may be used after the first week of life. Other suitable antibiotics include cefalexin (cephalexin), ceftriaxone or cefotaxime (cephotaxime). Treatment is continued for 10 days, when repeat microurine and culture are performed. Ultrasound examination together with a micturating cystourethrogram (MCU) are indicated in all neonates with proven urinary tract infection. Other investigations include radionuclide scan for functional imaging (MAG 3; see p. 237) and a DMSA scan, which delineates renal scarring or dysplasia and allows estimation of differential renal function (Gordon & Riccabona 2003). Severe reflux may be associated with renal scarring even in the absence of infection. Specimens of urine should be regularly checked during the first year of life to ensure that reinfection does not occur.

Renal mass

Normal kidneys, especially the right, may be just palpable in the newborn infant. If a renal mass is easily felt, the kidney is probably pathologically enlarged. Differentiation of the mass can be achieved using ultrasound. The causes of a renal mass are listed in Table 22.4.

Cystic disease of the kidneys

There are a great variety of cystic conditions of the kidney in the newborn. Congenital renal cystic diseases are a genetically and clinically diverse group of disorders with the common pathological finding of diffuse bilateral cystic structures without dysplasia. Many hereditary malformation syndromes are associated with renal cysts. They may be classified as follows (Becker & Avner 1995):

1 *Polycystic kidney disease.* Linkage analysis and positional cloning have led to advances in the isolation of the genes and gene products responsible for these conditions.

  (a) *Autosomal dominant polycystic kidney disease (ADPKD).* This is the commonest inherited renal disease, with an incidence of 1/200–1/1000. It was originally known as 'adult-onset PKD' because of the usual clinical presentation in the third to fifth

Table 22.4 Causes of a renal mass in the newborn period

Hydronephrosis (bilateral)
Pelvi-ureteric junction obstruction (unilateral)
Cystic disease of the kidneys
Renal vein thrombosis
Wilms' tumour (nephroblastoma)
Adrenal haemorrhage

decades, although the disease can manifest itself in utero or at any time thereafter. It may be diagnosed on perinatal ultrasound with the finding of enlarged or cystic kidneys. Clinically the disease can present along a spectrum, from the severe neonatal form with renal failure and Potter's syndrome, to the asymptomatic unilateral renal cyst found on renal ultrasound.

(b) *Autosomal recessive polycystic kidney disease (ARPKD).* Originally known as 'infantile PKD' because of its more common perinatal presentation, ARPKD can present at any time from in utero to adulthood. It is characterized by cystic dilatation of the renal collecting ducts and hepatic biliary dysgenesis with periportal fibrosis.

2 *Glomerular cystic kidney disease* (GCKD). Primary GCKD can be sporadic or inherited in an autosomal dominant pattern. It may present in the newborn with palpable enlarged cystic kidneys.

Cystic dysplasia of the kidneys

This can fall into two basic categories:

1 *Cystic dysplastic (multicystic) kidneys.* This is a sporadic condition producing a non-functioning kidney and is usually unilateral as bilateral cases are fatal. The kidney shows multiple large and small cysts. There is little or no renal function on the affected side and a unilateral cystic dysplastic kidney should be surgically excised in infancy. If bilateral, it is incompatible with life.

2 *Cysts secondary to obstruction.* This condition occurs as a result of obstruction to urinary outflow (e.g. posterior urethral valves).

Haematuria

In the first few days of life the presence of red cells in the urine is not uncommon, but after this haematuria is an important finding and must be further investigated. Table 22.5 lists causes of haematuria. Investigations include urinalysis, clotting studies, creatinine and ultrasound examination. Treatment depends on the underlying cause. Haematuria must be differentiated from the presence of urates in the urine, a benign condition that produces pink staining of the nappy/diaper.

Table 22.5 Neonatal renal disorders associated with haematuria

Acute tubular necrosis
Infection
Renal vein thrombosis
Bleeding disorders
Cystic renal disease
Obstructive uropathy
Tumours

Congenital abnormalities

Hypospadias

In this condition the urethral meatus opens onto the undersurface of the glans penis, the penile shaft or the perineum. It is one of the most common abnormalities of male infants, with an incidence of 1/350 male births. It may be classified as glandular, penoglandular, penile, penoscrotal or perineal, depending on the site of the urethral opening. Frequently there is a dorsal hood to the penis and a ventral curvature of the glans (chordee). Chromosome studies are indicated with undescended testes and severe penoscrotal or perineal lesions. Epispadias refers to the urethra opening on the dorsal surface of the penis.

Treatment

Mild types are repaired in a one-stage procedure in the first 6 months, but severe types require several staged operations. The infant must not be circumcised, otherwise definitive surgical treatment will be made more difficult.

Ectopia vesicae (bladder exstrophy)

This is a complex disorder of the abdominal wall, bladder and pelvis. The mucosa of the bladder herniates through a deficient lower abdominal wall. There is a deficient pelvic floor and wide separation of the pubic symphysis. It is more common in male than in female infants. In the male there is total epispadias, undescended testes and a deficient penis. In the female the two halves of the clitoris are separate and the vagina is duplicated.

The surgical management of this complex disorder is extremely difficult and continues over many years. Urinary continence is rarely achieved.

References

Becker N, Avner ED. Congenital nephropathies and uropathies. *Pediatr Clin N Am* 1995;**42**:1319–1329.

Gordon I, Riccabona M. Investigating the newborn kidney: update on imaging techniques. *Semin Neonatol* 2003;**8**:269–278.

Rudd PT, Hughes EA, Placzek MM, Hodes DT. Reference ranges for plasma creatinine during the first months of life. *Arch Dis Child* 1983;**58**:212–215.

Further reading

Avmer ED, Harmon WC (eds) *Pediatric Nephrology*, 5th edn. Baltimore: Lippincott Williams & Wilkins, 2003.

Haycock GB. Management of acute and chronic renal failure in the newborn. *Semin Neonatol* 2003;**8**:325–334.

CHAPTER 23

23 Gastrointestinal disorders

Development of the GI tract

The gastrointestinal (GI) tract develops 4 weeks after conception as a tube from mouth to cloaca. Part of the foregut differentiates into trachea and oesophagus, and disorders of development at this stage cause oesophageal atresia, usually with tracheo-oesophageal fistula. The lip is normally fused by 5 weeks and the palate by 8–9 weeks. The lower bowel initially opens into the yolk sac and later forms the vitello-intestinal duct. The midgut forms a loop, which protrudes from the abdominal cavity and then re-enters the abdomen after turning through 270°. Failure of the bowel to re-enter the abdomen causes exomphalos, and failure to twist leads to malrotation. During the sixth week of gestation a septum separates the cloaca into rectum and urogenital sinus. The gut then ruptures through the perineum to form an anus. The liver and pancreas develop from the gut endoderm at the same time as the duodenum is formed. The gut is fully differentiated by 20 weeks.

Functional development

The bowel develops functionally as follows.

Motility

Bowel motility is present from 16 weeks' gestation but is not fully functional until 36 weeks, and the passage of meconium *in utero* is rare under 34 weeks. Disorganized bowel motility in the last trimester makes functional intestinal obstruction or paralytic ileus not uncommon in premature infants.

Swallowing

In the second trimester the fetus begins to swallow, and hydramnios often occurs if the upper gastrointestinal tract is not patent by mid-pregnancy. Gastro-oesophageal reflux is common, especially in the preterm infant, because of low gastro-oesophageal sphincter pressures.

Carbohydrate absorption

Disaccharidase activity in the small bowel is low at term and gradually increases to mature levels by 10 months of age. In the preterm baby maltase is the first disaccharidase to reach reasonable activity, followed by sucrase and then lactase. Lactase deficiency is common prior to 30 weeks' gestation, with consequent lactose intolerance in these infants.

Fat absorption

Bile salts are essential for fat absorption but are themselves not readily absorbed. Fat malabsorption in the newborn may occur because of reduced bile salts. In infants below 1300 g birthweight, 70–75% of dietary fat is absorbed. Premature infants are better able to absorb polyunsaturated fats (present in excess in human milk) than saturated fats. Some degree of physiological steatorrhoea is therefore normal in preterm infants. Premature infants cope better with the absorption of medium-chain triglyceride fats than long-chain fatty acids.

Secretions

Gastric acid secretion does not occur to any significant degree before 32 weeks' gestation. Pancreatic secretions of lipase are adequate for dietary needs by full term, but trypsin is often deficient, resulting in relative protein malabsorption.

Malformations

Cleft lip

Cleft lip, with or without cleft palate, occurs in 1/1000 births and is more common in the male. It is usually of polygenic inheritance (rarely autosomal dominant) and has a higher frequency in some families. The risk of recurrence in subsequent pregnancies is about 3–5%. It is more common in the pregnancies of older mothers. It may be unilateral (70% on left side) or bilateral. Recurrence risk counselling is affected by whether the lesion is unilateral or bilateral, is associated with cleft palate, and if other first-degree relatives are affected. Cleft lip with or without cleft palate is associated with a broader pattern of altered morphogenesis in 35% of cases. Severe midline facial clefts are associated with intracranial anomalies, including holoprosencephaly, and are a feature of trisomy 13. Cleft lip and palate have been associated with maternal anticonvulsant therapy, and also occur in the fetal alcohol syndrome.

Management

The infant has an unattractive appearance and time must be spent with the parents talking to them about the condition. Photographs of treated cases showing the preoperative and postoperative appearances are particularly helpful in allaying parental anxieties (Fig. 23.1). There may be feeding difficulties, particularly if there is an associated cleft palate (see below).

Surgical treatment
Most surgeons prefer to repair the lip in the first 6–12 weeks of life, but very early closure in the first week is recommended by some.

Cleft palate

In 70% of cases cleft palate is associated with a cleft lip. The palate forms by fusion of the bilateral maxillary processes and the midline premaxilla. A variety of clefting abnormalities occur.
1 Complete cleft of the hard and soft palate, which may involve the alveolar margin. It may be unilateral, bilateral or involve the midline. Cleft palate may be associated with the Pierre Robin syndrome.
2 Submucous cleft. There is a bony defect completely covered by mucosa, and often a bifid uvula.
3 Simple cleft of the soft palate.

Pierre Robin sequence. This is the association of cleft palate (hard or soft) with micrognathia (Fig. 23.2). The small jaw allows the tongue to prolapse backwards, thereby obstructing the airway and leading to cyanotic spells. The infant should be nursed prone to prevent airway obstruction, and a special nursing frame to keep the head in the midline may be required. The jaw usually grows rapidly and the

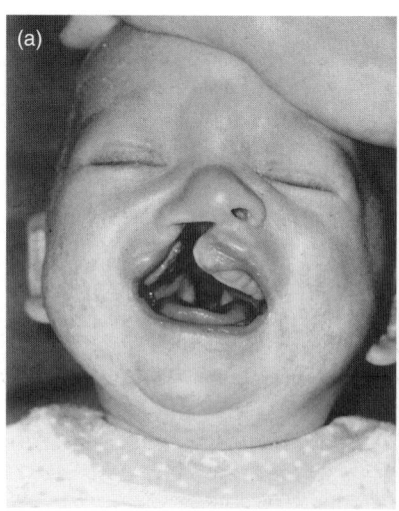
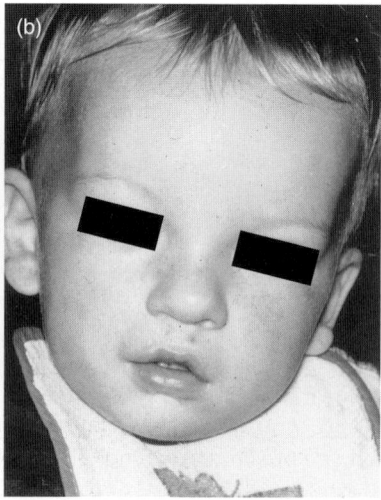

Figure 23.1 Cleft lip. At birth the infant has a right-sided cleft lip (a). The same infant following repair (b).

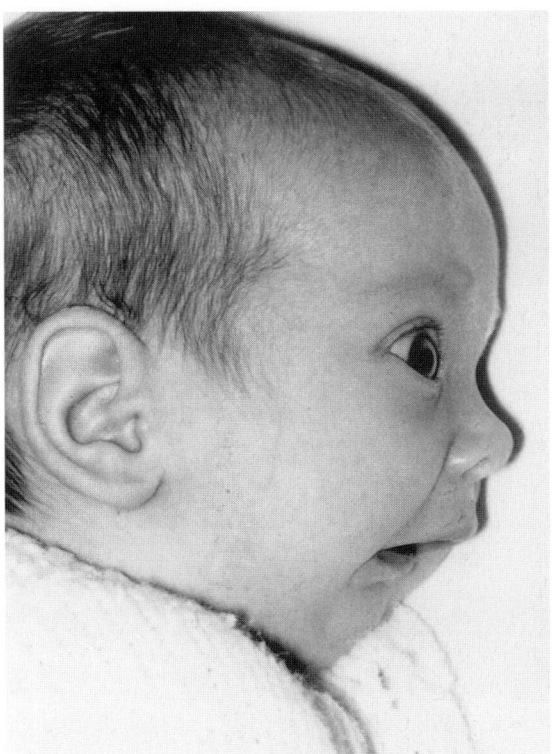

Figure 23.2 Pierre Robin syndrome showing micrognathia.

infant can then be fed with a bottle and gradually sat up. The cleft palate is treated surgically.

Clinical features

Feeding is usually a problem because the baby is unable to achieve adequate suction, with resultant regurgitation of milk through the nose. Aspiration of milk can cause recurrent pneumonitis.

Treatment

If feeding is difficult, a special teat may be required. Such devices include a lamb's teat (longer than usual), a flanged (Great Ormond Street) teat or a Maws' teat. The rubber flange acts as an artificial palate. The careful use of a squeeze bottle aids suction in many infants. In some cases the fitting of an acrylic dental obturator around the edges of the palate is helpful.

The surgical management of cleft palate requires the services of a plastic surgeon, an orthodontist, an ear, nose and throat (ENT) surgeon, and a speech therapist. If the alveolar ridge is involved, an orthodontist may make a series of plates to encourage appropriate bone growth. Surgical closure of the palate is attempted at 9–12 months before speech has developed.

Prognosis

The following problems are to be anticipated.

Speech and language
These problems include nasal escape and articulation. A speech therapist should always be closely involved in the management of these children.

Hearing
Eustachian tube function is usually impaired, predisposing the child to middle-ear infections. Regular hearing assessment and ENT supervision are essential.

Dental
Teeth development is often delayed and there may be malocclusion.

Local ulceration
Ulceration may be due to poorly fitting acrylic plates.

Intestinal obstruction

Complete or partial obstruction of the small bowel or colon may be suspected in the antenatal period or diagnosed in the neonate. Intestinal obstruction occurs in about 1/1000 babies and may be associated with maternal polyhydramnios. If more than 25 mL of fluid is aspirated from the stomach after birth, intestinal obstruction should be suspected. Occasionally, bile-stained amniotic fluid from intrauterine vomiting may be confused with meconium-stained liquor. There are a variety of types of congenital bowel obstruction (Table 23.1). Oesophageal atresia is discussed in Chapter 10. If the obstruction is high or complete, symptoms are present at or shortly after birth.

Clinical features

The infant presents with some or all of the following features:

Table 23.1 Types of intestinal obstruction in the newborn

Congenital	Acquired	Functional
Intrinsic		
Atresias –	Necrotizing enterocolitis	Hirschsprung's disease
oesophageal, duodenal,	Intussusception	
small bowel, colonic	Peritoneal adhesions	Meconium plug syndrome
Stenoses		
Anorectal malformation		Ileus
Meconium ileus		Peritonitis
Enteric duplications		
Extrinsic		
Volvulus		Intestinal pseudo-obstruction
Peritoneal bands		syndrome
Annular pancreas		
Cysts and tumours		
Incarcerated hernia		

1 Bile-stained vomiting. This is a very important sign that must not be ignored. A history of bile-stained vomiting demands immediate investigation as it suggests obstruction is below the second part of the duodenum. Sporadic bile-stained vomiting suggests partial obstruction caused by malrotation, duplication or annular pancreas.

2 Abdominal distension. This may not be prominent with a high obstruction:

3 Visible peristalsis.

4 Delayed passage of meconium. In cases of low obstruction there may be no passage of meconium at all. With a high obstruction meconium may be passed for a day or two. A changing stool is never seen with congenital bowel obstruction. Anal atresia should be recognized early at routine examination.

5 Dehydration. The infant may present with dehydration and collapse as the result of excessive vomiting.

Investigations and management

The following investigations and management options apply in cases of suspected intestinal obstruction.

1 Obstetric ultrasound as early as 17–19 weeks might reveal suspicious features such as polyhydramnios, 'double bubble' or echogenic bowel.

2 Initial abdominal X-rays should be plain films with infant in the supine and left lateral positions:
- duodenal obstruction shows a 'double bubble';
- distal obstruction shows a series of dilated air- and fluid-filled loops of intestine;
- meconium ileus usually has no air/fluid levels but sometimes a 'soap bubbles' appearance.

3 Withhold feeds, insert i.v. and nasogastric Replogle (double-lumen) tube.

4 Consult paediatric surgeon if obstruction confirmed or suspected.

5 If diagnosis is in doubt or meconium ileus suspected, a contrast enema is performed:
- microcolon suggests small bowel atresia or meconium ileus.

6 An upper gastrointestinal contrast study is performed if plain film and contrast enema are non-diagnostic.

Classification of intestinal obstruction

The causes of obstruction may be classified depending on the site of blockage (large or small bowel) or whether it is anatomical or functional. On occasions it is impossible to be sure of the diagnosis or even the level of obstruction, and laparotomy may be the only way of making a diagnosis in order to treat the condition effectively.

Anatomical obstruction

Pyloric stenosis

Vomiting (often projectile) is the predominant symptom and occurs between birth and 15 weeks, most commonly weeks 3–5. The vomitus contains partially digested milk but no bile. Gastric peristalsis may be seen. The condition is due to hypertrophy of the pylorus and a definite tumour can be felt on palpation. There is often a family history, and boys are affected four times more often than girls. The cause of the hypertrophy is not known, but may be related to stress in a genetically susceptible infant. Incidence is 1/1000 – 1/3000. The risk for subsequent siblings is about 7%. Preterm infants characteristically present 5 weeks after full enteral feeding is achieved.

Diagnosis is made by palpation of the upper abdomen during a test feed. Ultrasound examination reveals a characteristic 'doughnut' ring corresponding to the hypertrophied pylorus. Only rarely should radiological contrast studies be necessary.

Treatment is surgical following adequate restoration of electrolyte and fluid balance and correction of metabolic alkalosis. At surgery the muscle fibres of the hypertrophied pylorus are incised down to the mucosa. This is known as Ramstedt's procedure and is performed via a periumbilical incision or laparoscopically.

Duodenal obstruction

Complete duodenal obstruction presents early with vomiting, which will be bile stained if the obstruction is below the second part of the duodenum. Partial duodenal obstruction, such as occurs with malrotation, may be more difficult to diagnose, as vomiting may be intermittent and stools are passed (see below). Duodenal atresia may be due to either intrinsic or extrinsic obstruction.

Intrinsic causes
- Duodenal atresia – 50% are associated with Down syndrome but other associations include other bowel atresias, and cardiovascular and anorectal malformations.
- Duodenal stenosis – septum or membrane.

Extrinsic causes
Malrotation may cause the second part of the duodenum to be obstructed by Ladd's peritoneal bands. Annular pancreas may also cause extrinsic obstruction to the duodenum.

Diagnosis
A plain X-ray of the abdomen classically shows a 'double-bubble' appearance (Fig. 23.3) in duodenal atresia. If there is no air beyond this double bubble, then the diagnosis of duodenal atresia is certain and no further investigations are required. Small bubbles of air beyond the second part of the duodenum suggest an incomplete bowel obstruction and must be investigated further for malrotation.

Treatment
After resuscitation with fluids and electrolytes definitive surgical repair is performed. Postoperatively these infants often require prolonged total parenteral nutrition because of poor peristaltic activity across the anastomosis. Often the dilated proximal duodenum is tapered to reduce the duodenal dysmotility. Passage of a trans duodenoduodenostomy feeding tube may facilitate earlier enteral feeding.

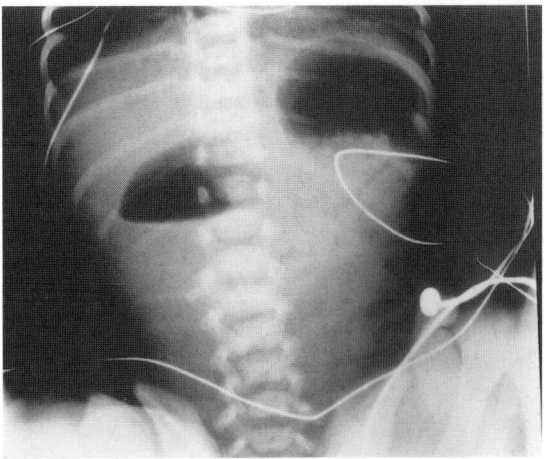

Figure 23.3 Duodenal atresia. Abdominal radiograph showing the 'double-bubble' appearance.

Malrotation (volvulus neonatorum)

This results from incomplete fixation and rotation of the bowel after it returns to the fetal abdominal cavity from the yolk sac between the eighth and tenth weeks of gestation. The three features of malrotation are:

1 the duodenojejunal junction is at or to the right of the vertebral column;

2 the ileocaecal junction is near the midline and higher than normal;

3 Bowel is abnormally fixed by avascular (Ladd's) bands, which cross the second part of the duodenum.

These abnormalities cause the small bowel mesentery, in which the superior mesenteric artery lies, to be abnormally mobile and to twist around its axis, leading to a volvulus with rapid impairment of gut blood flow. This may cause intestinal obstruction in one of two ways:

1 strangulation obstruction: the superior mesenteric artery supplying blood to the bowel is occluded;

2 Ladd's bands obstruct the second part of the duodenum.

Midgut volvulus can occur at any time but 80% of cases occur in the neonatal period or *in utero*.

Diagnosis

This lesion characteristically produces episodic obstruction with abdominal distension, bile-stained vomiting, pallor and a vague abdominal mass in an infant who was previously tolerating feeds well. The baby may rapidly proceed to shock.

Plain X-ray of the abdomen in the erect position may show a characteristic double bubble, but gas is seen beyond the duodenum. Contrast studies may show a corkscrew duodenum or an abnormally situated subhepatic position of the caecum. Ultrasound scan may show an abnormal relationship between the superior mesenteric artery and vein strongly suggestive of malrotation.

Treatment

Laparotomy needs to be performed urgently to untwist and relieve the volvulus. It may be difficult to exclude volvulus clinically and, in view of the rapidity with which bowel infarction occurs, an early laparotomy is advisable in suspected cases.

Jejunal atresia

Half of all intestinal atresias occur in the jejunum or ileum. Rarely they are associated with gastroschisis, intrauterine volvulus or meconium ileus.

The jejunum is the commonest site for intestinal atresia. Bowel atresias are probably due to in early fetal life. The atretic segment may be isolated or multiple. The diagnosis is often made on prenatal ultrasound examination. After birth the infant rapidly develops marked abdominal distension, and X-ray shows loops of dilated bowel with multiple fluid levels. Peritoneal calcification signifies the presence of meconium peritonitis. Treatment is by resection of the atretic segment, but sacrifice of grossly dilated bowel above the stricture may be necessary before primary anastomosis is possible.

Colonic atresia

Less than 10% of bowel atresias occur in the colon; they are probably due to a vascular accident in the mesentery during early pregnancy. The infant presents with low bowel obstruction, usually on the second or third day of life. A contrast enema shows a distal microcolon.

Anorectal malformations

An imperforate anus is a perineum without an anal opening. The commonest classification of anorectal malformations is shown in Table 23.2. The arrested development of the anus and rectum may be divided into high lesions (rectal deformities), intermediate and low lesions (anal deformities).

The incidence is 1/5000 live births. There is a slight preponderance of cases affecting male infants, in whom there is a higher incidence of the more serious rectal deformities, whereas in females the anal type is more common, with a stenotic ectopic orifice.

Clinical features

This condition should be obvious on examination. Other anomalies, such as genitourinary, vertebral, alimentary tract (especially oesophageal atresia), cardiac and central nervous system, must be carefully excluded. Anorectal anomalies may be one of the features of the VACTERL association (Vertebral,

Table 23.2 International classification of anorectal malformations (Stephens & Smith 1986)

	Female	Male
High (above levator ani)	Anorectal agenesis Rectovaginal fistula No fistula Rectal atresia	Anorectal agenesis Rectoprostatic fistula No fistula Rectal atresia
Intermediate	Rectovaginal fistula Rectovestibular fistula Anal agenesis	Bulbar fistula Anal agenesis
Low (below levator ani)	Anovestibular fistula Anocutaneous fistula Anal stenosis	Anocutaneous fistula Anal stenosis persistent cloaca

Anal, Cardiac, Tracheal, Esophagus, Renal and Limb defects).

Defecation and micturition should be observed in these infants. In the female all orifices must be carefully examined and probed for evidence of additional fistulous tracts. Most female infants will decompress their bowel spontaneously via a vaginal fistula. In the majority of males meconium will be seen in the urine owing to a rectovesical or rectourethral fistula.

Investigations
X-rays of the spine and sacrum will detect any vertebral or sacral anomalies. A cross-table plain X-ray is taken, with the pelvis elevated, after 24 hours of age, when adequate gas should have passed to the end of the bowel. A line drawn between the pubic symphysis and the sacrococcygeal junction constitutes the pubococcygeal line. Gas cranial to this line indicates a high rectal anomaly, whereas gas caudal to this line indicates an anal anomaly.

An intravenous pyelogram or ultrasound examination will reveal a renal anomaly in 25% of cases. A micturating cystourethrogram will demonstrate a rectovesical fistula and vesico-ureteric reflux. Low lesions have a good prognosis and can usually be managed with local reconstructive surgery of the anus.

Management and outcome
High lesions will require a colostomy in the neonatal period to decompress the bowel, followed by rectoplasty at 6–2 months of age. High lesions are generally associated with rectal incontinence after treatment. Before closure, a distal colostogram allows for the precise localization of fistula.

The results of surgery in intermediate or low atresia are somewhat better. Generally, about one-third will have normal anal continence, one-third will have acceptable continence with some soiling, and one-third will be totally incontinent. The avoidance of repeated urinary tract infections in males with rectovesical fistula is important. Long-term constipation is a common complication of this disorder.

Functional obstruction

Hirschsprung's disease (aganglionosis)
This condition results from the absence of ganglion cells in the plexus of Auerbach, which prevents orderly peristaltic activity through the bowel. It is the commonest cause of large bowel obstruction in the newborn and has an incidence of 1/5000. In 20% there are other associated diseases such as Down syndrome, Waardenburg syndrome, Smith–Lemli–Opitz syndrome or central hypoventilation syndrome. It is inherited as a polygenic disease with a recurrence risk within families of 12.5%. Hirschsprung's disease may result from mutations in several genes either singly or in combination. These mutations may give dominant, recessive or polygenic patterns of inheritance. There are two distinct types:
1 *Short aganglionic segment* (85–90%). This is the most common type, with a male to female ratio

of 4:1. It usually affects the rectum and sigmoid colon.

2 *Long aganglionic segment* (8–10%). This is rarer and has a 1:1 male to female ratio. This type is more commonly inherited in families.

Only 15% of patients with Hirschsprung's disease present in the newborn period.

Diagnosis

The most common presentation in the newborn period is with acute obstruction. The infant vomits and has a distended abdomen, with failure to pass meconium. Rectal examination may reveal an explosive gush of meconium, to be followed by progressive constipation and further signs of obstruction. In older infants chronic constipation may develop with 'spurious diarrhoea', which is not seen in the neonate. It may be difficult to distinguish Hirschsprung's disease from cystic fibrosis and meconium plug syndrome.

Management

Definitive management is surgical repair, but there are three alternatives for initial treatment:

- rectal irrigation;
- colostomy;
- primary repair.

Irrespective of whether repair is done using one or two operations, the classic operation is the 'pull through', consisting of excision of the aganglionic segment and pulling the normally innervated bowel down to the anus.

Meconium plug syndrome. This may occur with intrauterine growth restriction, Hirschsprung's disease, meconium ileus, or as an isolated condition. The infant fails to open his or her bowels in the first 24 h and may develop clinical and radiological signs of obstruction. A white plug of meconium is passed spontaneously or following rectal examination or contrast enema, and the signs of obstruction settle down. These infants require careful follow-up in order to detect those with Hirschsprung's disease or cystic fibrosis.

Necrotizing enterocolitis (NEC; see p. 254). This may develop acutely in infants with Hirschsprung's disease. This diagnosis must be considered in all infants with NEC.

Investigations

A plain X-ray of the abdomen may show dilated bowel loops and fluid levels, and lateral X-ray of the pelvis may show the air-filled cone. Contrast studies using barium or other agents may show the dilated normal bowel above a tapering transitional zone with distal microcolon. The definitive diagnosis is made by biopsy. This may be either a suction biopsy of the rectal mucosa and submucosa (less invasive), or a formal full-thickness strip biopsy of the bowel under a general anaesthetic. Histology reveals the absence of ganglia in the nerve plexus. Some centres use cholinesterase staining techniques to confirm the histological findings.

Treatment

In the neonate a colostomy is performed just above the site of transition, together with a biopsy to confirm that the stoma has been fashioned in normally innervated bowel. Rectosigmoidectomy is performed 3–6 months later, with closure of the colostomy at that time or at a third operation.

Meconium ileus

Ten to fifteen percent of infants with cystic fibrosis present with meconium ileus owing to pancreatic insufficiency with inspissated meconium. In about half, meconium ileus is complicated by ischaemia, volvulus, stenosis and malrotation, or meconium peritonitis with intraperitoneal calcification and pseudocyst formation, secondary to intrauterine perforation. Ninety percent of infants with meconium ileus have cystic fibrosis.

Diagnosis

Cystic fibrosis may present with an acute bowel obstruction, a meconium plug syndrome, or the infant may become acutely ill with sepsis and cardiovascular collapse.

A plain X-ray of the abdomen shows multiple fluid levels and typically a foamy pattern of air bubbles trapped around inspissated meconium. A Gastrografin enema shows a microcolon.

In the first month of life measurement of immunoreactive trypsin (IRT) on a heel-prick blood specimen is a very sensitive method for diagnosing cystic fibrosis, and can be used as a screening test. Unfortunately, after operation for meconium ileus the IRT level may rapidly fall despite the child having cystic fibrosis. For this reason, all neonates with signs of bowel obstruction should have an IRT measurement prior to surgery. Eighty percent of children with cystic fibrosis have the ☐F508 gene, which should be determined in all cases of meconium ileus. Definitive diagnosis of cystic fibrosis is by genetic probes as soon as the condition is suspected, or by sweat testing at 1–3 months of age.

Treatment

The decision as to whether the bowel obstruction is to be managed medically or surgically will be made by the surgeon. Management with Gastrografin enemas under fluoroscopic control may be initially diagnostic and subsequently therapeutic by softening the meconium so that it can be passed normally. Surgical decompression is often necessary in complicated cases, and is done in conjunction with Gastrografin washouts of the bowel. The baby with cystic fibrosis will also require lifelong treatment with appropriate antibiotics, chest physiotherapy, salt replacement, pancreatic extracts and fat-soluble vitamins. Genetic counselling is essential for this autosomal recessive condition.

Abdominal wall defects

Exomphalos (omphalocoele) and gastroschisis are discussed together as they are both eviscerations of gastrointestinal contents: an exomphalos emerges through the umbilicus, whereas gastroschisis is through a right paramedian abdominal cleft.

Exomphalos (omphalocoele)

Exomphalos occurs in 1/6000 births and is due to an embryological abnormality at 18 weeks of gestation, resulting in the bowel failing to re-enter the abdomen. The extra-abdominal bowel is covered by peritoneum and the umbilical cord is at the apex of the exomphalos. It is associated with other anomalies in 60–80% of cases, particularly when the defect is small. These include congenital heart disease, Beckwith–Wiedemann syndrome (exomphalos, large tongue and hypoglycaemia) or chromosomal disorders (trisomy 13, trisomy 18).

The diagnosis is often made on prenatal ultrasound examination after 14 weeks' gestation and elevated maternal serum α-fetoprotein, and fetal chromosome analysis is essential together with careful surveillance for other congenital malformations. On occasion, the peritoneal sac ruptures *in utero* and exposes bowel loops to amniotic fluid with resultant matting of bowel loops.

Management

At birth, sac and contents should be kept warm and moist by use of plastic wrap. A nasogastric tube is inserted, the stomach is decompressed and i.v. fluids commenced at 1.5 times maintenance rate. Operative repair is recommended within 2–4 hours after birth.

Small lesions, with abdominal defects of less than 5 cm, can generally be treated surgically with primary closure. Larger defects may be amenable to primary closure, but if this is not possible the eviscerated bowel is protected by a Teflon silo, which is progressively reduced in size to allow reduction of the hernia.

Frequently, the intra-abdominal compartment is too small readily to accommodate the bowel, and complications such as respiratory distress due to splinting of diaphragm, compression of vena cava, and renal failure, hypotension and bowel ischaemia, occur. Recently described is the use of a vacuum device to facilitate the reduction of bowel contents and wound healing for giant exomphalos.

Gastroschisis

Gastroschisis is the herniation of abdominal contents through an abdominal wall defect, usually to the right of the umbilical cord. In contrast to exomphalos, gastroschisis has no peritoneal covering and the bowel is loose within the amniotic cavity. Consequently, it becomes scarred and bound with adhesions, with resultant stenosis, strictures, atresias and poor intestinal motility. There is often intrauterine growth failure, possibly associated with a short bowel syndrome, failure to thrive and steatorrhoea.

The incidence of gastroschisis is increasing worldwide and is currently 1:3800 births in Australia. It is usually associated with young mothers of low gravidity. Unlike exomphalos, it is rarely associated with other congenital malformations. There is no satisfactory embryological explanation for gastroschisis, but a vascular lesion related to intrauterine interruption of the omphalomesenteric artery seems most plausible.

Management

At birth the bowel must be handled very carefully to avoid further trauma. It should be placed in a sterile saline-filled plastic bag to avoid hypothermia. Primary repair is possible if the defect is small, but repair becomes more difficult when there is massive evisceration. A silo may be necessary before the abdomen can be fully closed. For selected cases, reduction of the gastroschisis can be successfully undertaken in the intensive care nursery shortly after birth, without general anaesthesia, by a paediatric surgeon. Following abdominal repair severe respiratory embarrassment may occur as the result of diaphragmatic splinting secondary to raised intra-abdominal pressure. Prolonged mechanical ventilation is often required postoperatively.

Unlike in exomphalos, the bowel tends to show prolonged dysfunction in the absence of any anatomical abnormality. This may require long-term total parenteral nutrition.

Necrotizing enterocolitis (NEC)

NEC is the most important acquired bowel abnormality occurring in the newborn period. It is defined as an inflammatory disease with ulceration and sometimes perforation of the bowel. It most commonly affects the terminal ileum or sigmoid colon. The radiographic appearance of intramural gas (pneumatosis intestinalis) is generally considered confirmatory evidence of the disease. A definitive diagnosis can only be made at autopsy or on pathological examination of surgical specimens.

NEC is much commoner in very low birthweight (VLBW) infants (approximately 5% of these), but is generally less commonly seen in the UK and Australia than in the USA. The incidence varies between 0.2 and 3/1000 births. If NEC occurs in full-term infants, causes of gut ischaemia such as congenital heart disease, perinatal asphyxia,

Hirschsprung's disease or an endocrine disorder, must be sought. The overall mortality is 25–30%, higher in infants <28 weeks' gestation, and surgery is required in 25–50% of survivors.

Pathogenesis

The cause of NEC is unknown, but there are three main predisposing factors (Weaver 1997).
1 *Mucosal injury.* This may occur as a result of immaturity of the mucosal defences or as a complication of abnormal blood flow to the gut mucosa, as occurs in:
 (a) asphyxia;
 (b) patent ductus arteriosus, which is twice as common in babies who develop NEC than in controls;
 (c) polycythaemia;
 (d) severe intrauterine growth restriction with evidence of compromised blood flow on antenatal Doppler studies (absent or retrograde diastolic flow);
 (e) umbilical venous and arterial catheter use;
 (f) cyanotic heart disease;
 (g) a complication of Hirschsprung's disease due to local mucosal ischaemia.
2 *Enteral feeds.* NEC is very rare in babies who have received no enteral feeds. The risk of NEC may be due to the effect of milk on bacterial proliferation, or the volume of feed. NEC is also more common where hyperosmolar feeds and formula feeds rather than breast milk are used. Although the leucocytes and immunoglobulins in breast milk are thought to protect an infant from this disease, NEC occasionally occurs in exclusively breastfed infants. Recent studies suggest that NEC occurs more commonly in at-risk babies when the volume of feeds is increased rapidly over the first few days of life.
3 *Infection.* Although infection is probably not the direct cause, some enteric organisms predispose to the development of this condition. Many organisms have been implicated, including coliforms, staphylococci, clostridia and rotavirus.

Mucosal injury by one of the above mechanisms allows secondary invasion of gas-producing bacteria, which causes pneumatosis coli. A schema to illustrate this process is shown in Fig. 23.4.

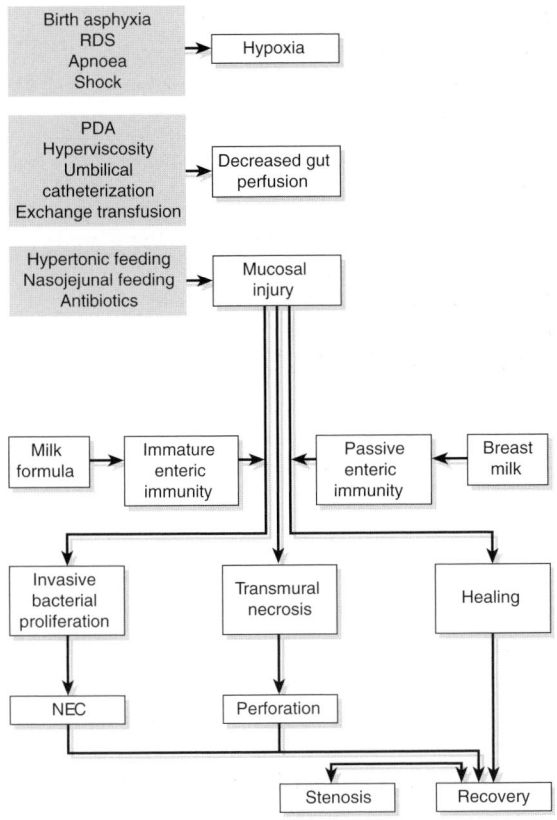

Figure 23.4 Schema for the development of NEC.

Clinical features

The early signs of NEC are often non-specific, with lethargy, apnoea, bile-stained aspirates and failure to maintain body temperature. These features are common in preterm infants, but the early cessation of feeding under these circumstances may prevent the progression to full-blown NEC. The signs may progress to include abdominal distension, blood and mucus in the stool, and circulatory collapse. Apnoea, bradycardia, shock, poor urine output and metabolic acidosis are commonly seen in severe cases. Complications of the disease include:

1 DIC (disseminated intravascular coagulation);
2 septicaemia in 33% of cases;
3 bowel perforation with a localized abscess or generalized peritonitis;
4 bowel obstruction;
5 gangrenous bowel;

6 lactose intolerance and malabsorption in the recovery period;
7 relapse after commencing oral feeds;
8 intrahepatic cholestasis relating to inflammatory bowel disease and total parenteral nutrition.

The severity of NEC is staged using Bell's criteria (Table 23.3). Fifty percent of survivors have long-term complications such as relapse (10%), intestinal stricture, short bowel syndrome and intrahepatic cholestasis.

Investigations

The main avenues of investigation in cases of NEC are:

1 *Erect and cross-table lateral abdominal X-rays.* These may show distension of bowel loops only. Later a foamy gas pattern (pneumatosis intestinalis, Fig. 23.5), portal vein gas, pneumoperitoneum, fluid levels or free peritoneal fluid may be seen on abdominal films.
2 *Full blood count.* This shows a neutropenia or neutrophilia, a shift to the left of the leucocytes, toxic granulations in the neutrophils and thrombocytopenia.
3 *Microbiological investigation.* Faeces and blood are examined and cultured. Many Gram-positive and Gram-negative organisms have been associated with NEC, but the most frequent isolates are *Clostridium* sp. and *Klebsiella* spp. Faeces should also be sent for viral studies and examination for rotavirus, as this agent has been incriminated in the pathogenesis of some cases of NEC.

Management

Prevention

Various strategies have been suggested to reduce or eliminate the risk of NEC. These include:

1 Antenatal steroids. These have shown a dramatic effect in reducing the risk of NEC. This is most likely to be related to the reduced risk of respiratory distress syndrome (RDS) and the lower likelihood of gut ischaemia secondary to this.
2 Delay in milk feeding in high-risk babies. Babies delivered early because of severe intrauterine growth restriction, particularly when there has been retrograde flow on antenatal Doppler

Table 23.3 Modified Bell's Staging Criteria for Necrotizing Enterocolitis

Stage	Systemic signs	Intestinal signs	Radiological signs	Treatment
I: Suspected				
A	Temperature instability, apnoea bradycardia	Elevated pregavage residuals, mild abdominal distention, occult blood in stool	Normal or mild ileus	NPO, antibiotics × 3 days
B	Same as for IA	Same as for IA, plus gross blood in stool	Same as for IA	Same as for IA
II: Definite				
A: Mildly ill	Same as for IA	Same as I, plus absent bowel sounds, abdominal tenderness	Ileus, intestinal pneumatosis	NPO, antibiotics × 7–10 days
B: Moderately ill	Same as for I, plus mild metabolic acidosis, mild thrombocytopenia	Same as I, plus absent bowel sounds, abdominal tenderness, abdominal cellulites, right lower quadrant mass	Same as for IIA, plus portal vein gas, with or without ascites	NPO, antibiotics × 14 days
III: Advanced				
A: Severely ill, Bowel intact	Same as for IIB, plus hypotension, bradycardia, respiratory acidosis, metabolic acidosis, disseminated intravascular coagulation, neutropenia	Same as for I and II, plus signs of generalized peritonitis, marked tenderness, and distention of abdomen	Same as for IIB, plus definite ascites	NPO, antibiotics × 14 days, fluid resuscitation, inotropic support, ventilator therapy, paracentesis
B: Severely ill, Bowel perforated	Same as for IIIA	Same as for IIIA	Same as for IIB, plus pneumoperitoneum	Same as for IIA, plus surgery

NPO, nil per os.

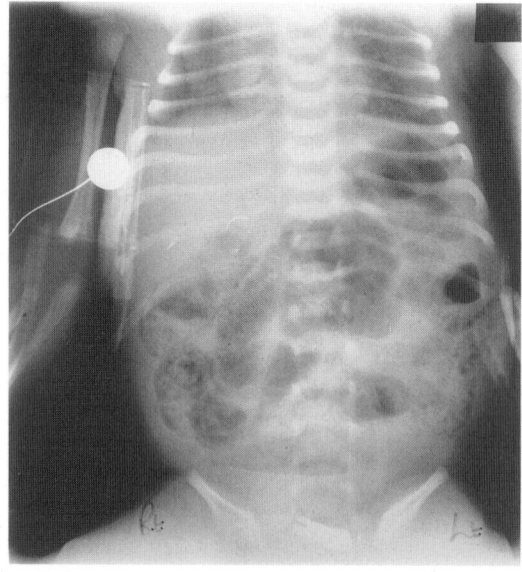

Figure 23.5 Radiological appearance of NEC. The bowel shows extensive intramural gas (arrowed).

assessment, appear to be at increased risk of NEC. Delaying the introduction of any milk feed in these babies for the first 5 days is advisable and when introduced it should be increased only slowly at 1–2 mL/kg/day.

3 Breast milk is also known to confer a reduced risk of NEC compared with formula feeds. In one controlled study, the risk of NEC was six times higher in the formula-fed group than in the breastfed premature infants (Lucus & Cole 1990). Small volumes of breast milk and breast milk mixed with formula also appear to lower the risk.

4 Oral antibiotic therapy. This has been shown to reduce the risk of NEC in a number of small studies (Bury & Tudehope 2006), but this is not recommended at present because of the risk of antibiotic resistance.

5 Oral immunoglobulin (IgA and IgG). This has been suggested to reduce the risk of NEC, but the results of a larger randomized controlled study did not support this finding.

6 The preventive role of enteral probiotics and pre-biotics is currently under investigation.

Therapy

Great caution should be exercised when the infant is given milk. At the first sign of gastrointestinal intolerance feeds are stopped in order to rest the bowel. Total parenteral nutrition is started for at least 10 days and broad-spectrum antibiotics given (gentamicin, ampicillin and metronidazole), or third-generation cephalosporins for 7–10 days. Fluid, electrolyte and acid–base disorders must be corrected. Transfusions with fresh whole blood and correction of coagulopathy may be necessary.

Infants with proven NEC are best managed conservatively. The indications for surgical intervention include:

1 free air in the peritoneum, indicating bowel perforation;

2 clinical deterioration during conservative management – this should be carefully assessed with a view to surgical intervention;

3 failure to improve on medical management.

Care must be taken in transfusing babies following acute NEC because the T-antigen on red cells may cause massive haemolysis. Use of low titre T-antigen blood for transfusion is recommended in some units.

Surgical intervention includes peritoneal drainage or formal laparotomy. The former may be done under general anaesthetic or in the newborn unit with a cannula under local anaesthesia.

Laparotomy is best done in a specialist neonatal surgical centre. Fashioning an ileostomy in a healthy bowel with peritoneal drainage is usually the best form of treatment, and necrotic bowel is often not resected as a primary procedure. A second laparotomy may be necessary when the baby has recovered from the acute NEC.

Complications

Short bowel syndrome

This is a major problem in babies with very extensive NEC. If the bowel is too short (<40 cm in a full-term baby) or if the ileocaecal valve has been surgically resected along with a significant amount of ileum, then the baby may be left with too little bowel for normal absorption. Some centres undertake long-term total parenteral nutrition at home for this condition. Small bowel transplantation is successful in selected cases and is available on a supraregional basis in many Western countries.

Stricture

This occurs in approximately 15% of infants following NEC; the descending colon is the most commonly affected site.

Lactose intolerance

This is caused by damage to the brush border of the mucosa, with sloughing of the disaccharidases. This condition arises in 5–10% of infants after NEC. Semi-elemental formulas are recommended when the gut is rechallenged after recovery from extensive disease.

Recurrence

This occurs in 10% of babies, and Hirschsprung's disease must be considered as an aetiological factor.

Rectal bleeding

Blood and mucus in the stool is a common finding in the neonatal period, but the sight of blood on the nappy of a newborn infant is alarming for a mother. It is important to distinguish whether the blood is fresh or altered, confined to the outside of the stool or mixed throughout. Other symptoms, such as constipation, abdominal distension or pain, may assist with the diagnosis.

Common causes of blood in the stools include:

1 Sallowed maternal blood.

2 Rectal or anal fissure from thermometer, rectal examination or severe constipation.

3 NEC.

4 Benign haemorrhagic colitis. This is one of the commonest causes of blood in the stool. It is usually associated with mucus and occurs most commonly in formula-fed infants. It may be due to cows' milk protein intolerance and recurs when cows' milk protein is reintroduced in the feeds.

5 Malrotation, intussusception.

6 Meckel's diverticulum and bowel duplication with ectopic gastric mucosa.

7 Gastroenteritis: human rotavirus, *Shigella* spp., *Salmonella* sp., enteropathogenic *Escherichia coli*.

8 Rectal polyp.

9 Haemorrhagic disease of the newborn.

The clinical history and examination will elucidate many of the above causes. Apt's test will distinguish fetal from maternal blood. Plain X-rays of the abdomen may confirm NEC or may suggest malrotation. Faecal cultures and examination of the stool for human rotavirus or other infectious agents will confirm the clinical diagnosis of gastro-enteritis. The ectopic gastric mucosa in a bleeding Meckel's diverticulum or bowel duplication may be demonstrated with a technetium radioisotope scan. The bleeding and prolonged prothrombin time in an infant with haemorrhagic disease of the newborn are corrected by a dose of vitamin K, 1 mg intramuscularly.

Most infants with blood and mucus in their stool will settle spontaneously without any obvious cause being found on investigation.

References

Bury RG, Tudehope DI. Enteral antibiotics for preventing necrotizing enterocolitis in low birth weight or preterm infants. *Cochrane Database of Systematic Reviews* 2006: (1) CD 000405.

Cass DT. Unravelling the pathogenesis and molecular genetics of Hirschsprung's disease. *Semin Neonatol* 1996;**1**:211–217.

Lucus A, Cole TJ. Breast milk and neonatal necrotising enterocolitis. *Lancet* 1990;**336**:1519–1521.

McDonnell M, Wilkinson A. Necrotizing enterocolitis – perinatal approach to prevention, early diagnosis and management. *Semin Neonatol* 1997;**2**:291–296.

Stephens FD, Smith ED. Classification, identification and assessment of surgical treatment of anorectal anomalies. *Pediatr Surg Int* 1986;**1**:200–205.

Weaver LT. Digestive system development and failure. *Semin Neonatol* 1997;**2**:221–230.

Further reading

Altman PR, Stylianos S. Paediatric surgery. *Pediatr Clin N Am* 1993;**40**(6).

Lloyd DA. Neonatal surgery. *Semin Neonatol* 1996;**1**(3).

Wilkinson AR, Tam PKH. Necrotizing enterocolitis. *Semin Neonatol* 1997;**2**(4).

24 Skin disorders

Cutaneous lesions are present at birth in 8% of newborn infants. They are immediately obvious, attract attention and may cause considerable concern. Sometimes they are part of a neurocutaneous syndrome where there are skin markers of brain disease. Examples presenting in the neonatal period include Sturge–Weber syndrome, neurofibromatosis and incontinentia pigmenti.

Cutaneous lesions in the newborn can be classified in the following major groups:

1 vascular birthmarks;
2 epidermal naevi;
3 pigmented birthmarks;
4 ichthyotic disorders;
5 blistering and bullous disorders;
6 miscellaneous.

Vascular birthmarks

Vascular birthmarks may be classified as either haemangiomas or vascular malformations. Older descriptive terminology, such as 'cavernous', 'strawberry' and 'naevus flammeus', should be avoided.

Haemangiomas

These vascular tumours are characterized by rapid endothelial growth followed by slow involution. Approximately 30% are present at birth as a blanched area or a telangiectatic patch. The majority appear during the first month of life, and grow rapidly over the next 5 months (Fig. 24.1). Slow involution subsequently occurs over the next 5–10 years.

Superficial haemangiomas deep in the dermis, subcutaneous fat or muscle produce a bluish colour in the overlying skin.

The majority of haemangiomas do not require treatment. Oral corticosteroids commenced during the rapid growth phase in the first 5 months of life are very effective in slowing growth and hastening resolution but there may be a resurgence after cessation of treatment. Indications for treatment with corticosteroid include lesions that interfere with vital functions, 'edge structures' (e.g. eyelids, nares, philtrum, lips or pinnae), those associated with high cardiac output failure, and extensive facial lesions. Bleeding is rarely a problem, even after trauma, but large lesions around limb girdles may be associated with thrombocytopenia, intravascular coagulation and severe bleeding (Kasabach–Merritt syndrome).

Vascular malformations

These represent structural anomalies, are present at birth, grow in proportion to the infant's growth, and in general do not have a tendency to resolve.

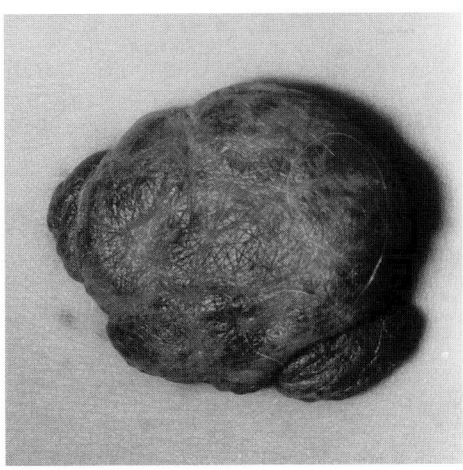

Figure 24.1 Vascular haemangioma.

Capillary malformations

Fine capillary haemangiomas, which are deep red in colour and blanch with pressure, occur on the glabella, upper eyelids, upper lips and nape of the neck. They are of no significance and tend to fade during the first 6 months.

Larger, flat, deep, purple-red ('port-wine') lesions may occur on any part of the body. Those in the distribution of the trigeminal nerve may be associated with retinal and intracranial haemangiomas, requiring ophthalmological follow-up (Fig. 24.2). Association of this type of lesion with vascular malformation of the ipsilateral meninges and cerebral cortex is termed the Sturge–Weber syndrome and requires neurological assessment. The skin manifestations may be treated with cosmetic cover creams or by pulsed dye laser in later infancy.

Epidermal naevi

These birthmarks presenting at birth or in the first few months of life represent proliferation of keratinocytes or cells of the skin appendage. They are

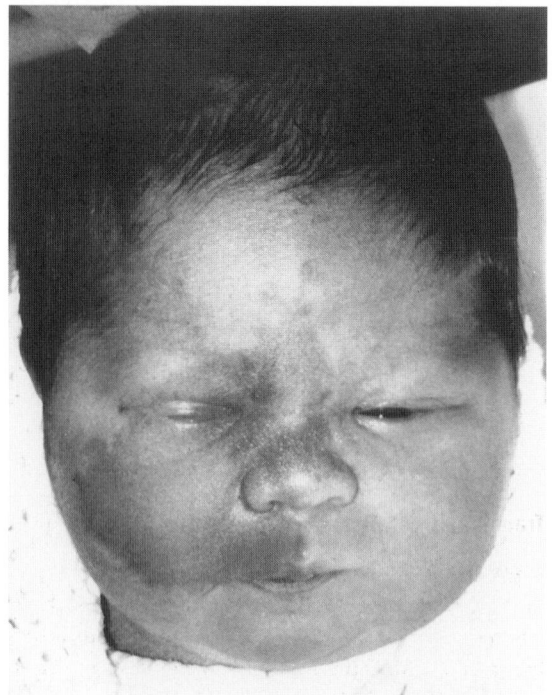

Figure 24.2 Port-wine stain affecting the maxillary region.

rare lesions that may involve any area of the skin, including the oral cavity. On the scalp and face they are often yellowish because of a prominent sebaceous gland component. Trunk and limb epidermal naevi are scaly, flat or raised, varying in colour from black or brown to pale grey, with plaque or linear streak distribution. Treatment with topical retinoic acid or oral retinoids is generally unsatisfactory. Excision may be indicated for small and linear lesions and for irritating and cosmetically troublesome naevi.

Hyperpigmented and hypopigmented birthmarks

These must be differentiated from the skin lesions of generalized disorders, such as neurofibromatosis and tuberous sclerosis (neurocutaneous syndromes), which usually appear after birth.

Congenital hyperpigmented patches

These common pale or dark-brown macular or flat hypermelanotic patches may be solitary or extensive, involving large areas of the trunk or limbs. They must be differentiated from the *café au lait* spots of classic neurofibromatosis, which are occasionally present at birth. Treatment consists of cosmetic cover creams, or plastic surgery for smaller lesions.

Congenital melanocytic naevi

These are collections of melanocytes in the epidermis, dermis or both. Most are not present at birth, but when present they appear as raised verrucous or lobulated lesions of various shades of brown to black (Fig. 24.3). They vary in size and may have blue or pink components, often growing long black hairs. They grow in proportion to the infant's growth. Controversy exists about the risk of malignant change. Lesions over the lower spine may be associated with a tethered spinal cord (see p. 208). Large or multiple lesions may be associated with benign or, rarely, malignant proliferation of melanocytes in the leptomeninges, demonstrated by magnetic resonance imaging (MRI). Small lesions are easily removed surgically; for larger lesions plastic procedures may be possible.

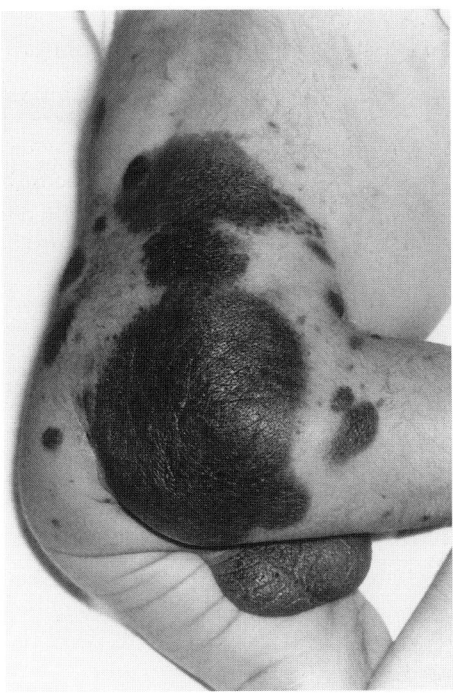

Figure 24.3 Congenital melanocytic naevus involving the buttock and loin.

Mongolian spots

These are flat, blue or slate-grey lesions comprising collections of melanocytes in the dermis. They are seen in the majority of oriental and black infants. In white infants there is usually a background of Mediterranean origin. Single or multiple, they occur particularly in the lumbosacral area, less often on the shoulders, back or other areas, and tend to fade with age. These lesions should not be confused with non-accidental injuries and they do not require any intervention.

Congenital hypopigmented patches

These are pale areas of reduced cutaneous melanin varying in size from a few centimetres to large areas covering the trunk and limbs. They do not involute. Similar lesions occur in incontinentia pigmenti, a rare genetic neurocutaneous condition affecting females and associated with multiple abnormalities, especially of the eye, skeleton and central nervous systems.

Ichthyotic disorders

These are a rare group of skin disorders where the skin at birth resembles fish scales. There are several varieties.

Ichthyosis vulgaris

This is an autosomal dominant disorder and other members of the family may have a history of atopy. It rarely causes problems in the newborn period and is best treated with an aqueous ointment.

Recessive X-linked ichthyosis

This condition only affects males and is associated with placental sulphatase deficiency. Unrecordable oestriol measurements during pregnancy should alert the clinician to this possibility in male infants.

Collodion baby

The most severe form of this group of disorders is the collodion baby (Fig. 24.4). At birth the infant looks as if he or she has instead of skin a dry plastic-like membrane, which cracks easily. These infants often later develop lamellar ichthyosis, but some may have no persistent skin abnormality. It is likely that the collodion baby, and the more severe harlequin fetus, represent a heterogeneous pathological group.

Blistering and bullous disorders

These constitute a wide group of unrelated disorders characterized by blistering of the skin. They can be divided into transient and chronic disorders (Table 24.1).

Transient

Erythema toxicum (urticaria neonatorum)

This appears in the first few days of life as multiple vesicles. The vesicles are differentiated from infection by a macular base and the presence of multiple eosinophils within the vesicular fluid. No treatment is necessary.

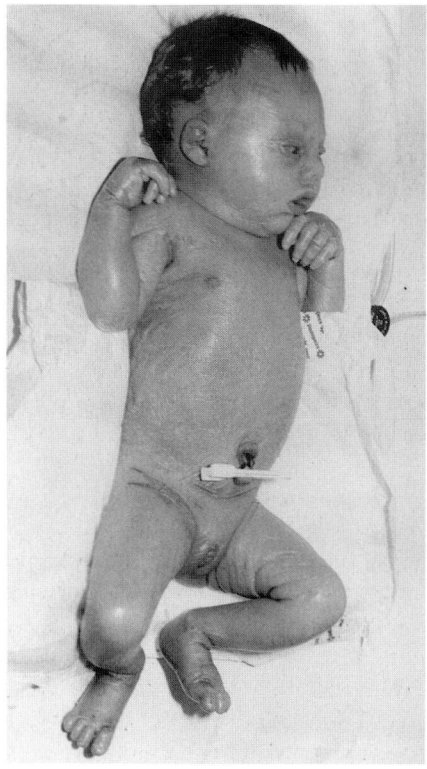

Figure 24.4 Newborn infant with collodion skin. Six weeks later the skin appeared entirely normal.

Table 24.1 Classification of blistering and bullous disorders affecting the neonate

Transient	Chronic
Erythema toxicum	Epidermolysis bullosa:
Congenital candidiasis	Non-scarring
Impetigo neonatorum	Scarring
Toxic epidermal necrolysis	

Candida vesicles

These are usually associated with oral candidiasis and may rarely be present at birth. Diagnosis is by the identification of hyphae or budding spores from the blister. Treatment is by topical nystatin or miconazole.

Impetigo neonatorum (pemphigus neonatorum)

This term is used to describe staphylococcal bullous lesions appearing on the second or third

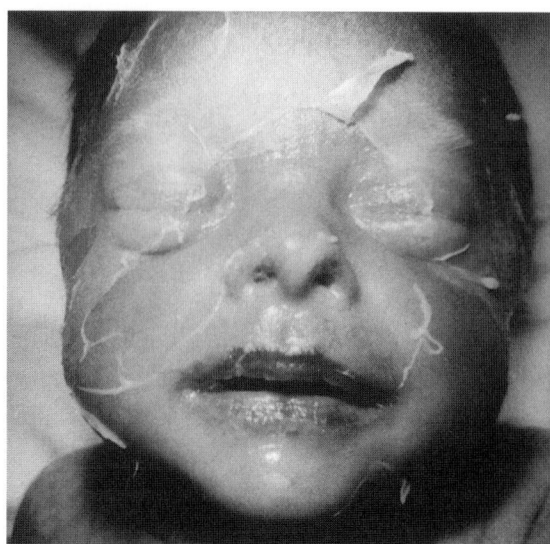

Figure 24.5 Toxic epidermal necrolysis ('scalded skin syndrome').

day of life. The pustules develop on an erythematous base and are often seen on the neck, axillae or groin. The infant may show signs of systemic infection. Intravenous flucloxacillin should be given while culture from the pustules is awaited, as the condition may spread quickly.

Toxic epidermal necrolysis (scalded skin syndrome; Ritter's disease)

This condition is characterized by generalized erythema accompanied by fever and irritability, which is followed within a few hours by the formation of flaccid bullae filled with serous fluid. Sheets of epidermis can be stripped away, revealing a raw, oozing surface (Nikolsky's sign) (Fig. 24.5). This clinical picture is most commonly associated with a *Staphylococcus aureus* infection (phage type 50 or 71), although sometimes no infectious aetiology can be established.

Treatment is with systemic flucloxacillin. The large denuded areas of skin must be treated like a severe burn, requiring isolation to prevent secondary infection, and careful fluid and electrolyte management.

Chronic

Epidermolysis bullosa includes a group of conditions in which blistering or bullous eruptions occur at birth or are seen in the first week of life in response to mechanical trauma. They can be divided into scarring and non-scarring forms.

Non-scarring (epidermolysis bullosa simplex)

This is a relatively mild form and is inherited as an autosomal dominant condition. The soles, toes and fingers are most often affected. Blisters may be present within minutes of delivery. A more severe form, inherited as an autosomal recessive condition, may heal to leave atrophic areas. Differentiation is only possible on electron microscopy. The non-scarring types tend to improve by puberty, but lesions frequently become secondarily infected.

Scarring (dystrophic) forms

These conditions may be inherited as either autosomal dominant or recessive disorders. These blisters often occur early and are deep. The recessive form is usually more severe and the gastrointestinal tract may be involved. The scarring is often extremely destructive, with loss of nails, the formation of ugly scars and contractures, fusion of digits, and sometimes digit or limb amputations.

Management

This will depend on the individual case, but the parents should be encouraged to ensure that the child's lifestyle is as normal as possible. Nevertheless, the avoidance of mechanical trauma, hot baths and high temperatures is important. Genetic counselling will be necessary.

Miscellaneous

Cutis marmorata

This represents a normal physiological reaction to cold commonly seen in the neonate and young infant. The bluish mottling usually exhibits a characteristic reticulated pattern on the trunk and extremities. It is symptomless and transient, requiring no treatment.

Aplasia cutis congenita

This presents as a focal absence of skin at birth. Most often the lesions are on the scalp in the midline, but they can occur on the trunk or extremities.

Prevention of infection in cases of ulceration and surgical skin grafting (for larger defects) may be required.

Cutis laxa

Congenital cutis laxa (generalized elastolysis) is an inherited disorder, and affected infants have diminished resilience of the skin, which hangs in folds. This condition is not associated with joint laxity and increased bruising as seen in cases of Ehlers–Danlos syndrome. Further, in Ehlers–Danlos the skin is hyperelastic but snaps back to normal resiliency and does not hang in redundant folds when released.

Harlequin colour change

This refers to a differential colour change commonly seen during the first few days of life in preterm but also in term infants. It occurs with axial rotation: when the infant is lying on its side the upper part of the body is paler than the lower half, which is normal or reddish in colour. It may last for seconds or minutes and requires no treatment.

Acrodermatitis enteropathica

This is due to zinc deficiency. The classic tetrad consists of diarrhoea, apathy, alopecia and a vesicular bullous rash around the mouth and anus. Excellent results can be achieved with oral zinc therapy.

Neonatal eczema (atopic dermatitis)

Eczema is a common problem after 2 months of age but is unusual in the newborn. Management consists of avoiding potential allergens, including soap and cows' milk. Moisturizing creams and emulsifying ointment should be used in the bath. Severe cases may require 0.5% hydrocortisone cream in urea base, antipruritics, and occasionally hospitalization for intensive nursing care.

Seborrhoeic dermatitis

This is a chronic inflammatory disease of the skin and scalp occurring in all paediatric age groups, especially early infancy. Crusting and scaling of the scalp (cradle cap) may be the initial and only manifestation. It may spread to the face, neck, behind the ears, axillae and napkin area. Treatment consists of the use of moisturizing creams, regular shampooing and steroid creams for severe cases.

Ectodermal dysplasia

This is an abnormality affecting the skin, sweat glands, hair and nails. It is divided into hidrotic and anhidrotic (sweating and non-sweating) forms.

Hidrotic form

Affected children have hyperkeratosis of the hands and feet, sparse hair and hypoplastic or absent nails. The teeth are usually normal. This form does not present in infancy. In contrast to the anhidrotic form the infected child has the ability to sweat.

Anhidrotic form

The most serious problem with this form is the inability to sweat, which may cause hyperpyrexia. The skin is thin, the hair is sparse, and when the first dentition appears the teeth are peg-like. It is usually inherited as an X-linked recessive trait and males are most severely affected.

Neonatal lupus erythematosus (NLE)

Babies born to mothers with systemic lupus erythematosus (SLE) (especially those with positive anti-SSA/Ro or anti-SSB/La) often present with transient skin lesions and congenital heart block. The skin lesions are primarily annular and papulosquamous and are widespread, but most commonly seen on scalp and face (in butterfly fashion affecting the periorbital and malar areas). Sun exposure precipitates or aggravates these lesions. Treatment includes protection against sunlight and topical steroids.

Further reading

Feilchenfeld LF, Frieden IJ, Esterly NB. *Textbook of Neonatal Dermatology*, W.B. Saunders, Philadelphia, 2001.

Frieden IJ. Special Symposium. Management of Haemangiomas. *Paediatr Dermatol* 1997;**14**:57–83.

Rogers M. The significance of birthmarks. *Med J Australia* 1996;**164**:618–623.

Rutter N. The newborn skin. *Semin Neonatol* 2000; **5**(4);271–332.

Schachner LA, Hansen RC (eds) *Pediatric Dermatology*, 2nd edn. Edinburgh: Churchill Livingstone, 1995.

Weinburg S, Prose NS, Kristal L. *Color Atlas of Paediatric Dermatology*, 3rd edn. New York: McGraw-Hill Professional, 1997.

25 Multiple births

The incidence of multiple births was first studied by Hellin in 1895. Following this work the Hellinic law was described, which stated that the incidence of twins was 1/89 pregnancies and of triplets $1/89^2$ (1/7921) and quadruplets $1/89^3$ (1/704 969). There was a decreased incidence of dizygotic twinning in industrialized countries from 1960 to 1976 possibly related to pollutants and a decrease in sperm quality.

With the advent of assisted reproductive technologies for infertile couples the incidence of multiple fetus pregnancies is progressively rising.

There are three levels of artificial reproductive technology (ART):

1 Ovulation induction with a variety of drugs, the most commonly used being clomiphene.

2 *In vitro* fertilization (IVF). Eggs are collected, fertilized *in vitro* and replaced into the reproductive tract. This includes intracytoplasmic sperm injection (ICSI), which is now widely used for male infertility.

3 Embryo transfer into the uterus or zygote intrafallopian transfer (ZIFT).

The Australian rates of multiple pregnancy for assisted reproductive technology (ART) in 2003 were:

Hyperstimulation of ovarian follicles with clomiphene	8%
Hyperstimulation of ovarian follicles with gonadotrophins	20%
Intracytoplasmic sperm injection (ICSI)	21.8%
Gamete intrafallopian tube transfers (GIFT)	28%
In vitro fertilization (IVF)	21.8%

From all pregnancies in Australia the rates of twin pregnancy were 1 in 37, triplet pregnancy 1 in 945 and quadruplet pregnancy 1 in 17 700.

In the UK the incidence of multiple births has fallen in recent years as legislation has restricted the number of embryos that can be implanted to one, or at most two in exceptional cases. This has not occurred in other countries where regulation of IVF is more lax.

Antenatal diagnosis of multiple gestation

In industralized countries with routine antenatal care and ultrasound assessment the birth of undiagnosed twins is a rare event. Antenatal diagnosis enables assessment of chorionicity, and detection of malpresentation and complications of multiple gestation. The 'twin peak' sign of dichorionic twin placentas is best detected in the first trimester.

Determination of zygosity

In 44% of twins zygosity is not easily assessed. An approach to determination of zygosity is provided in Fig. 25.1.

Sex
Twins of different sexes must be dizygotic.

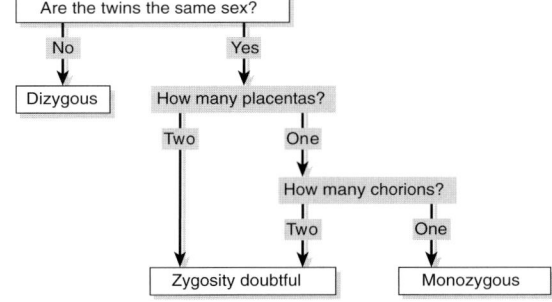

Figure 25.1 Determination of the zygosity of twins.

Placenta

Monozygotic twins who divide before the sixth day after fertilization have separate chorions. They may share the same placenta or have separate placentas. Those who divide later will always have only one chorion and either one or two amniotic cavities. Their placentas will be fused. About one in four like-sexed twins who are dichorionic are monozygotic, but determination of zygosity is not possible without DNA testing.

Parental counselling

Counselling of parents regarding the zygosity of their multiple births may be of benefit in terms of rearing practices, concordance of 70–90% with medical conditions and donation for solid organ transplant. The medical profession is notorious for imprecise counselling, and multiple birth support groups have requested that zygosity testing is provided as a routine service in cases of multiple births regardless of the high cost of DNA testing.

Zygosity

Dizygotic twins

Dizygotic (DZ) twins develop when two separate ova are fertilized. Previously 60% of twins were dizygotic but since the success of ART programmes from 1980 about 80% are dizygotic. Factors influencing the increased rate of dizygotic twinning other than ART are maternal age 35–39 years, high parity, tall stature, periconceptual folate and familial factors (increased risk $\times 4$ if mother, or $\times 2$ if sister is a DZ twin).

Monozygotic twins

Twins are monozygotic (identical) when one ovum is fertilized and then splits during the first 14 days to produce two identical embryos. The monozygotic twinning rate is constant throughout the world at 3–4/1000 pregnancies, and is not influenced by heredity. The ensuing twins are identical and they usually share the same chorionic membrane.

Of all naturally conceived twins, 40% are monozygotic, and of all monozygotic (MZ) twins, 63% are monochorionic diamniotic, 33% are dichorionic diamniotic with either separate or fused placentas, and 4% are monochorionic monoamniotic. The overall incidence of 4/1000 is not influenced by ethnicity, maternal age, nutritional status or environmental factors. Artificially conceived multifetus pregnancies contain MZ twins in 6–10% of cases. There is fivefold increased risk of monozygotic twinning of an IVF embryo.

Complications of twin pregnancy

Discordant growth rates

Normally both twins will continue to grow at the rate of a singleton fetus until 30 weeks' gestation, after which growth restriction may occur. As the number of fetuses increases from twins to triplets to quadruplets, the gestational age at which birthweight first falls below that of a singleton fetus also decreases. Twins have birthweights similar to singletons up to 30 weeks, but thereafter are below singleton levels; similarly, birthweights in triplets deviate from the singleton curve at 27–28 weeks, and in quadruplets at approximately 26 weeks. In addition, as the fetal number increases the rate of individual fetal growth in the third trimester decreases. Thus, the further the multiple gestation advances and the higher the fetal number, the more individual birthweights will differ from singleton values. Twins usually grow at nearly identical rates, the mean intertwin birthweight difference being 11%. Small for gestational age (SGA) infants have been reported in 24–40% of twin gestations. In one study, 13% of twin gestations resulted in one SGA fetus and 9.4% of gestations resulted in two SGA fetuses. Monozygotic twins grow less well than dizygotic twins, and major discrepancies in weight are commoner in monozygotic twins. Causes of discrepancy are poor insertion of the cord into the placenta in one twin, and in dichorionic twins poor placentation of one twin. The commonest cause is fetofetal transfusion (see below).

Disappearing twin phenomenon

Ultrasound studies in the first weeks of pregnancy have shown that up to 50% of pregnancies found to contain twins in the first 8 weeks of gestation absorb one conceptus and continue as singleton pregnancies. This has been referred to as the 'disappearing twin' phenomenon. Rarely, the dead twin is not resorbed and fetus papyraceous ensues. It is suggested that the disruption to the surviving twin as a result of the early fetal loss of the co-twin predisposes the baby to cerebral palsy, but there is currently little direct evidence for this.

Fetus papyraceous

This occurs if one twin dies early in the first trimester and becomes mummified. The other twin continues to grow normally. There is a strong association with the occurrence of embolic phenomena (from the dead fetus) affecting the surviving twin. Multicystic encephaloleukomalacia and multiple cutis aplasia have been reported in the surviving twin.

Conjoined twins (Siamese twins)

Conjoined twins occur in 1/100 000 pregnancies, and the condition is often incompatible with life (Fig. 25.2).

Prematurity

The incidence of premature delivery in twin pregnancies is 20–30%, and the incidence is greater in higher-order multiple pregnancies. Fifty percent of twins weigh less than 2500 g at birth. Premature birth relates to increased intrauterine volume, premature rupture of the membranes and third-trimester bleeding.

Malpresentation

Twins may present in the uterus in many ways, some of which predispose them to trauma:

Vertex and vertex	45%
Vertex and breech	40%
Breech and breech	10%
Vertex and transverse	3%
Breech and transverse	1.5%
Transverse and transverse	0.5%

Locked twins may occur as a result of unstable lies and cause obstruction to delivery.

Congenital malformations

The incidence of major malformation is 2%, and of minor malformation 4%. It is often stated that monozygotic twinning results from a chance

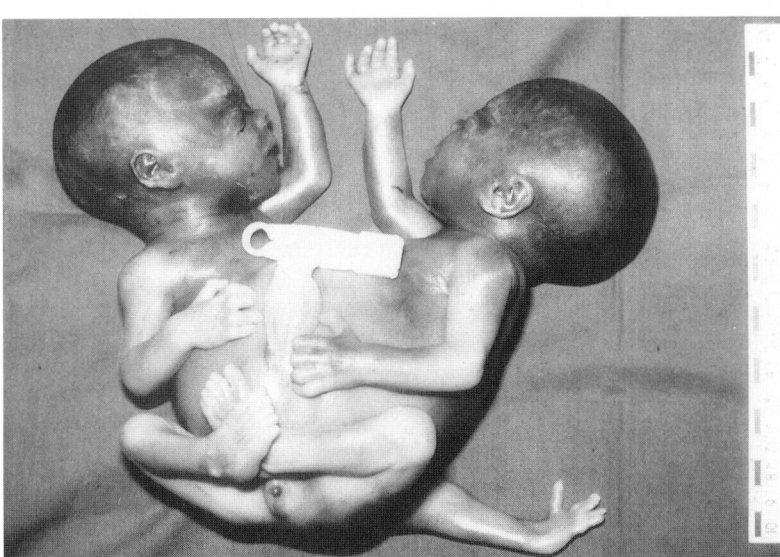

Figure 25.2 Conjoined twins attached from chest to buttocks.

teratogenic event. Malformations due to the event of twinning itself are conjoined twins, amorphous twins, sirenomelia, holoprosencephaly, neural tube defects and anencephaly. Other malformations result from vascular interchange between monozygotic twins, and include acardia in one twin, disseminated intravascular coagulation (DIC) from embolization, with defects such as microcephaly, hydranencephaly, intestinal atresia, cutis aplasia and limb amputation.

Postural deformities

Deformations such as talipes and hip dysplasia result from intrauterine crowding and are equally common in monozygotic and dizygotic twins.

Twin-to-twin transfusion (TTTS)

This occurs in monozygotic twins with a shared placenta. It is recognized in the neonatal unit by either discordant growth (>20% birthweight difference), which is referred to as chronic TTTS, or a haemoglobibn difference $\geq 5\,g/dL$ (acute TTTS). More recently, TTTS has been diagnosed antenatally in the mid-trimester by one twin showing oligohydramnios (the donor twin) and the other polyhydramnios (recipient twin). In its most severe form one twin with very severe oligohydramnios becomes 'stuck' and immobile. Fetal medicine specialists now recommend scanning all monochorionic twins every 2 weeks to detect discordant amniotic fluid volume. Fetal treatment includes serial amniocentesis, septostomy and laser ablation of surface interconnecting vessels on the placenta. A randomized clinical trial has shown reduced mortality and improved neurological outcome in the twins treated by laser ablation compared with other methods.

In the neonate rapid treatment of the anaemic twin may be necessary (see p. 193), and the plethoric twin may require a dilutional exchange transfusion (see p. 200). An acute twin-to-twin bleed may cause severe hypotension in one twin, which may lead to cerebral infarction and subsequent cerebral palsy (see below).

Infection

This occurs much more commonly in the first twin and probably relates to premature rupture of the membranes of the first amniotic sac.

Asphyxia

The second twin is more vulnerable to asphyxia than the first twin. This is related to delayed delivery, cord prolapse, placental separation and malpresentation. The second twin, if SGA, is also more at risk of respiratory distress syndrome (RDS) and hypoglycaemia. Asphyxia is more common in twins than singletons owing to increased rates of prematurity, operative delivery and malpresentation.

Respiratory distress syndrome (RDS)

Overall, there is an 8.5% incidence of RDS in twins, with 29% of preterm twins being diagnosed as having RDS. The increased incidence in the second twin probably relates to birth asphyxia rather than a difference in lecithin to sphingomyelin (L/S) ratios.

Neurological morbidity

Twins are overrepresented in populations with cerebral palsy (5–10% in most studies), particularly spastic diplegia. Probable antecedents are premature birth, growth restriction, birth trauma, asphyxia and intrauterine demise of one twin. The risk of a twin developing cerebral palsy is 5–6 times higher than in a singleton pregnancy, and the risk in a triplet is 17–20 times higher than in a singleton. Typical rates of cerebral palsy per thousand births are singleton 2.3, twin 12.6 and triplet 44.8. This risk is particularly increased where there is the death of a monozygotic co-twin *in utero*. In all such cases the brain of the surviving twin must be carefully examined with ultrasound or magnetic resonance imaging (MRI) to detect evidence of cerebral infarction (most probably periventricular leukomalacia). The mechanism for this is that the twins share a placental circulation. When a co-twin dies, the mixing of the blood supplies means that the falling blood pressure of the dying twin will cause the surviving twin to become transiently hypotensive, with resultant cerebral injury. It is estimated that the risk of cerebral palsy in a surviving monozygotic twin whose co-twin dies is 12 times greater than when both twins survive.

Impact of assisted reproduction on multiple gestation

The past decade has seen an expansion in therapeutic options available to the 8–12% of couples who experience difficulty in conception. In 1978, Edwards and Steptoe pioneered *in vitro* fertilization, and many spin-off technologies such as intracytoplasmic sperm injection (ICSI) and zygote intrafallopian transfer (ZIFT), have followed. Associated with ovulation stimulation and the new technologies there has been a dramatic increase in multiple births – not just twins, but triplets and higher multiples – placing extraordinary demands on neonatal intensive care units. The incidence appears to be falling again where the number of transferred emryos has been restricted.

Prognosis

The perinatal mortality rate is much higher for multiple pregnancies than for singletons, with a fivefold increase for twin and 14-fold increase for triplet pregnancies for birth, stillbirth and neonatal death. Similarly, twinning is markedly overrepresented in neonatal morbidity. The mortality rate for the second twin is considerably higher than that for the first. At the Mater Hospital, multiple births represent 3.8% of all births but contribute 18.8% of admissions to the intensive care nursery, and 29.6% of all neonatal deaths.

Parents need a great deal of support and advice with the care of their twins or triplets. The mother particularly needs encouragement to breastfeed her infants. Voluntary community groups, such as the Twins Club and Twins and Multiple Birth Association, may be helpful in providing support and counselling.

FOCAL POINTS AND EVALUATION

- The 'success' of ART programmes has altered the natural balance between monozygotic and dizygotic twinning.
- There should be tight regulation of ART programmes especially with number of embryos transferred.
- Ascertainment of chorionicity by ultrasound scanning in the first trimester determines obstetric management.
- Placenta should be routinely sent for pathological examination for all same sex twins.
- Multiple births have increased risks of perinatal death, neonatal morbidities and neurosensory disabilities compared with singletons of the same gestational age.
- Although multiple births represent 3.8% of all births they contribute 18.8% of admissions to neonatal intensive care and 29.6% of all neonatal deaths.
- Care during pregnancy and of the newborn should be undertaken in a level II or III hospital.

Further reading

Blickstein I, Shinwell ES. Multiple births. *Semin Neonatol* 2002;7(3):167–256.

Bryan EM. *The Nature and Nurture of Twins*. London: Baillière Tindall, 1983.

Harrison MR, Evans MI, Adzick NS. *The Unborn Patient. The Art and Science of Fetal Therapy*, 3rd edn. W.B. Saunders, Philadelphia, 2001.

Noble E. *Having Twins and More*. Houghton Mifflin, Boston 2003.

Waters AD, Dean JH, Sullivan E. *Assisted Reproduction Technology in Australia and New Zealand* 2003. AIHW National Perinatal Statistics Unit, University of NSW. Sydney, 2006.

CHAPTER 26

26 Organization of perinatal services and neonatal transport

Organization of perinatal services

In recent years, highly regionalized models for delivery of perinatal services have been developed. The goals of highly regionalized perinatal services are to prevent costly duplication of services, improve outcomes with high critical mass and provide cost-effective models of perinatal care.

Regionalization of perinatal care is based on the following premises:
- prospective risk assessment;
- prompt recognition of unanticipated problems;
- appropriate graded levels of matched obstetric and neonatal care;
- ready availability of transport teams, equipment and vehicles;
- perinatal outreach education for clinical staff.

Clinical governance
Clinical governance is a framework through which health organizations are accountable for continually improving the quality of their services and safeguarding high standards of care by creating an environment in which excellence in clinical care will flourish. There is corporate accountability for clinical performance.

Clinical governance involves safety, quality management, improvement, assurance and control, and is consumer focused and continually proactive. The tertiary perinatal team has a strong focus on quality management improvement, risk reduction, clinical audit, evidence-based practice, ethics and research using systematic reviews.

The role of neonatal networks
Collaboration with a National Neonatal Network audits outcomes, provides benchmarking standards, develops clinical indicators, provides standardized guidelines and policies, and facilitates research through critical mass.

Organization of perinatal care

Levels of neonatal care in the UK were proposed by the British Paediatric Association and the British Association for Perinatal Paediatrics, and are divided into three categories (British Association of Perinatal Medicine 2001). Similar levels of care have been defined by the Sub Specialty Services Subcommittee of the Australian Health Ministers Advisory Council (1990).

Description of neonatal services

Neonatal intensive care is a coordinated effort by healthcare providers in a defined geographical region to intervene in the reproductive process so as to make available to every neonate a level of medical care commensurate with the perceived risk of neonatal death or serious morbidity.

The integration of neonatal and obstetric services into a perinatal programme offers the best opportunity for prevention and treatment.

A neonatal intensive care unit should provide care for all babies born in a district or region, and babies requiring intensive care are referred to the intensive care nursery. Facilities for neonatal surgery and cardiology should be available in regional neonatal intensive care units.

Neonatal units in the UK are classified according to the intensity of the care they provide and are described as follows.
- *Level 3 units* provide the whole range of medical neonatal care but not necessarily all specialist services such as neonatal surgery. This requires one-to-one specialist nursing per cot.

- *Level 2 units* provide high-dependency care and some short-term intensive care as agreed within the network. This requires one trained nurse to two babies.
- *Level 1 units* provide special care but do not aim to provide any continuing high-dependency or intensive care. This term includes units with or without resident medical staff. The requirement is for one nurse to every four babies.
- *Normal care* is care given by the mother substitute, with medical or neonatal nursing advice if needed.

Level 3 intensive care

This should be provided for the following babies:

1 a baby receiving any respiratory support via a tracheal tube and in the first 24 hours after withdrawal of such support;

2 one receiving nasal continuous positive airway pressure (NCPAP) for any part of the day and less than 5 days old;

3 one below 1000 g current weight and receiving NCPAP for any part of the day and for 24 hours after withdrawal;

4 a baby less than 29 weeks' gestational age and less than 48 hours old;

5 one requiring major emergency surgery, for the preoperative period and postoperatively for 24 h;

6 a baby requiring complex clinical procedures:
   - full exchange transfusion;
   - peritoneal dialysis;
   - infusion of an inotrope, pulmonary vasodilator or prostaglandin, and for 24 hours afterwards;

7 any other very unstable baby considered by the nurse in charge as needing one-to-one nursing;

8 a baby on the day of death.

Level 2 high dependency

This should be provided for the following babies:

1 ones receiving NCPAP for any part of the day and not fulfilling any of the criteria for intensive care;

2 babies below 1000 g current weight and not fulfilling any of the criteria for intensive care;

3 ones receiving total parenteral nutrition;

4 babies having convulsions;

5 babies receiving oxygen therapy and below 1500 g current weight;

6 ones requiring treatment for neonatal abstinence syndrome;

7 ones requiring specified procedures that do not fulfil any criteria for intensive care:
   - care of an intra-arterial catheter or chest drain;
   - partial exchange transfusion;
   - tracheostomy care until supervised by a parent.

8 babies requiring frequent stimulation for severe apnoea.

Level 1 special care is provided for all other babies who could not reasonably be expected to be looked after at home by their mother.

Neonatal units in Australia and New Zealand

These are classified according to the intensity of the care they provide, and are described as follows.

Level 1 hospitals (50–400 deliveries per annum). These provide services for uncomplicated maternity and newborn patients >36 weeks' gestation. The mature infant nursery provides basic life supports, receives back transfer from level 2 hospitals, and establishes networks with level 2 and level 2 perinatal services.

Level 2 hospitals (400–2000 deliveries per annum). These provide services for low- and medium-risk pregnancies and for babies >32 weeks' gestation. The special care nursery (SCN) is staffed by neonatal nurses, and a paediatric registrar and consultant, and can provide stabilization of preterm and sick infants prior to neonatal retrieval. The overall requirement for level 2 cots is 4.25/1000 births.

Level 3 hospitals (usually >3000 births and >10 000 births in catchment area). These provide services for low-, medium- and high-risk obstetrics, and have a maternal fetal medicine unit and a full range of ventilation options. The staff include neonatal nurses, neonatal registrars and a consultant, and there is access to a full range of paediatric subspecialties. These units may be located in obstetric hospitals, in general hospitals or in children's hospitals. The cot requirement is at least 1.2–1.5/1000 live births (all cots are potentially assisted ventilation) and there is a nurse:patient ratio of 1:2, or 1:1 for unstable infants.

Level 4 hospital. This is a term that is sometimes used to describe services provided to neonates requiring paediatric subspecialty care (e.g. those with complex metabolic and/or cardiac conditions, and surgical cases). Units at paediatric referral centres provide level 4 neonatal services.

Developments in perinatal services

The development of perinatal services and changes in clinical practice have included:

1 the development of specialist perinatal units to concentrate expertise and utilize high-cost services efficiently;

2 collaborative antenatal and perinatal management of high-risk pregnancies;

3 emphasis on *in utero* transfer of high-risk pregnancies to tertiary-level hospitals to optimize perinatal management;

4 coordinated neonatal transport of sick and premature newborns from peripheral hospitals to level 3 neonatal intensive care units;

5 the application of technological developments in the areas of fetal monitoring, prenatal diagnosis and neonatal intensive care.

Normal care. This is care given in a postnatal ward, usually by the mother under the supervision of a midwife or doctor but requiring minimal medical or nursing advice.

All maternity units must provide normal care for babies. A district general hospital with a consultant obstetric unit should provide special care facilities, and approximately 6% of infants will require this type of care.

Models of care

Ideally mother and baby should be kept together as much as possible so that models of care for babies with special needs, such as neonatal abstinence syndrome (NAS), infants of diabetic mothers, marginal prematurity 35–36 weeks, intravenous antibiotics and jaundice requiring intensive phototherapy, should be predominantly provided by parents.

Health area networks for delivery of neonatal services should be developed to oversee a continuum of care between level 1, 2 and 3 hospitals and community-based primary health facilities.

Transport *in utero*

The ideal time to transfer a potentially sick infant is *in utero*, if the problem can be anticipated. High-risk pregnancies should be transferred before delivery, and a high-risk fetus should be transferred *in utero* to a unit with perinatal intensive care facilities. In all cases there must be consultation with the receiving hospital before transfer. Unfortunately, not all neonatal problems can be recognized from an at-risk pregnancy, and some women are unwilling to be transported before delivery.

The rationale for transporting sick or low birthweight (LBW) neonates to special care or intensive care nurseries is based on the premise that specialized units reduce mortality and improve outcome, and that these advantages outweigh the risk of transport and physical or social disadvantages for the family. The incidence of intraventricular haemorrhage in infants born in a referring hospital after *in utero* transfer appears to be lower than in a similar group of outborn babies.

Neonatal transport

The decision to transfer a sick neonate will depend on the expertise of the intensive care nursery, the safety of travel and the facilities available at the hospital where the baby was born. Discussion with a neonatal paediatrician may obviate the need for transport or provide advice on the best methods of transfer. Personnel from the neonatal emergency transport service can assist with the decision on whether transfer is necessary.

Consideration should be given to the transfer of the following infants to special care or intensive care nurseries:

1 gestational age <30 weeks;

2 respiratory distress of early onset or persisting more than 4–6 h;

3 oxygen requirement >50% or associated apnoea, meconium aspiration or suspected pneumonia;

4 apnoeic episodes;

5 convulsions;

6 depression following birth asphyxia;

7 jaundiced infant in need of exchange transfusion;

8 bleeding;

9 surgical conditions;

10 congenital heart disease;

11 severe or multiple congenital abnormalities;

12 need for special diagnostic or therapeutic services;

13 'unwell' infant with lethargy, poor perfusion, oliguria, etc.

Preparation for transport

The infant should be resuscitated and his or her condition stabilized prior to transport. While awaiting transfer the referring hospital should provide the following care:

1 The infant is kept warm (ideally servocontrolled to a skin temperature of 36.5°C). Bubble plastic may help to reduce heat loss.

2 The infant is given sufficient oxygen to maintain oxygen saturation in the normal range (90–98%). If blood gas analysis is available, the arterial oxygen tension should be maintained at 50–80 mmHg (6.7–9.7 kPa).

3 Ensure a clear airway by adequate suction.

4 Ensure adequate respiration.

5 Make frequent observations of temperature, heart rate, respiratory rate, blood pressure and blood sugar by reagent stick.

6 Follow procedures for surgical patients:
  (a) attention to fluids and electrolytes;
  (b) intravascular volume;
  (c) special requirements.

7 Intravenous dextrose with maintenance of blood glucose >2.5 mmol/L.

8 Prostaglandin E1 (PGE1) infusion if possibility of duct-dependent cyanotic heart disease (see p. 185).

Principles of stabilization

The amount of stabilization required prior to departure depends on the baby's condition and the rate of progress of the disease. It is also influenced by the distance to be travelled, the duration of the journey and the mode of transport.

It is important not to waste time, power, oxygen or air. Always use the nursery or ambulance utilities where possible. Staff must be aware of the difficulties of detecting and correcting problems in transit, and must ensure appropriate stabilization before transport.

Principles of transportation

These include:

1 Complete resuscitation and stabilization of the infant prior to transport.

2 Procedures such as insertion of an intravenous line or umbilical artery catheter, intubation, mechanical ventilation and polaroid or digital photography of the baby for the mother are performed prior to transport if indicated.

3 The baby is not fed during transport and the stomach is aspirated prior to leaving the referring hospital. The gastric tube remains *in situ*.

4 Frequent gastric and pharyngeal suction is necessary to prevent aspiration.

5 An intravenous (i.v.) line with 10% dextrose is set up prior to transfer to prevent hypoglycaemia.

6 If oxygen is necessary, it should ideally be warmed and humidified.

7 The percentage of inspired oxygen should be measured with an oxygen analyser or oxygen blender.

8 A headbox should be used if greater than 30% inspired oxygen is necessary.

9 Oxygenation should be monitored continuously by either pulse oximetry or transcutaneous Po_2.

10 Monitoring of temperature, heart rate and respiration rate is essential, and monitoring of blood pressure is desirable.

Important decisions to be made

1 Intubation: the decision whether or not to intubate is influenced by factors relating to the particular baby, such as diagnosis, current condition and likely course, size and gestational age, and transport factors, such as the nature of the trip and operational conditions. If in doubt contact the receiving neonatologist.

2 Exogenous surfactant administration, by either referring or retrieval staff, is to assist with stabilization of a critically ill infant or one on high ventilator pressures.

Individual neonatal emergency transport systems need to develop their own protocols.

Before leaving

Before the transfer commences the referring hospital should provide the following:

1 perinatal history sheet, completed in detail;
2 signed parental consent for the infant's transfer and treatment;
3 copies of relevant records and results of tests, including X-rays;
4 10 mL of clotted blood from the mother to allow accurate cross-matching prior to surgery or exchange transfusion;
5 cord blood if available;
6 placenta if available.

Choice of vehicle

On the UK mainland infants are generally transferred by the road ambulance service. Occasionally, a fixed-wing aircraft (civil or RAF) is necessary for transportation overseas or over longer distances. In Australia there is usually a range of options, including road ambulance (up to 100–150 km), helicopter (up to 250 km) and fixed-wing (>200 km). The choice of vehicle depends on availability of vehicles and aircraft, distance, degree of urgency, weather conditions and other factors. Each transfer is considered individually on its merits.

Who should accompany the baby?

A neonatal nurse experienced in transport should accompany babies over 1500 g who are not critically ill. The attending doctor, registrar or resident should escort babies with apnoea or convulsions, or spontaneously breathing infants with respiratory distress who require oxygen. A neonatal retrieval team is usually necessary for infants of birthweight less than 1500 g and those requiring mechanical ventilation. It is desirable, but not always practicable, that the mother should be transported with her baby to promote bonding. Careful monitoring of the baby's heart rate, respiratory rate, temperature and blood pressure should be continued during transport.

Surgical problems

Babies with surgical lesions may have special problems, which depend on the nature of the case.

Diaphragmatic hernia. These babies must not receive bag-and-mask ventilation. If mechanical ventilation is necessary, it should be through a carefully positioned endotracheal tube. If possible, very high ambient oxygen environments are preferable to ventilation because of the risk of pneumothorax. The stomach must be frequently aspirated via a nasogastric tube. Correct any acidosis before departure and consider paralysis if the baby is hypoxic.

Oesophageal atresia with tracheo-oesophageal fistula. Feeding is absolutely contraindicated in these infants. The infant is nursed prone with the body elevated to 30° from the horizontal, and frequent suctioning with an indwelling nasopharyngeal tube is essential to empty the blind-ending upper pouch. Limit crying with the use of a pacifier.

Exomphalos/gastroschisis/myelomeningocoele. The eviscerated lesions should be wrapped in a sterile plastic bag to prevent heat and fluid losses from evaporation and excessive cooling. The infant is nursed on the surface opposite to the lesion. Reposition the bowel if it appears to have impaired blood supply. Assess perfusion and give colloid if necessary.

An indwelling open nasogastric tube is placed in the stomach and aspirated intermittently. An intravenous infusion is desirable. Moist packs are contraindicated as they quickly become cold and lead to hypothermia.

Bowel obstruction. Fluid and electrolyte disturbances should be corrected prior to transport and continuous nasogastric suction maintained throughout. The infant should be nursed prone or lying on his or her right side with the head up.

Pierre Robin sequence/choanal atresia. In these conditions an adequate airway must be established for the infant, both while awake and when asleep. The infant is nursed in the prone position and an oropharyngeal airway strapped in place. In some cases a long nasopharyngeal tube is positioned with tip just above the epiglottis. Continuous observation of respiratory pattern, skin colour and oxygen saturation is required.

Transport equipment

Various safeguards should be observed when providing and organizing the equipment.

1 *Quantity.* A minimum of two sets of equipment are required for any one geographical area to allow for breakdown, maintenance, concurrent calls and twin transportation.

2 *Safety requirements.* The equipment should satisfy all areas of safety regulation and other statutory requirements.

3 *Transport incubators.* These must provide a neutral thermal environment under a wide range of external temperatures and environmental conditions. There must be good lighting and visibility and easy access. Incubators must be capable of operation from a mains source, aircraft (24> V d.c.) and road vehicle (10–13 V d.c.) power. Most transport systems have an air compressor.

4 *Monitoring equipment.* Monitoring of temperature, heart rate, inspired oxygen concentration and oxygen partial pressure and/or saturation is essential. Blood pressure monitoring is desirable.

5 *Respiratory support.* Independent supplies of oxygen and medical air are required to provide controlled inspired oxygen concentrations from 21% to 100%. Ideally, inspired gases should be heated and humidified. Inhaled nitric oxide is now available for ventilators on transport incubators.

6 A mechanical ventilator able to provide intermittent positive pressure ventilation (IPPV) and continuous positive airway pressure (CPAP) is required. A suitable hand-operated ventilator system, consisting of bag and mask with manometer, must be available as a back-up to mechanical ventilation.

7 *Suction.* Suction equipment must have an independent power supply, and negative pressure must be controlled and adjustable. Oral suction mucus traps must be available as back-up.

8 *Infusion pumps.* Infusion by a constant-rate pump is required for intravenous and/or intra-arterial infusion. Battery-operated syringe infusion pumps delivering a constant flow are used.

Emergency equipment

Several items of equipment are essential to deal witih emergencies.

1 Equipment for emergency intubation: laryngoscope, endotracheal tubes with introducers, tape.

2 Equipment for emergency insertion of a chest tube: intercostal catheter, Heimlich one-way flutter valve.

3 Equipment for emergency insertion of an umbilical arterial catheter.

4 Drugs for resuscitation, such as adrenaline (epinephrine), sodium bicarbonate, calcium gluconate and plasma. Special drugs include surfactant, Prostaglandin E1 [prostin] (PGE) and anticonvulsants.

Other equipment

Other miscellaneous items of equipment include:

1 Digital camera.

2 Paediatric stethoscopes.

3 Blood glucose meter and strips.

4 Prostaglandin E1 (PGE1).

Transport vehicles

Transport vehicles should be dedicated neonatal ambulance vehicles; these are desirable for large services where retrievals exceed 150 per annum. The vehicles must meet national passenger safety standards, and have adequate seating with safety restraints for staff. Adequate lighting and internal climate control are necessary. A fixed positive mounting system is required to restrain the transport system. Tolerable noise and vibration levels are an essential prerequisite. External communication should be available to allow the team to be directly connected to any telephone number at any stage of the transfer.

Aerial transport

Transfer by aeroplane or helicopter has several unique problems.

1 Any air flight, even in a pressurized cabin, decreases ambient pressure with resultant expansion of gases in body cavities. This is particularly relevant in infants with pneumo-thorax, lung cysts or trapped gas in the bowel or the peritoneal cavity. Pain may occur as a result of expansion of air in the facial sinuses in larger infants.

2 Inspired oxygen is decreased owing to the rarefied atmosphere.

3 Noise and vibration may lead to loss of the gag reflex and promote vomiting, with resultant aspiration.

4 Difficulty with illumination, observation and especially auscultation of the heart and lungs.

The role of a neonatal transport service

An integral part of a successful neonatal transport programme is frequent communication with personnel in the referring nursery, and especially with the mother. The infant should be transferred back to the referring nursery at the earliest possible time.

A coordinated neonatal transport service organizes retrievals and return transfers of infants back to the base hospital, and is also involved with consultation services and education for outlying practitioners. It provides an active role in the coordination of all neonatal transport facilities, utilization of perinatal facilities and outreach education.

It plays a pivotal role in the coordination and utilization of perinatal facilities. The selection and standardization of transport facilities involves liaison with all transport providers. There is also a commitment to audit, research and quality assurance.

Care of parents

The transport team must be sensitive to the needs of the parents during this stressful period. They must introduce themselves to parents and explain the nature of the transport, treatment and likely prognosis. Parents are encouraged to touch their baby and are offered a Polaroid photograph. An information booklet about the tertiary hospital is provided, and informed consent for transfer and care must be obtained.

Relationships with referring hospital and staff

The retrieval staff must be sensitive in relating to referral hospital personnel: they should never, either directly or by implication, criticize the referring doctor's management. Smooth communication and relationships between referring and receiving units are essential for effective regionalization of care. Staff should involve ambulance officers with equipment needs and educate them about the infant's condition. A debriefing with referring staff is an essential component of quality management improvement.

PRINCIPLES OF MANAGEMENT

- Health area networks of perinatal services oversee:
  - a continuum of care between level 1, 2 and 3 hospitals and primary health centres;
  - the integration of midwifery, obstetric and neonatal services into a perinatal programme that offers the best opportunity for prevention and treatment.
- The ideal time to transfer a potentially sick or preterm infant is *in utero*.
- The decision to transfer a sick neonate depends on the expertise of the intensive care nursery, and the safety of transport and facilities available at regional centres.
- Ensure appropriate stabilization before transport because it is difficult to detect and manage problems during transport.
- The extent of stabilization of a neonate prior to transport depends on the baby's condition, the rate of progress of his or her disease, and operational conditions of transport.

Further reading

Australian Health Ministers Advisory Council. Sub Specialty Services Subcommittee. *Guidelines for Level Three Neonatal Intensive Care.* Canberra: Australian Institute of Health, 1990.

Bowman ED, Levi SM, McLean AJ, Presbury FE (eds) *Stabilization and Transport of Newborn Infants and At-Risk Pregnancies*, 4th edn. Melbourne: Newborn Emergency Transport Service, 1998.

British Association of Perinatal Medicine. *Standards for Hospitals Providing Neonatal Intensive and High Dependncy Care (2nd edn) and Categories of Babies Requiring Neonatal Care* (www.bapm.org/documents/publications/hosp_standards.pdf).

Field D. Neonatal transport. *Semin Neonatol* 1999;**4** (4):217–287.

Jaimovich DG, Vidyasagar D (eds) *Handbook of Pediatric and Neonatal Transport Medicine*, 2nd edn. Philadelphia: Hanley & Belfus; St Louis: Mosby, 2002.

CHAPTER 27

27 Discharge and follow-up of high-risk infants

Parents whose babies have had a prolonged stay in hospital will be anxious about the discharge of their babies. Ideally, the mother and father should 'room in' with their baby, or at least sleep in the hospital in close proximity to baby for some days and nights prior to discharge, so that they can gain confidence and learn to care for their previously sick or preterm infant. Prior to discharge the parents will need advice on feeding, iron and vitamin supplementation, introduction of complimentary food, immunizations, etc. An information booklet on these subjects may be issued to the parents. A full discharge summary should be sent to the infant's general practitioner and referring paediatrician/obstetrician at time of discharge. Parents should have a copy of the discharge summary. The summary should highlight ongoing care at discharge and need for follow-up. Preterm parent support groups can provide support to parents when the child is in hospital and advice for the transition into the home.

Feeding advice

Feeding of the low birthweight (LBW) infant is discussed in Chapter 6. The frequency of feeds depends on the maturity and neurological integrity of the infant, but 3–4-hourly feeds are usually necessary on discharge from the neonatal unit. The mother should be encouraged to demand-feed her baby, but feeds should not be more than 5 h apart during the day. Artificially fed infants are usually transferred from a preterm 'ready to feed' formula to a term formula before discharge.

Iron

Term infants receive sufficient iron from breast milk until about 6–9 months of age. Although the iron content in breast milk is low (0.5 mg/L), the absorption is excellent. The term infant being fed on iron-fortified formula receives sufficient iron until 5–6 months, at which time iron-containing foods such as cereals, vegetables, eggs and meat should be started. Although the preterm infant needs supplemental iron from 3 months of age, whether breastfed or not, for convenience iron therapy is commenced in hospital on day 28, with 30–50 mg/day of ferrous sulphate paediatric mixture.

Additional folic acid is only necessary if the infant has a haemolytic disease (particularly important for babies with rhesus isoimmunization).

Vitamins

Term infants probably receive adequate vitamins in their breast milk or vitamin-fortified breast-milk substitutes. However, preterm infants and other ill infants will require extra vitamins, especially D and C. Parenteral nutrition fluids and human milk fortifiers contain both water- and fat-soluble vitamins. Preterm infants with inadequate vitamin C intake often have an immaturity of the enzyme phenylalanine hydroxylase and may develop transient tyrosinaemia. A multivitamin preparation such as Dalivit, Pentavite or Abdec should be commenced in weeks 3–4 of life and continued until 6–12 months. Sick and extremely preterm infants receive multivitamins in parenteral nutrition infusion, and oral supplementation can wait until the baby is on full enteral feeding.

Fluoride

Fluoride drops are recommended in areas where the water supply is not fluoridated. The dose is four drops per day in the first year of life, eight drops per day from 1 to 2 years and 15 drops per day or 1 tablet after 2 years of age. It is important to adhere to this dosage schedule as excessive fluoride may cause tooth staining as a result of fluorosis. Fluoride drops should preferably be given in water rather than milk to permit better absorption.

Immunization

Details of the immunization schedules in the UK and Australia are shown in Tables 27.1 and 27.2. The current recommendations advise starting the immunization programme when the infant is 2 months of actual age, rather than age corrected for prematurity.

Contraindications to pertussis immunization

There are some circumstances in which pertussis immunization should be deferred or withheld.

Table 27.1 Immunization routinely given in the UK during infancy

Vaccine and route	Content	Age at administration
BCG in selected groups (see text) Intradermal	BCG (bacille Calmette–Guérin)	In neonatal period
Triple i.m. injection 1	Diphtheria (D) Tetanus (T) Acellular pertussis (aP)	2, 3 and 4 months
Triple i.m. injection 2 (DTaP/IPV/ Hib)	Inactivated polio vaccine (IPV) Haemophilus influenzae type B (Hib) Meningitis C	2, 3 and 4 months
MMR i.m. injection	Measles Mumps Rubella	Around 13 months

1 Immunization should be temporarily withheld if the child is suffering from any acute illness. Minor infections without fever or systemic upset are not reasons for withholding immunization.

2 A history of severe local or general reaction to a previous dose.

3 An evolving neurological abnormality or uncontrolled epilepsy: immunization should be deferred until the child is assessed by a paediatric neurologist.

A family history of allergy is not a contraindication, nor is a perinatal or family history of fits, provided the child has not had an acute encephalopathic illness within 7 days. Children with evolving neurological conditions may be immunized when the condition has become stable.

Pertussis vaccine in most countries is now acellular, with much lower complication rates than its predecessor the cellular vaccine.

Special vaccine circumstances

BCG (bacille Calmette–Guérin)

In Britain BCG is reserved for babies at risk for tuberculosis (TB) and is given by intradermal injection during the early neonatal period. Indications include:

- All infants living in areas of TB prevalence.
- Infants with parents or grandparents born in a country with a high TB prevalence.
- Babies born to previously unvaccinated recent immigrants from high-risk countries.

Surveys in British children have shown that this vaccine is over 70% effective, with protection lasting at least 15 years.

In Australia, high-risk groups, such as Asian or Aboriginal neonates, are given 0.1 mL BCG vaccine intradermally in the first week of life.

Hepatitis B

Infants born to mothers who are hepatitis B surface antigen (HbsAg)-positive should receive passive immunization with 100–200 IU of hepatitis B immunoglobulin and active immunization with 10 µg of hepatitis B vaccine as soon after birth as possible, and again at 1 and 6 months (see also p. 65). Hepatitis B immunization for infants of <2000 g birthweight should be delayed until 1 month or just prior to

Table 27.2 Australian recommendations for immunisation of premature and term infants

Chronological age	Birth weight		
	<1500 g	1500–2000 g	>2000 g
Birth	HepB*	HepB*	HepB*
2 months	DTPa-hepB, HiB, 7vPCV, OPV[†]	DTPa-hepB, HiB, 7vPCV, OPV[†]	DTPa-hepB, HiB, 7vPCV, OPV[†]
4 months	DTPa-hepB, HiB, 7vPCV, OPV[†]	DTPa-hepB, HiB, 7vPCV, OPV[†]	DTPa-hepB, HiB, 7vPCV, OPV[†]
6 months	DTPa-hepB, &vPCV, OPV[†] plus extra dose Hib	DTPa-hepB, &vPCV, OPV[†]	DTPa-hepB, &vPCV, OPV[†]
7 months	Measure anti HBs antibody, If <10 mIU/mL, give further dose HBV vaccine at 12 months	Measure anti-HBs antibody, If <10 mIU/mL, give further dose HBV vaccine at 12 months	
12 months	MMR, Hib plus extra HepB if indicated[†]	MMR, Hib plus extra HepB if indicated*	MMR, Hib

DTPa-hepB, acellular diphtheria, tetanus and pertussis; OPV, polio vaccine; PCV, pneumococcal conjugate vaccine; MMR, measles mumps rubella.

* Clinicians may elect to postpone the first dose of HepB vaccine until 2 months of age (and give at 2, 4, 6, 12 months) in extremely premature babies (<1 kg) or those with suspected coagulopathy – unless mother is HepBsAg +ve when HepB vaccine must be given at birth.

[†] OPV schedule should be initiated on discharge from hospital.

hospital discharge. Infants of birthweight <1000 g should be immunized when they weigh a minimum of 2000 g or when they are 2 months old.

Modification to immunization schedule for preterm infants

Generally, preterm infants are immunized according to their actual postnatal age and not their corrected age. Some extremely preterm infants are still too unstable to receive diphtheria-pertussis-tetanus (DPT), Hib (*Haemophilus influenza* type B) and polio at 2 months, and immunization needs to be deferred for some weeks. Preterm infants should receive paracetamol (20 mg/kg) and may require separate monitoring for 24–48 h after injection because of the high risk of apnoea. Acellular pertussis vaccine has not been shown to reduce the incidence of apnoea in extremely preterm infants. In the UK inactivated polio vaccine (IPV) is now given routinely by injection rather than oral polio vaccine, which carried a very small risk of producing vaccine-associated paralytic polio. If oral Sabin (polio) vaccine (a live attenuated virus) is given to preterm infants it is preferable for this to be given on the morning of discharge so that there is no risk to other infants from the excretion of virus in stools.

Growth

The maternal and child health clinic or the general practitioner should follow the growth of preterm and high-risk infants during the first year of life and plot length, weight and head circumference on appropriate percentile graphs.

The use of charts allows accurate assessment of these important parameters of physical growth. As a guide, term infants usually double their birthweight by 5 months and treble it by 1 year. The head circumference usually grows about 1 cm a month for the first 6 months, and then 0.5 cm a month for the next 6 months. Most babies increase their length by 20–30 cm (or 50%) in the first year of life.

Postnatal development

There is great variability in infant development. The rate of progress is influenced by many factors, including gestational age, nutrition, intercurrent illness, environmental stimulation and emotional support. Milestones in development can be considered in four groups: social, speech and language, gross motor and fine motor. The ages for the acquisition of these skills and milestones are approximate and there are wide variations between normal babies. Table 27.3 summarizes some of these important milestones. If there is evidence of significant developmental delay or cerebral palsy, the child should be referred to a child development centre for more comprehensive assessment by a multidisciplinary team. The totality of handicapping conditions in very low birthweight (VLBW) infants relates to corrected postnatal age and is illustrated in Fig. 27.1.

Definitions

Great care must be taken to use the terms 'handicap', 'impairment' and 'disability' correctly, so that comparisons can be made between different centres. The following are the internationally accepted World Health Organization (WHO) definitions.

Impairment

Any loss or abnormality of psychological or anatomical structure or function.

Disability

Any restriction or lack of ability (resulting from an impairment) in performing an activity in the manner or within the range considered to be normal.

Handicap

A disadvantage for an individual arising from a disability that limits or prevents the fulfilment of a role that should be normal for that individual.

Table 27.3 Milestones in development. Note that ages are very approximate and there are wide variations between normal babies

Age	Social	Speech and language	Gross motor	Fine motor
1 month	Quietens when talked to	—	Holds head up momentarily	Fists clenched at rest
2 months	Smiling with good visual interest	Listens to bell	Chin off couch when prone	Hands largely open
3 months	Follows objects through 180°	Vocalizes when talked to	Weight on forearms when lying prone	Holds objects placed in hands
4 months	Laughs aloud	—	Pulling to sit: no head lag	Hands come together
6 months	Imitates	Localizes sound	Lying prone, pushes up on hands	Reaches for objects
7 months	Feeds him/herself with biscuit	Makes four different sounds	Sits unsupported	Transfers from hand to hand
9 months	Waves bye-bye	Says 'Mama'	Stands holding on	Pincer grasp
12 months	Plays 'pat-a-cake'	2–3 words	Walking unsupported	Gives objects
15 months	Drinks from a cup	4–5 words	Climbs up stairs	Tower of two cubes
18 months	Points to three parts of body	8–10 words	Gets up and down stairs	Tower 3–4 cubes
21 months	Dry (mostly) during day	two-word sentences	Runs	Scribbles circles
24 months	Puts on shoes	2–3-word sentences	Walks up and down stairs	Tower 6–7 cubes
2½ years	Recognizes colours	Knows full name		Copies with pencil
3 years	Dresses and undresses fully	Tells stories		Copies with pencil

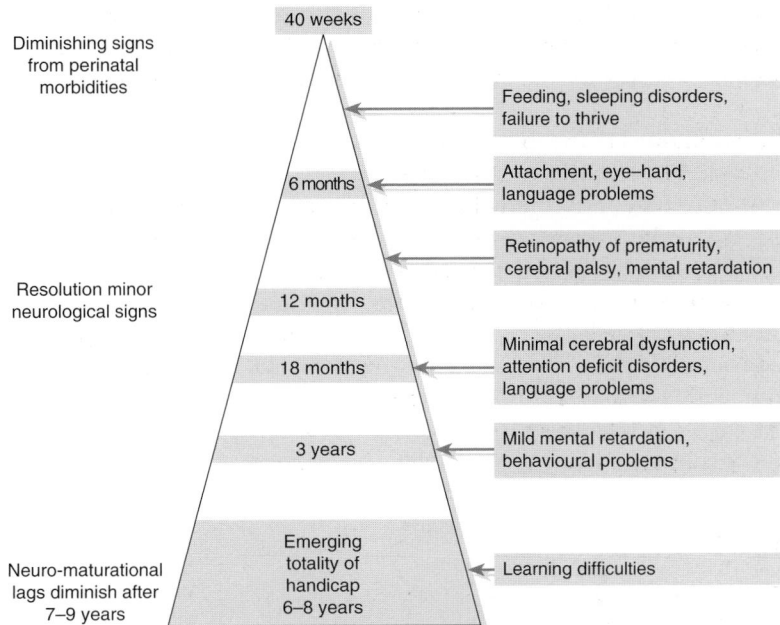

Diminishing signs from perinatal morbidities

Resolution minor neurological signs

Neuro-maturational lags diminish after 7–9 years

40 weeks

Feeding, sleeping disorders, failure to thrive

6 months

Attachment, eye–hand, language problems

Retinopathy of prematurity, cerebral palsy, mental retardation

12 months

18 months

Minimal cerebral dysfunction, attention deficit disorders, language problems

3 years

Mild mental retardation, behavioural problems

Emerging totality of handicap 6–8 years

Learning difficulties

Figure 27.1 Corrected postnatal ages at which disabilities become evident in VLBW infants.

Specialized follow-up clinics

The follow-up of high-risk infants is a continuation of neonatal intensive care and an integral part of it. The benefits of following up high-risk infants in specialized clinics include:

1 early diagnosis of problems enables early intervention and perhaps a better long-term prognosis;

2 evaluation of the perinatal factors that have an adverse effect on outcome, with subsequent modification of methods of delivery of perinatal intensive care;

3 evaluation of the long-term prognosis of high-risk populations of infants;

4 assessment of a cost-benefit analysis for perinatal intensive care.

Infants who are at risk for chronic handicapping conditions should be followed in special multidisciplinary clinics or by their paediatrician. Categories of infant that should be considered for specialized follow-up include:

1 those who were mechanically ventilated in the neonatal period;

2 VLBW infants (less than 1500 g birthweight);

3 those with severe perinatal asphyxia;

4 those with intracranial haemorrhage;

5 those with neonatal convulsions;

6 those with abnormal neurological examination at discharge;

7 infants who had major surgery.

Service, audit/quality assurance, research and education

Following high-risk children in a multidisciplinary follow-up clinic has several purposes.

Service role

Follow-up is considered an integral part of assuming responsibility for high-risk infants and provides early identification of developmental disability, reassurance to parents, psychosocial support and referral for appropriate treatment. Debate exists whether the multidisciplinary clinic personnel should provide treatment or merely have an evaluation role in follow-up of high-risk cohorts. The provision of healthcare by the clinic team gives greatest assurance of both a low attrition rate and an effective system of healthcare delivery.

Audit role

Multidisciplinary follow-up provides ongoing surveillance of morbidity, enabling evaluation of the impact of changes in obstetric and neonatal care on quality of survival of VLBW infants. Many advances in clinical practice have emanated from longitudinal cohort evaluation.

Research role

Follow-up programmes are expensive, require patience and perseverance, take several years to complete before research findings are available, and run the risk of being outdated because current neonatal practice has changed.

Educational role

The clinic provides an excellent multidisciplinary resource for teaching allied health professionals and medical and nurse clinicians about child development and the needs of families of high-risk infants.

Follow-up of preterm infants

The assessment of growth in preterm infants must always take into consideration the number of weeks of prematurity. Growth and development should be assessed according to the corrected age:

$$\text{Corrected age} = \text{postnatal age} - \text{number of weeks infant is preterm}$$

Data supporting this biological model suggest that, for infants less than or equal to 28 weeks' gestation, correction should be continued for 4 years; in those 29–31 weeks for 2 years; those 32–34 weeks for 1 year; and in those 35 weeks and beyond no correction is made for gestational age.

Growth

The healthy preterm baby who is appropriate for gestational age (AGA) should grow at the same rate as a term infant, with the same growth patterns as low birthweight infants; that is, regains birthweight at 2 weeks postnatal age and then accelerates, so that by the expected date of delivery the infant will be close to the expected weight of a term infant. At follow-up the height, weight and head circumference will be at or just below the 50th percentile for postconceptual age.

Growth failure often occurs in small for gestational age (SGA) and sick preterm infants, who receive inadequate nutrition for the first 4–6 weeks after birth. In this latter group linear and head growth virtually cease, and even when adequate nutrition is established growth may remain suboptimal. The SGA infant usually loses little, if any, weight in the neonatal period and then rapidly gains weight to reach his or her potential growth percentile. This growth spurt may not be maintained, and a permanent deficit in somatic growth persists into childhood.

Growth of head circumference is often difficult to interpret in preterm babies. This is partly due to the scaphocephalic head shape. For 3–4 weeks after birth, growth in head circumference is suboptimal at about 0.2 cm/week; then follows a period of rapid head growth (catch-up brain growth spurt) at about 1 cm/week for 1–2 months; the head then grows at the normal rate of 1 cm/month for the first 6 months and then 0.5 cm/month for the rest of the first year of life.

Common problems identified in preterm infants at follow-up are shown in Table 27.4.

Developmental outcomes

Long-term outcomes can be difficult to predict in the newborn period. Most preterm infants admitted to the neonatal unit grow and develop to be healthy, normal children. Some infants, however, develop significant disability – intellectual deficits, movement problems including cerebral palsy, and visual and/or hearing impairments.

- Examples of major disability: blindness, deafness requiring hearing aids, inability to walk without assistance, or a low level of intellectual abilities. Table 27.5 shows expected major disability rates from one large neonatal intensive care unit.
- Examples of less severe disability: short sightedness requiring correction with glasses, weakness on one side, clumsiness, learning difficulties, behavioural problems.

Predictors of outcome

Some of the major risk factors for survival are:
- birthweight;
- gestational age;

Table 27.4 Complications in the first year of life in preterm infants

Medical

Respiratory	Nasal congestion
	Exacerbation of bronchopulmonary dysplasia
	Recurrent wheezing
	SIDS
Cardiac	Patent ductus arteriosus
	Ventricular septal defect
Ophthalmic	Retinopathy of prematurity
	Strabismus
	Myopia
Auditory	Sensorineural hearing loss
	Conductive dysfunction
Surgical	Inguinal hernia, umbilical hernia, undescended testes, hydrocoele
Growth	Failure to achieve genetic growth potential
Gastrointestinal	Vomiting, gastro-oesophageal reflux, constipation, colic

Neurological deficits

Major	Spastic diplegia/ hemiplegia/ quadriplegia,
	hypotonia, hydrocephalus, microcephaly, moderate to profound global delay
Minor	Ataxia, incoordination and clumsiness
Miscellaneous	Child abuse, neglect, deprivation, behavioural disturbances, emotional disturbances, failure to thrive

Table 27.5 Representative rates of disability in survivors analysed by gestational age (data from Mater Mothers' Hospital, South Brisbane

Gestation at birth (weeks)	Disability in survivors (%)	
	Major	Any
23	40	50
24	30	40
25–26	20	30
27–28	10	15
More than 28		10

- retinopathy of prematurity – stages 3–5;
- moderate/profound sensorineural hearing loss.

Issues to consider when interpreting published outcome studies on preterm infants include:

- What is the denominator? Studies that include babies alive in the labour ward compared with studies that report a denominator of only babies admitted alive to the neonatal unit may be associated with a 50% difference in outcome at the extremes of prematurity.
- Reported by gestational age or birthweight?
- Survival rate/approach to resuscitation at limit of viability.
- Hospital-based or geographic population?
- Proportion of outborn babies.
- Correction for preterm birth.
- Attrition rate.
- Duration of follow-up.
- Outcomes measured/classifications of disability.
- Approach to untestable children.

Long-term outcome for extremely preterm infants compared with term control children

Compared with their full-term peers, extremely preterm children tend to achieve lower levels of physical and intellectual performance.

- Studies consistently find mean IQs for ELBW infants are 0.7–1.0 SD less than term controls.
- Subtle cognitive deficits include lower scores in maths, reading, spelling, English, visual short-term memory and executive function independent of IQ.
- Dyspraxia (clumsiness) particularly in ball skills (kicking and catching) and fine motor control, is more common in ELBW infants.

- inborn vs outborn status;
- sepsis (early or late onset).

Predictors of adverse outcome prior to discharge in VLBW infants are:

- periventricular haemorrhage – grade 2/3 complicated by hydrocephalus or grade 4;
- cystic periventricular leukomalacia (especially bilateral occipital cysts);

The use of magnetic resonant imaging (MRI), spectroscopy and cranial volumetric assessment to predict long term outcome require further longitudinal research;

- School performance – functioning below grade level (34–56% in various studies vs 2–21% in controls) and repeating a grade (in 23% vs 11% in controls).
- Attention deficit, hyperactivity disorders in premature infants relative risk (RR) of 2.64 (95% confidence interval (CI) 1.85–3.78).

However, the majority of preterm infants rate their quality of life as high and they are less likely to participate in risk-taking behaviours such as heavy alcohol consumption and illicit drug use.

Further reading

Illingworth RS. *The Development of the Infant and Young Child. Abnormal and Normal*, 8th edn. Edinburgh: Churchill Livingstone, 1983.

Johnson A. Long term follow-up of neonates. *Semin Neonatol* 2000;**5**(2):87–178.

NHMRC. Special risk groups: Preterm babies. *The Australian Immunisation Hand book* (9th edn) p. 28. Canbera, ACT: NHMRC, 2004.

Pickering *et al. Red book immunization in special clinical circumstances. Report of the Committee of Infections Disease* (27th edn). Elk Grove Village, IL: American Academy of Pediatrics, 2006.

Salisbury D, Ramsay M, Noakes K. *Immunisation Against Infectious Disease.* London: Department of Health; The Stationery Office, 2006.

Internet resource

Department of Health. NHS immunization information (www.immunisation.org.uk).

CHAPTER 28

28 Parent–infant attachment and support for parents experiencing perinatal loss

Parent–infant attachment

Following important observations in the 1970s by Klaus and Kennell (1982), it is now well accepted that a powerful parent–infant attachment ('bonding'), especially in mothers, has usually been established by the time of birth. Moreover, the research showed that little attention had been given to the possible effects on parents of the death of an infant who had had little or no opportunity for life. Since then there has been considerable literature on perinatal death, revealing that the care of recently bereaved parents leaves much to be desired. Thus, an understanding of the parent–infant bonding process can help the doctor and other healthcare providers to minimize the devastating effect of perinatal loss, and also to understand the effects of prematurity and congenital abnormality on a family.

For mothers a bond is formed quite early in pregnancy, stimulated by hormonal changes, psychological preparation and fantasies about the unborn child. 'Nesting' behaviour is manifested by the preparation of a nursery and the purchase of baby clothes. For the father the attachment process is less recognizable during the pregnancy but heightens with the birth, enhanced by an involvement with the delivery and handling of the baby. A sense of pride and hope for the future ensues.

Steps in attachment

The actual process by which attachment bonds are formed is unknown, but the time periods listed below are believed to be essential to this process. The strength of the attachment during these stages may vary from one woman to the next.

1 Planning the pregnancy.
2 Confirming the pregnancy.
3 Accepting the pregnancy.
4 Onset of fetal movements (quickening).
5 Accepting the fetus as an individual.
6 The birth process.
7 Seeing the baby.
8 Touching the baby.
9 Caretaking.

Most research, however, has concentrated on early contact in the immediate postnatal period. Extrapolation from animal research has proposed that there is a 'maternal-sensitive' or 'maternal-critical period', which is the optimal time for a bond of affection to develop between a mother and her infant. Although there is little doubt that the importance of this immediate postnatal period has been overemphasized in humans, this knowledge had major benefits for hospital practice. Some mothers are unable to achieve strong attachment without consistent contact. Failure to bond can result in rejection and resultant problems with child abuse, neglect and deprivation of nutrition, love and affection.

Parents learn to love their infant at varying times during the pregnancy and after birth. Parents 'bond' to their adopted babies, yet there has been no 'maternal-critical period'. It is apparent that humans differ from other animals in their patterns of bonding.

After birth a mother initially demonstrates attachment to her baby in several ways.
1 She is able to establish eye contact with the infant, who is in a state of arousal after birth.
2 If she is left alone with her naked infant, she may touch each part of the body with her fingertips.
3 A mother becomes overprotective of her infant in the first few days after delivery and becomes anxious

285

about crying and minor difficulties. This anxiety may appear excessive to hospital staff and family around her.

4 Babies may mimic the facial expressions of their parents, e.g. protrude their tongues.

5 Breastfeeding may be used to comfort and pacify the infant.

Management factors that promote attachment

The parents together plan the pregnancy and attend antenatal educational and physiotherapy classes. The antenatal preparation of breasts and nipples will assist with subsequent breastfeeding. The father should support the mother during labour and witness the birth of the baby. Unless the baby is ill, the mother and baby should be permitted to respond to each other in their own time and manner. Unnecessary separation of infant and mother must be avoided. The infant should 'room in' with the mother for 24 h of the day and be taken out to the nursery at night only if the mother is ill, or if other mothers are being disturbed. Breastfeeding on demand, even at night, should be actively encouraged. However, if a mother fails in her attempts to breastfeed or does not wish to do so, she must not be made to feel inadequate or guilty or told she is an unnatural mother. Successful bottle feeding is much better than unsuccessful breastfeeding.

Risk factors for failure to produce attachment

Mothers who plan their pregnancies have good expectations of the outcome, breastfeed their babies and rarely subsequently maltreat them. Some of the risk factors that may have an adverse effect on bonding and render the family 'at risk' for child protection concerns are listed below.

During pregnancy
1 Unsupported pregnancies.
2 Where the father was unfaithful or deserted the mother during pregnancy.
3 Frequent pregnancies with excessive workload.
4 Maternal depression during the pregnancy.
5 Loss of an emotionally significant person in relation to the pregnancy, e.g. the maternal grandmother,

grandfather, a loved sibling, a child of the mother or even a close friend, especially when the mother was somewhat isolated.
6 Conception during a period of marital conflict.

During labour and delivery
1 Being left alone and afraid in the labour ward, or when the mother perceived the staff as unconcerned.
2 When the birth itself was more painful or prolonged than was expected.
3 When breastfeeding was thrust upon the mother by the staff.
4 When the mother was unable to see the child after delivery, without explanation, or was told that the baby was damaged.
5 When the mother herself was damaged as a result of the birth.
6 When the father exhibited more interest in the infant than in his partner.

In the neonatal and postnatal period
1 Prematurity.
2 Congenital malformations.
3 Critically ill infants requiring neonatal intensive care.
4 Postnatal depression.

Rejection is more likely to occur when the infant has problems in the perinatal period or requires neonatal intensive care. There is a discrepancy between the idealized, perfect baby and the real baby: under these circumstances the parents require careful counselling and support.

Failure of bonding or attachment

When bonding fails there is rejection or non-acceptance of the child. This may result in problems for both the child and the mother.

Long-term problems in the child
1 *Child abuse.* Several studies have shown that preterm infants are overrepresented among abused children. Approximately 30% of battered children are premature, yet the overall incidence of prematurity is 8%.
2 *Non-organic failure to thrive.* Failure to thrive without organic cause is sometimes due to neglect or deprivation. Studies have revealed a fourfold increase

among preterm infants and babies who require prolonged hospitalization in the newborn period.

3 *Temper tantrums, infant colic, feeding problems, sleeplessness and vomiting.* Behavioural and feeding disorders are more common when an affectional bond has not been formed.

4 *Inadequate personality and poor interpersonal skills.* Infants who have been deprived of love and affection may subsequently have emotional and personality disturbances. They may become abusing or neglecting parents as adults, and so the cycle may repeat itself.

Problems in the mother
1 Hesitant, clumsy handling of the baby.
2 Anxiety states and depression.
3 Mother states that 'the baby belongs to the hospital or nursing staff'.
4 Feelings of inadequacy, disappointment, failure, deprivation and anger.
5 Mother may complain that the baby does not bond with her.

Care of parents of critically ill infants

The modern intensive care nursery is a bewildering and frightening place for the parents of a recently delivered premature or sick infant. These parents often have feelings of extreme frustration, stress, guilt and helplessness and must be counselled sensitively. The total care of the high-risk neonate must include the parents. The approach to the parents is discussed in a chronological manner, from antenatal clinic through to discharge and follow-up.

Antenatal contact

Women with high-risk pregnancies should be introduced, prior to delivery, to a 'baby doctor', whom they will probably meet after the baby is born. It is also helpful to the parents if they have the opportunity to visit the neonatal intensive care unit prior to delivery, so that they are aware of the sights that will greet them when they first enter to see their own baby. They might benefit from receiving an introductory book describing the nursery care and staff, and an introduction to a support group for parents of preterm babies or babies with a specific congenital anomaly.

Labour ward

When condition of the baby permits, the baby should be given to the mother for suckling and skin-to-skin contact for as long as possible. The baby should be suctioned, dried and warmed prior to being handled by the mother. Even if the baby is critically ill, his or her condition should be explained and the mother should see the baby. The open visiting policy of the nursery should be explained to the parents.

Intensive care nursery

When the baby's condition is stable, the mother and father should come into the nursery to see and touch their baby. Careful explanations are given regarding abnormal signs (retractions, bruising, etc.) and equipment (monitors, incubators, respirator, umbilical arterial catheter, etc.).

Before entering the nursery the parents will take off their coats, watches, rings, etc. and roll up their sleeves to above the elbows. They will be instructed on hand-washing, and in some units will wear overgowns. Having adopted this careful technique, there is no evidence that parental visiting and handling of premature infants have influenced the incidence of bacterial infection or even colonization. The organisms that parents harbour are less virulent and exhibit less antibiotic resistance than the commensal organisms of hospital staff.

There is every reason for the parents to be intimately involved with their critically ill infant from the outset. The premature infant has enough physiological problems already without adding attachment problems to the list. The parents are informed that they may visit or ring the nursery 24 h a day, and that both parents will be kept informed of the baby's progress. Consideration should be given to providing a pamphlet explaining the intensive care nursery and encouraging the parents to become actively involved in their child's care. A digital photograph may help the mother to accept her baby for the day or two before she is able to visit the nursery. Occasionally, the baby may be placed in a port incubator and taken to the mother.

Parents' first visit to the intensive care nursery

Parents should be greeted and welcomed to the nursery. Again, the equipment should be carefully explained. It is most important for the mother to be able to establish eye contact with her baby, and if appropriate the goggles used with phototherapy may be removed. Often the mother will have to look through the porthole to establish an *en face* position with her infant (i.e. align her head with her baby's). Some parents are very apprehensive of handling, and usually state that their baby is too fragile to touch.

The nursing staff must work through this anxiety with the parents and encourage them to touch, fondle and caress their baby. Once the parents realize that their baby can actually see them, respond to their voices and can be pacified by them, their attachment grows.

Parents' subsequent visits to the intensive care nursery

The parents should be encouraged actively to participate in their baby's care. They derive great satisfaction from holding the gavage syringe, changing napkins and sponging the baby. Although in an incubator, the baby can usually come out for a brief cuddle, or skin-to-skin ('kangaroo') care, provided care is taken to maintain body temperature and the patency of all attached tubes. This may even be possible when baby is receiving assisted ventilation.

Most mothers are only too happy to express their breast milk for their baby. The 28-week gestation infant needs the milk from his or her mother's breasts. It is remarkably well tolerated, considering the immaturity of the gastrointestinal tract at that gestational stage, and may decrease the incidence of necrotizing enterocolitis (NEC) and infection. The mother will need a great deal of empathy and support from staff members to continue breast expression for the 8–10 weeks before her infant will be able to suckle. The role of maternal milk in feeding the very low birthweight (VLBW) infant is

discussed on p. 82. Breastfeeding should be encouraged while the mother is in hospital, so that the benefits of colostrum may be obtained.

Babies as individuals

Notes attached to the baby's bed should be encouraging to the parents, for example 'Mum is to feed me at 3 pm. I am looking forward to my first breast-feed. Love Billy'.

The parents are asked to provide the staff with the baby's name as soon as possible. An artist can then write the name in large print on the incubator. The baby should be referred to as 'Billy' or 'Susie' where possible, and *never* as 'it'.

Appropriate decorations and mobiles, which may help parents adjust to a long hospital stay, can be attached to incubators. Parents are encouraged to use the pastoral care personnel of the hospital, or else to bring their own minister of religion to baptize or administer rites to the baby.

How is my baby doing?

The staff should answer this question in a realistic but optimistic way. Never should an unduly pessimistic attitude be conveyed, as this will only encourage detachment from the child. It has been shown that even if the baby dies, the parents gain from having attached to their child. Their grief is physiological and appropriate. It is difficult to grieve appropriately for someone you have never known. When asked the above question, it is often useful to ask the parents how *they* think the baby is getting on. Caution should be exercised when making predictions about outcome, and a problem-orientated approach to the baby should be avoided. It is easy for the parents to become involved with the intricacies of oxygen therapy and oxygen tension, rather than the baby as a whole.

The social worker

The social worker plays an important role in the intensive care nursery. She or he should be introduced to the mother at the first visit and help to prepare her for the difficult period ahead. The social worker provides support, investigating the attitudes of parents towards the child, and at the same time may uncover social and economic problems. At times the social worker acts as the 'case manager' providing the continuum of care that can be difficult to achieve with nursing and medical rostering. Consideration should be given towards keeping a parental contact chart recording telephone enquiries, visits and the specific involvement of parents during these visits. This helps with communication, especially between nursing shifts.

Babies transferred from other hospitals

Parents of babies transferred from other hospitals into the intensive care nursery have unique problems. Prolonged parent–infant separation is common. If possible, the mother should be transferred along with the baby; but this may separate mother from her husband and other children. If the mother cannot be transferred, emailed digital photographs and daily progress reports should be provided. Whenever possible, the baby should be transferred back to the referring hospital for recovery care. Many tertiary perinatal hospitals have temporary accommodation facilities for 'out of town families' of high-risk infants.

Preparation for discharge

Once the need for intensive care has passed, the baby will still need monitoring, incubator care and gavage feeding. This can be a very frustrating time for the parents, who have already experienced so much. Early discharge for LBW babies can safely be practised and may promote attachment. Babies have been discharged to an optimal home situation with birthweights below 1600 g, provided they are feeding well, the mother is handling competently, they are gaining weight steadily and adequate follow-up can be maintained.

Caring for parents of an infant who dies

Birth and grief – a paradox

A birth is an event that is usually associated with joy and excitement. It is preceded by planning, expectations, dreams and hopes. For most people,

having a baby brings with it changes in the family structure that affect each family member in a different way. The nine months of the pregnancy are filled with adjustments in role for the mother, father and siblings, and with an awareness that a new life is growing within the mother. Grandparents and members of the extended family share in the preparations and hopes. In many families there may be ambivalent feelings. Perhaps the pregnancy was unplanned or unwanted, or the siblings may be reluctant to share their parents with a new baby.

Whatever the hopes and feelings, the news that the baby is dead comes as an unexpected catastrophe. For parents who have experienced miscarriage or a stillbirth, the fact that they have never known the baby can make their loss seem even more unreal and difficult to accept. When the baby survives for a short time, the parents have had an opportunity to experience their child as a living being.

Some of the common characteristics of normal grief are outlined below. The stages of grief are not necessarily in this order, and occupy a variable period of time. Culberg (1972) has suggested that a normal grief reaction lasts 6–9 months, although the most intensive phase lasts from 1 to 6 weeks.

1 'Shock'.
2 Emotional release.
3 Utter depression, loneliness and isolation.
4 Physical symptoms, e.g. choking, dyspnoea, empty feeling, weakness, fatigue, insomnia, loss of appetite.
5 Panic – about their own worth and the safety of other children.
6 Guilt.
7 Anger.
8 Inability to return to normal activities.
9 Overcoming grief.
10 Readjustment of life.

Management of parents of critically ill babies

Parents of critically ill children will all have their own special difficulties to overcome. However, guidelines of proven value in decreasing pathological grief and promoting normal reactions are given below.

1 The parents are encouraged to visit the nursery and handle the baby.

2 There should be frank discussions with the doctor regarding the chance and quality of survival of the infant.

3 Parents of critically ill babies should be visited by the hospital priest or chaplain and asked if they would like to have their child baptized.

4 Once death is imminent the parents are encouraged to cuddle the baby, who may die in their arms. Occasionally, this may even occur outside the nursery, and in some instances the infant may be taken home if this is the parents' wish.

5 The parents should, if possible, be permitted to express their emotions and feelings without the use of sedation.

6 If the mother is in the postnatal ward, she is offered the privacy of a single room and discharged early.

7 The staff should discuss death, autopsy and funeral arrangements with the parents at the earliest opportunity.

8 A health visitor or social worker may visit the parents at their home if this is thought to be desirable.

9 Preliminary autopsy results are discussed with parents as soon as they are available.

10 A follow-up appointment is made 8 weeks after the death to discuss the autopsy findings and causes of death, and for counselling for further pregnancies.

In spite of these attempts to support the parents, the death of a newborn infant, whether sudden or expected, imposes a severe stress on the family. A longitudinal prospective study of bereaved parents (Vance *et al.* 1991) has shown that parental distress, as manifested by anxiety and depression, is greatest at 6–8 weeks. Although the timing of the follow-up appointment should not be changed, those who carry out the interview should be aware of this.

Bereavement counsellors and perinatal loss support groups

Beneficial support, additional to that provided by doctors, nurses and social workers, can be provided by trained bereavement counsellors or by other parents who have experienced and recovered from perinatal loss, for example, the Stillbirth and Neonatal Death Support Group (SANDS). Invaluable support may also be provided by books (e.g. Kubler-Ross 1977) and resource packages (e.g. Murray 1993) that help parents to understand the grieving process.

Developmental care for high-risk infants

Rationale

ELBW infants are particularly vulnerable to the potentially noxious stimuli of the neonatal intensive care unit (NICU) environment, including light, noise, frequent disturbances and painful procedures. They react to the noisy and well-lit environment of many NICUs with variability of blood pressure, ventilatory requirements and oxygen saturation as well as behavioural disorganization. These disturbances may have both short- and long-term adverse effects on outcome.

The pattern of brain growth from conception through to the end of the second year of postnatal life can be seen in Table 28.1.

Recent research in animals, including humans, has developed the concept of a critical period for sensory development. This concept is based on a finite time during late fetal life or early neonatal life for critical neurosensory development, which is driven or influenced by stimuli with the potential to set patterns that affect capacity through to adult life. Figure 28.1 shows a time for neurosensory development.

What is developmental care?

Developmental care refers to interventions on babies receiving intensive care designed to minimize the

Table 28.1 The pattern of brain growth and development

Timing of exogenous/stimulation role	
Somataesthic (touch, temp, pain)	<24 wks
Position and movement	<24 wks
Chemosensory (smell and taste)	25–26 wks
Auditory	30–31 wks
Vision	Near term

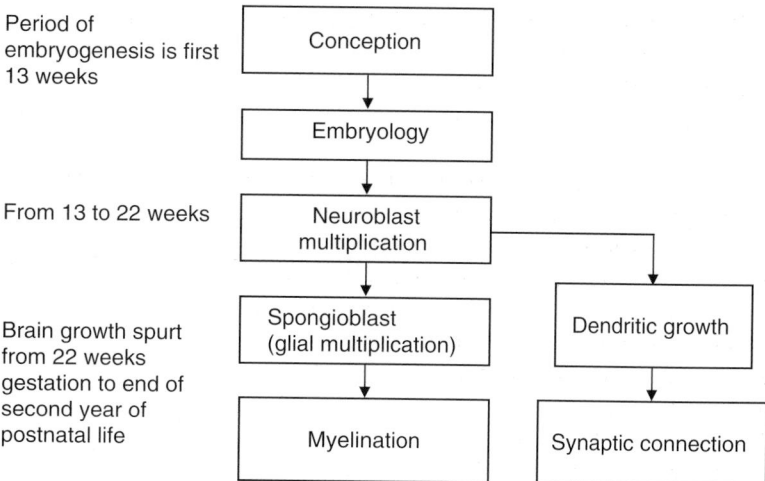

Figure 28.1 Neurosensory development.

Period of embryogenesis is first 13 weeks

From 13 to 22 weeks

Brain growth spurt from 22 weeks gestation to end of second year of postnatal life

Conception → Embryology → Neuroblast multiplication → Spongioblast (glial multiplication) → Myelination

Dendritic growth → Synaptic connection

stress of the NICU environment. Elements consist of control of external stimuli (vestibular, auditory, tactile), clustering of nursery care activities and positioning or swaddling to provide a sense of containment.

Developmental care is based on a programme involving careful positioning, which includes the provision of boundaries (nests), minimization of light and sound, optimal parental contact (especially skin-to-skin contact, massage and cuddle), cue-based care, procedural support and pain management. Skin-to-skin (kangaroo) care, in which the infant is placed unclothed on the mother's or father's bare chest, was originally developed in Bogotà, Columbia, to maintain temperature regulation in preterm infants. Kangaroo care has been shown to provide a number of benefits to both parents and babies. A Cochrane systematic review details the benefits to mothers in terms of sense of competence and some short-term benefits, including a decrease in nosocomial infection and subsequent reduction in respiratory tract infection, and promotion of breastfeeding.

The development of motor and behavioural responses in the preterm infant may be enhanced by positioning and handling techniques. This should not be considered as something extra being done to or for the infant but rather a special way of performing the everyday caregiving activities.

Developmental care or interventions should suit the needs of the individual infant with respect to their medical, motor and behavioural states. Any intervention should involve the parents to facilitate bonding and confidence in preparation for caring for their infant at home.

A neonatal individualized developmental care and assessment programme (NIDCAP) provides a preassessment to design the care package, behavioural observation and developmental care. Heiderlese Als developed the NIDCAP programme in Boston in 1986, and this has been accepted in many industrialized countries. Only small randomized trials comparing NIDCAP with conventional care of preterm infants have been conducted to date and long-term benefits are yet to be proven.

The NICU environment should be modified to limit exposure of ELBW infants to stresses, by lowering ambient light, reducing noise, clustering caregiving periods and procedures to allow periods of uninterrupted sleep, and using positioning aids to promote containment.

The physical layout of nurseries should consider the developmental needs of babies (baby-centred design), and the needs of families (family-centred design) and yet be functional for provision of clinical care. Recent design guidelines have been established for Australia and New Zealand, the UK and the USA.

Caterina Braun described the 'hospitalization syndrome' when there is a severe interruption of parent–infant interaction as having a critical impact on behaviour and resultant in deficits in speech, behaviour, personality development, intellectual and social capacity and mental disturbance.

Pain in newborn infants

Organizations have commissioned interdisciplinary teams to incorporate regulatory directives and results of scientific investigation into institutional practice guidelines and standards for care. Despite these initiatives surveys of physicians and nurses continue to suggest that pain in the neonatal population is under-addressed and under-managed.

Three common misconceptions have influenced the clinical approach to neonatal pain:
- Newborns do not have the neurological substrate for the perception of pain.
- Newborns do not remember pain and if they do it has no adverse effects.
- It is too dangerous to administer anaesthesia or postoperative analgesia to newborn infants.

These beliefs have recently been refuted by the following observations:
- Newborn infants subjected to noxious stimuli have immediate hormonal, physiological and behavioural responses.
- Pain in the neonatal period has long-term consequences with studies demonstrating both in pre-term and healthy term infants that it diminishes subsequent behavioural response to pain.

Clinical staff, especially neonatal nurses, need to be able to detect positive infant behaviours and negative or stress behaviours. An overriding principle is that no baby of any age should have to undergo any painful procedure without any support. Options consist of swaddling, sucking, skin-to-skin contact with mother or breastfeeding, sedation or sucrose.

The principles of management of pain in neonates consist of prevention where possible, environmental protection from noxious stimuli, behavioural methods such as breastfeeding and glucose feeding, pharmacological agents for pre-emptive analgesia and pharmacological therapy for ongoing pain.

PRINCIPLES OF MANAGEMENT

- Tertiary hospitals should develop management strategies to promote the attachment of parents to their sick and preterm infants.
- Opportunistic psychosocial assessments should be done on families for whom there are child protection concerns.
- The intensive care nursery should be designed to the needs of parents and babies, and staff should support unrestricted parental visiting.
- The compassionate care of parents who have suffered a perinatal loss involves a skilled multidisciplinary team approach.

References

Culberg J. Mental reactions of women to perinatal death. In: Morris N. (ed.) *Psychosomatic Medicine in Obstetrics and Gynaecology* 3rd edn. Karger, New York, 1972; pp. 326–329.

Klaus MH, Kennell JH. *Parental–Infant Bonding*, 2nd edn. St Louis: C.V. Mosby, 1982.

Kubler-Ross E (ed.) *On Death and Dying*. London: Tavistock Publications, 1977.

Murray J. *An Ache in Their Heart* [self help kit]. Brisbane: University of Queensland, Department of Child Health, 1993.

Royal Australasian College of Physicians (Paediatrics and Child Health Division). Guidelines statement: Management of procedure related pain in neonates. *J Paediatr Child H* 2006;**42**:S31–S39.

Vance JC, Foster WJ, Najman JM *et al.* Early parental responses to sudden infant death, stillbirth or neonatal death. *Med J Australia* 1991;**155**:292–297.

Further reading

D'Apolito KC. State of the science: procedural pain management in the neonate. *J Perinat Neonat Nurs* 2006;**20**(1):56–61.

Boyle FM. Mothers Bereaved by Stillbirth, Neonatal Death or Sudden Infant Death Syndrome. Aldershot: Ashgate, 1997.

CHAPTER 29

29 Ethical issues in the treatment of critically ill newborn infants: decision-making in the care of the newborn infant

Ethics is the science of morals; the branch of philosophy concerned with human character and conduct. Ethical issues arise in the interactions of persons that involve the welfare or freedom of humans. They occur when one person or group of persons acts in ways that affect the welfare of another person or group of persons.

In the practice of medicine the best course of action is generally determined by humanist values (intrinsic value of human life).

The very core of medicine is the respect for human life and the attempts to sustain and improve it. Life-sustaining treatment decisions for newborn infants are typically made in an environment of scarce resources and where the medical, ethical and personnel implications are complex and often ambiguous. Terminology such as 'sanctity of life', 'quality of life', and 'ordinary or extraordinary means' are unduly simplistic and usually unhelpful.

Principles of ethical reasoning

Four major principles of ethical reasoning are particularly relevant to making decisions about newborn infants:

1 *Beneficence* (discontinuing futile treatment). The traditional medical ethic is to act in ways that benefit the patient and do no harm to the welfare or freedom of the patient. In many cases, however, the institution or continuation of treatment aimed at sustaining life is futile. Futile treatment is not likely to prevent death or serious compromise to the patient. There are difficulties in assessing futility but medical determinations must be made so that treatments that offer no benefit and serve to prolong the dying process should not be employed.

2 *Non-malificence* (burdensome treatment). The primary ethical injunction for the doctor is 'First do no harm' [*primum non nocere*]. In making a decision to withhold or withdraw life-sustaining medical treatment the principle of non-malificence would require withholding treatment where it can be said that it harms the patient. This occurs when the treatment itself is an intolerable burden to the patient.

3 *Autonomy*. The patient has the legal right and ethical autonomy to refuse life-sustaining treatment and be allowed to die. The neonate has never been competent and therefore decision-making is based on the patient's 'best interests'. Generally the parents have the authority and responsibility to make decisions on behalf of their baby. The two rationales for giving the parents the responsibility are 'bearer of responsibility' and 'best advocate' grounds.

4 *Equity or distributive justice*. Doctors have an obligation to distribute benefits and burdens equally and where differential treatment is given, to explain the reasons for this based on widely accepted criteria. This principle might mean that in some cases the patient's best interests should not or need not be the sole determining criterion.

Decision-making

Several approaches to decision-making have been described.

1 *Wait-until-certainty approach*. In an aggressive treatment environment almost every infant who is thought to have any chance to survive has full treatment commenced and continued until it is clear that treatment should be withdrawn. The advantage of this approach is that it avoids the death of any infant who might have a good outcome, but at the cost of some infants for whom dying might be prolonged or who might survive with severe handicaps. This aggressive approach is understandable in societies where consumer rights, individualism and litigation are prevalent.

2 *Statistical approach.* This approach draws on the accumulated evidence in order to establish categories of patients for whom treatment should be withheld or withdrawn. This approach seeks to avoid 'creating' severely impaired children, even though this may be at the expense of the deaths of some infants who might have a good outcome. This approach has been widely adopted in the Netherlands and some Scandinavian countries.

3 *Individualized approach (prognostic decision-making).* Treatment is initiated on any infant who has a chance of survival but the patient is continually assessed to determine whether this treatment is in the child's best interests. A determination to withdraw treatment is made earlier than in the 'wait until certainty' approach. For example, applying this approach to a 25-week, 750-g infant with respiratory distress syndrome (RDS) who develops a grade IV intraventricular haemorrhage (IVH) may enable the experienced physician to recommend withdrawal of treatment.

Antenatal diagnosis

A paradigm shift has occurred in the last two decades in ethical decision-making in perinatal medicine. In previous decades ethical decision-making usually occurred after the unexpected birth of an infant with a major congenital anomaly. However, most pregnant women now have biochemical and ultrasound screening (nuchal fold thickness) in the first trimester and almost all have ultrasound assessment at 17–19 weeks' gestation for congenital anomalies. In developed countries most major congenital anomalies are diagnosed antenatally before 20 weeks' gestation. Parents receive full multidisciplinary counselling and are supported in their decision-making process. A clinical care plan is

developed and frequently a case manager supports the family.

The role of the Institutional Ethics Committee (IEC)

Institutions and neonatal service providers usually establish general principles and a process for ethical decision-making. The IEC may have a role to play in treatment decisions on 'imperilled' newborn infants, particularly in a Catholic hospital. The IEC also has an important proactive role in ethical decision-making for obstetric and fetal patients but less so for commencing, continuing, withholding or withdrawing treatment in a neonate.

The roles of an IEC can be summarized as follows:

1 Develop and ratify institutional guidelines.
2 Act as an advisory and consultative body.
3 Staff education.
4 Disseminate information.
5 Absolve the attending physician from the decision-making process when necessary.
6 Resolve differences of opinion.

There are no algorithms readily available that one can follow simply each time an ethical dilemma arises: rather, one must work through a complex series of moral, religious, cultural and legal issues to reach an acceptable conclusion (Freed & Hageman 1996).

Good ethics can only be exercised if the medicine practised is correct. Good ethics requires accurate medical facts; not even sound ethical reasoning will rescue a decision based on false assumptions. With the advances in medical technology has come a greater public awareness of neonatal intensive care.

Common neonatal ethical dilemmas

Most neonatal ethical dilemmas fall within the following four areas.

When not to resuscitate at birth. Unfortunately, junior physicians are often in the acute situation and may not have the relevant knowledge to make such a decision. Institutional guidelines are necessary to cover all situations. Mistakes can undoubtedly be made in those first few vital seconds, and if there is any doubt one must err on the conservative side of resuscitation. A decision can be reversed later on. Currently recommended indications for failure to resuscitate at birth would include very few conditions:

1 anencephaly;

2 other severe central nervous system malformations;

3 multiple absence of sense organs;

4 absence of fetal/neonatal heartbeat for more than 10 minutes.

Infants with conditions such as suspected chromosomal anomalies (triploidy, trisomy 13 and trisomy 18), perinatal lethal renal disease and lethal skeletal disorders should probably be resuscitated and then fully assessed and investigated so that a rational decision can be made with all relevant information available.

'How small is too small?' – When not to resuscitate on gestational age or birthweight criteria (Fig. 29.1). Human nature being what it is, we are straining to push back the frontiers of viability (technological imperative) to improve our statistics, and tend to accept death as failure.

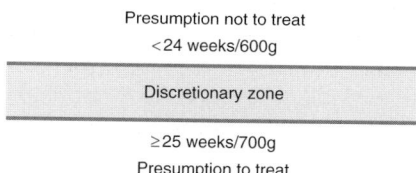

Figure 29.1 How small is too small? Or when not to resuscitate on birthweight or gestational age criteria.

Hospitals should develop guidelines based on their own survival and outcome data. An approach could be to attempt resuscitation on all infants over 600 g and/or ≥24 weeks' gestation, and for selected infants between 500 and 600 g, depending on past obstetric history, the likelihood of infection, birth trauma and severity, initial asphyxia and parental wishes. Present indications suggest that infants less than 600 g and of an appropriate weight for gestational age and those less than 24 weeks' gestation and with fully fused eyelids are unlikely to survive even with intensive care in centres of neonatal excellence. Survival rates for extremely low birthweight infants admitted to intensive care nurseries in 2004 in Australia and New Zealand are shown in Table 29.1 (Abeywardana 2007).

Saying that the neonatologist will attempt full resuscitation and subsequent intensive care for all infants >24 weeks' gestation and/or >600 g does not mean that the obstetrician must necessarily do everything possible for all these pregnancies, as he or she has two people to consider, not just the neonate. At times there will be a dichotomy in the aggressiveness of care between obstetrician and neonatologist.

Major congenital malformations. These can be considered under several categories.

1 Severe but not life-threatening abnormalities. These babies will be given all appropriate medical and nursing care to promote survival and minimize later disability.

2 Lethal abnormalities (e.g. anencephaly, trisomy D, E, encephalocoele). These babies receive good nursing

Table 29.1 Survival to discharge by gestational age and birthweight for live born infants

Gestational age (weeks)	% Survival to discharge		Birthweight group (g)	% Survival to discharge Australia and New Zealand 2004*
	Australia and New Zealand Data 2004*	UK data†		
22	20		<500	36
23	41	11	500–749	67
24	63	26	750–999	88
25	76	44	1000–1249	96
26	83	–	1250–1499	97
27	92	–		

*The data for Australia and New Zealand refer to 2004 and only include babies admitted to NICUs.

†UK national figures for survival to estimated date of delivery after extremely premature birth. Costeloe *et al.* 2000.

care to keep them comfortable, warm, free from hunger and relieved of pain. No active means are taken to shorten life. At times these babies are discharged home under the parents' care. Parents and family receive ongoing counselling and support.

3 Potentially lethal conditions that may be associated with severe handicap. Examples include:

(a) neural tube defects (myelomeningocoele, hydrocephalus, encephalocoele);

(b) birth asphyxia with evidence of severe hypoxic-ischaemic encephalopathy.

Life support measures may be instituted while the infant is fully assessed and all necessary information obtained. Parents are progressively counselled so that they are fully aware of the clinical condition, including the sequelae and the management options available.

Withdrawal of life supports. The situation regarding possible withdrawal of life supports arises under different circumstances.

1 Clear-cut cases (e.g. confirmation of bilateral renal agenesis, trisomy 13 or 18, triploidy, irreversible cervical cord injury). To continue ventilation for these lethal conditions would be futile and under the circumstances would constitute 'extraordinary care'.

2 Irreversible brain death following hypoxic-ischaemic injury.

3 Preterm infant with progressive bronchopulmonary dysplasia, grade IV cerebroventricular haemorrhage or posthaemorrhagic hydrocephalus.

These cases may be clear cut when the infant can be recognized as dying despite maximal assistance, and death seems inevitable.

The question of whether life support systems should be withdrawn for an extremely low birthweight (ELBW) infant demonstrating a large cerebroventricular haemorrhage with intraparenchymal extension is a frequent dilemma.

Selective withdrawal of neonatal intensive care

Reasons for considering withdrawal include:

1 Prognosis too bad:

(a) short-term survival;

(b) long-term outcome.

2 Therapy too burdensome.

The decision-making process involves:

1 Accurate and complete medical facts:

(a) subspecialist consultation;

(b) scientific documentation.

2 Consultation with hospital ethicist (if available) or independent consultant.

3 In-depth case conference: medical-moral-ethical discussion.

Parents in the decision-making process

Although parents are usually the best-qualified advocates for their infant, they should not shoulder the burden entirely but rather a shared decision should be made.

All 'proxy decision-makers', whether they be parents, physicians or courts of law, must be fully informed and cognizant of the relevant facts. Whatever approach is adopted it is vital that the process is made transparent and that the physician communicates clearly with parents and other members of the healthcare team.

The hospital and the State recognize their responsibility to provide appropriate care for all newborn infants. Usually, with ongoing open and frank communication between clinical staff and parents, there is agreement of full neonatal intensive care as to whether continuation or withdrawl, is in the baby's best interests. The decision to initiate treatment or to withhold treatment is a medical one and therefore one for the doctor to make; the decision to consent or refuse treatment is, in the first instance, for the parents to make in the best interests and as advocate for their child.

It is rare for there to be major disagreement between clinical staff caring for the baby and parents, provided that there are careful and repeated discussions between all parties. Tape recording of conversations has been shown to be a useful way to give the parents time to reflect on what was said. A major dispute between clinicians and family represents a failure in communication.

However, in the unusual situation of conflict when parents prefer no active treatment, the wishes of the parents may be overridden to sustain life. The reverse situation (i.e. parents wishing the continuation of life supports and medical staff wishing to withdraw) occasionally arises and must be handled compassionately.

Circumstances in which parents' wishes might be overruled, or when parents are incapable of decision-making

It is not the doctor's role to override the wishes of parents, particularly when their decision is arrived at after careful consideration and reflection. Often religious beliefs have a very strong influence on their decision and it may be helpful to engage religious advisers in the conversation provided the family is happy with this.

Where major dispute arises there are three possible courses of action. The first is to ask another neonatologist from a different hospital to give an independent opinion. Discuss this with the family and ask them whether they will agree to this as a way forward. Secondly in hospitals with clinical ethical committees the case may be reviewed by them and advice given.

In the UK the courts become involved in the rare cases where there remains a major disagreement about the continuation of care. This usually arises when the parents feel that care should be continued and the clinical staff feel that care is not going to save the baby's life or where survival will involve significant pain or suffering. The court will make a decision on the basis of an independent assessment of the evidence.

Exchange transfusion or urgent blood transfusion for infants of parents of the Jehovah's Witness faith raise particular problems. In the UK the child is made a ward of court so that life-saving treatment can be given against the parent's wishes.

Role of the case conference

A suggested approach to deal with issues regarding the withdrawal of life support is the case conference. This involves all relevant staff (medical, nursing, allied health, pastoral care) and parents to work through the complex series of medical, social and ethical issues.

Purpose of conference

A case conference can serve several purposes.
1 It ensures staff are comfortable with the decision.
2 It enhances communication between staff.

3 It can develop a future care plan:
  (a) further information (investigation);
  (b) time frameworks.
4 Provides guidance for counselling parents.
5 Maps out a process for withdrawal of life supports.
6 Enables staff to understand the decision-making process.
7 Gives an opportunity for all opinions to be expressed.

Communication of withdrawal of life support

The decision to withdraw life support entails several procedures that must be followed.
1 The attending physician clearly annotates the medical facts in the chart.
2 At times a second neonatologist is consulted and their opinion is documented in the chart.
3 Rarely the hospital ethics committee is convened if there is ethical uncertainty.
4 The decision-making process is annotated in the chart.
5 The decision is communicated to relevant persons, e.g. charge nurse, director of nursing, medical superintendent.
6 Cases with unique aspects are documented in detail and archived by the ethics committee.

Care of parents

The care and support of the parents is a necessary part of the decision-making process and its aftermath.
1 The parents, preferably together, receive progressive counselling from the neonatologist.
2 Ongoing support is provided by nursing staff, social workers and pastoral care staff.
3 Parents are informed of the case conference and are counselled afterwards.
4 Life and death decisions are made jointly by the neonatologist and the parents – the final decision is parental.

References

Abeywardana S. *Australian and New Zealand Neonatal Network 1997*. Sydney: AIHW National Perinatal Statistics Unit, 2007.

Costeloe K, Hennessy E, Gibson AE, Marlow N, Wilkinson AR. The EPICure study: Outcomes to dischage from hospital per infants born at the threshold of viability. *Pediatrics* 2000;**106**,659–671.

Freed GE, Hageman JR (eds) Ethical dilemmas in the prenatal, perinatal and neonatal periods. *Clinics in Perinatology* 1996;**23**.

Further reading

Catholic Health Australia. *Cost of Ethical Standards.* Canberra, ACT: Catholic Health Australia Inc., 2001.

Dickenson D. *Ethical Issues in Maternal–Fetal Medicine.* Cambridge: Cambridge University Press., 2002.

Goldsworth A, Silverman W, Stevenson DK *et al.* (eds) *Ethics and Perinatology.* New York: Oxford University Press, 1995.

Where possible a procedure should be witnessed at least twice and then performed under supervision before it is attempted without supervision. In ill infants some of these procedures may be potentially harmful, even when performed by experienced staff. Ensure that all equipment is prepared and that both the operator and assistants are familiar with the procedure. Maintain adequate thermal care during the procedure and ensure that adequate analgesia and anaesthesia have been provided except for emergency situations. Do not persist beyond three failed attempts – seek a colleague's help or take a break and try again.

Bag-and-mask ventilation

It is important for any nurse, midwife or doctor who is involved in the delivery or care of newborn infants to learn how to use a bag and mask for emergency assisted ventilation. The most commonly used bags on labour wards and in neonatal units are Laerdal bags (Fig 30.1). These are self-infanting bags and

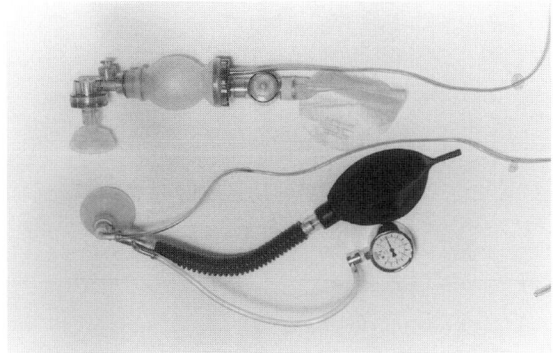

Figure 30.1 Laerdal (upper) and anaesthetic bagging systems with Laerdal face masks.

have pressures-relief safety valves which can be overridden when necessary. Most units now use a T-piece system (Tom Thumb circuits) which seems to be more effective in tidal volume delivery, and come with facilities to set up peak pressure and positive and expiratory pressure (PEEP.)

Laerdal bag. This is self-inflating with a blow-off valve set at $40\,cmH_2O$. It is easy to deliver high-pressure inflation to the baby's lungs with this bag, with inspired O_2. Oxygen flow only occurs when the bag is compressed or the baby inspires with the face mask applied. For free O_2 flow to the baby's nostrils disconnect the bag from the delivery valve Palme *et al.* 1985.

There are several different types of face mask in different sizes to suit premature and full-term infants. Choose a face mask that fits snugly over baby's mouth and nose but does not overhang the chin or cover the eyes. Round masks with a cushioned rim are preferable as it is easier to make a tight seal.

Technique (Fig. 30.2)

1 Place infant supine with neck extended (sniffing position), on a firm surface, and aspirate the airway.
2 Place face mask firmly over the nose and mouth with an O_2 flow rate of 4 L/min.
3 Hold face mask on firmly (but do not occlude nares) and hold the jaw forwards.
4 Inflate at a rate of about 30–40 breaths/min with a T or Y-piece (easier and better) or a self-inflating bag.

Make sure there is good chest wall movement, good air entry on auscultation of the lungs, and improvement in the infant's colour. If chest wall movement is poor, check position of the neck and that the airway is clear. Frequently, the insertion of

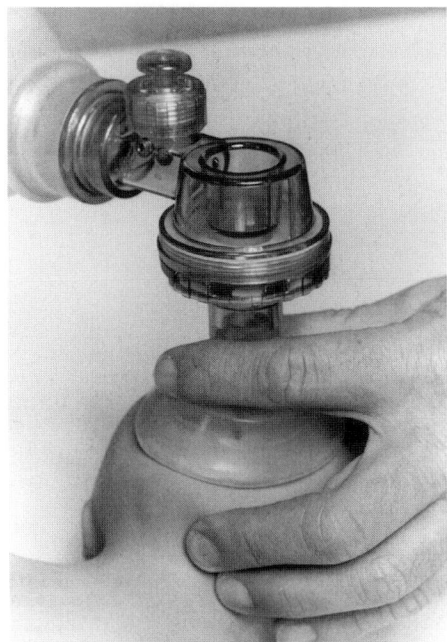

Figure 30.2 Bag-and-mask ventilation. Note fingers extending neck and holding mask securely.

an appropriate infant pharyngeal airway (Guedel) will improve air entry. The bag should be inflated only sufficiently to produce good chest wall movement. Damage can be done to the infant's lungs by overvigorous bagging. If there is no improvement in condition after inflation for 1–2 min, the infant will need intubation.

Intubation of the trachea

Endotracheal intubation is universally performed using an uncuffed tube (uniform-diameter tube). These tubes are designed for prolonged intubation and intubation of infants less than 1.5 kg birthweight. Use sizes 2.5, 3.0 and 3.5 mm for infants weighing 1.0, 2.0 and 3.0 kg, respectively. Premedication with suitable analgesia and sedation (such as morphine, atropine and suxamethonium) should always be used except for emergency resuscitation. A suitable muscle paralysing agent such as suxamethonium or atracurium can also be used to facilitate intubation. DO NOT paralyse the baby unless an experienced neonatologist is present, you

are confident that the airway can be maintained and hand ventilation is adequately provided until the tube has been inserted properly.

Orotracheal intubation

1 Select tube size and insert the introducer almost to the end of the tube and bend it slightly. Check laryngoscope, suction apparatus, bag, mask and adaptor. Prepare a means to secure the endotracheal tube once it is in place.
2 Place baby on a firm surface, suck pharynx and nares and ventilate by bag and mask for 30 s.
3 Place baby's head in 'sniffing' position by extending the neck by traction under the infant's jaw. Ensure the face is in the midline. An assistant may press directly on the cricoid cartilage to push the glottis up into view.
4 Pass laryngoscope blade gently along right side of mouth and pull tongue and epiglottis forward by exerting traction parallel to the handle of the laryngoscope (*not* by tilting the blade upwards) (Fig. 30.3).
5 Aspirate the airway again and pull the laryngoscope blade back until the epiglottis and vocal cords come into view (Fig. 30.4).

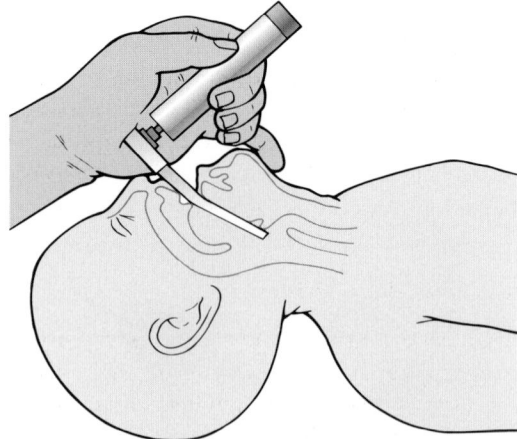

Figure 30.3 Laryngoscopy. The laryngoscope blade displaces the tongue and lifts the epiglottis anteriorly to expose the cords. (Reproduced with permission of Baillière Tindall.)

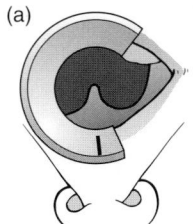 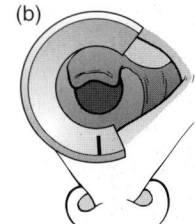 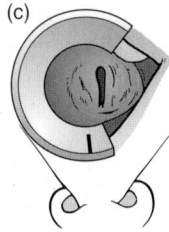

Figure 30.4 The stages of intubation. Visualization of the uvula and oropharynx (a). The epiglottis is seen with the oesophagus beyond it (b). The cords are seen (c).

Table 30.1 Recommendations for neonatal intubation

Infant's weight (g)	Tube diameter (mm)	Distance (cm)	
		Nasal tube (anterior nares to mid-trachea)	Oral tube (lip to tip)
500–750	2.5	7.5	6.5–6.8
750–1250	2.5	8.5	6.8–7.3
1250–2000	3.0	9.5	7.3–8.0
2000–3000	3.5	10.5	8.0–9.0
3000–4000	3.5	11.0–12.0	9.0–10.0

6 Pass endotracheal tube about 2 cm beyond the vocal cords (a slight 'give' can sometimes be felt as the tube passes into the larynx, *but no force is needed for insertion*), remove the introducer and apply gentle insufflation of the lungs. Table 30.1 gives the approximate distance for tube insertion, but the position of the tip of the tube should always be checked radiologically at least after initial intubation. It should be situated 0.5 cm above the carina or mid-trachea.

Tube position can also be confirmed clinically by equality of breath sounds (ideally compared under the axillae), no large leak, good symmetrical excursion of chest wall and appropriate physiological response in heart rate, respiratory rate and oxygen saturation.

Disposable end-tidal CO_2 detectors are now available to confirm that the tube is in the trachea.

Nasotracheal intubation

Nasal intubation is not normally used for emergency intubation but many units prefer this for long-term intubation (and ventilation) as fixation is more satisfactory. Therefore, this is mostly carried out as an elective procedure.

1 Select tube and check Magill's forceps. An introducer is not used. Visualize the back of the mouth with a laryngoscope.

2 Endotracheal tube is gently passed down the right nostril until it just appears behind the soft palate.

3 The tip of the endotracheal tube is picked up by the Magill's forceps and placed gently between the vocal cords. The assistant pushes the tube down the trachea as the operator guides it with Magill's forceps.

Fixation of the endotracheal tube

Each unit has its own methods for securing an endotracheal tube. It is most important that the tube is fixed securely onto the face to avoid accidental extubation, and also to ensure that the infant's sensitive skin is not traumatized by the procedure.

Taping the tube (Fig. 30.5)
Most units prefer to apply a plastic guard ring around the outside of the endotracheal tube and then suture this to the tube by silk thread penetrating both the ring and the tube. Care must be taken not to narrow the lumen of the tube by the suture, so that suction cannot be easily performed. The plastic guard ring may then be plastered to the upper lip or attached at either end to a bonnet over the infant's head (Fig. 30.6).

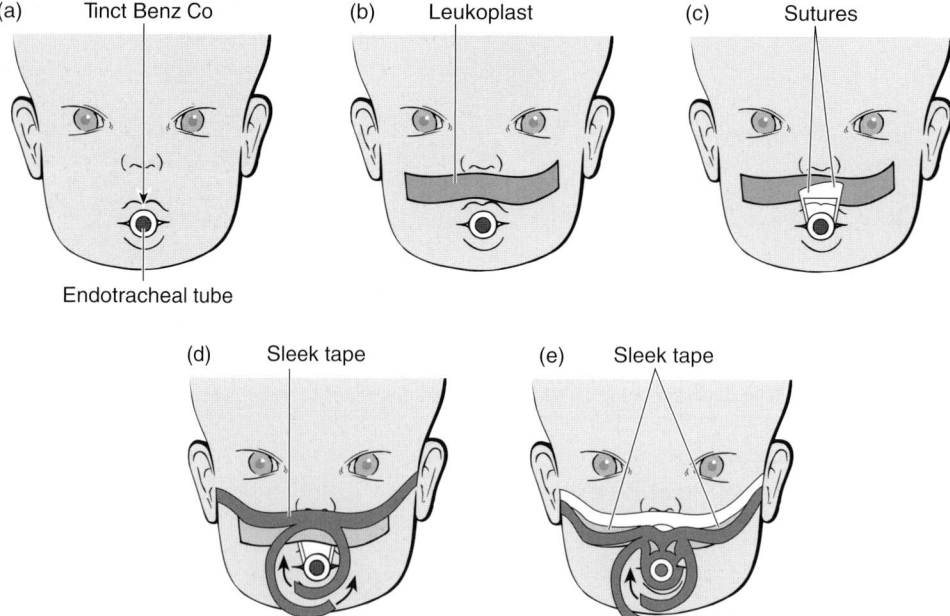

Figure 30.5 A method of fixing the endotracheal tube for long-term ventilation. This can be used for oral or nasal tubes.

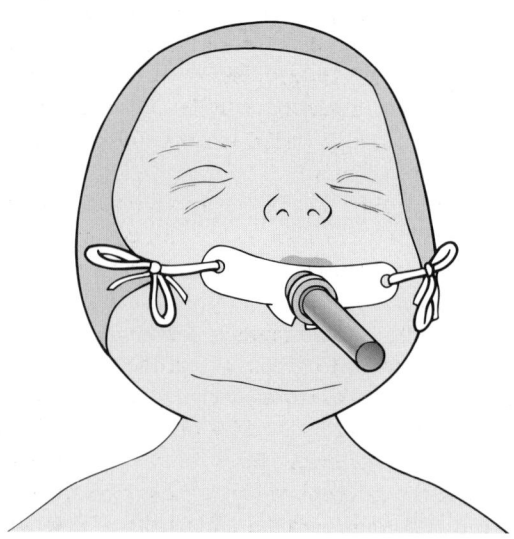

Figure 30.6 Alternative method for fixing the endotracheal tube using a plastic flange tied to the infant's bonnet. A suture is inserted through the cuff of the flange and the tube to secure it.

Routine endotracheal tube care

Individual units must develop their own protocols to look after a baby who is intubated and ventilated in order to minimize complications such as blockage due to secretion, accidental displacement or dislodging (especially during procedures such as X-ray or scans). Active chest physiotherapy is only required when positioning and suction methods fail to maintain a clear chest. There is no *a priori* reason to advocate routine change of an endotracheal tube (ETT).

Extubation procedure

This should be a planned procedure and one peformed only after careful assessment of baby's suitability for extubation. Despite this careful judgment, a baby may not tolerate extubation and require reintubation, and hence there should be a resuscitation trolley at hand. Prophylactic treatment with aminophylline or caffeine, and post-extubation switch to nasal continuous positive airway pressure (CPAP) (especially in low birthweight babies) may aid successful extubation and reduce the need for reintubation. Individual units must develop their own protocols.

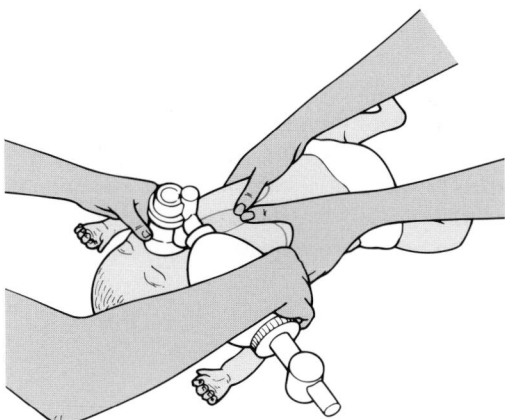

Figure 30.7 External cardiac massage over the lower third of the sternum. Simultaneous ventilation is also necessary as shown.

External cardiac massage

This is necessary in cases of cardiac arrest or severe bradycardia not responding to suction, oxygenation and ventilation.

1 The hands are placed around the chest with the fingertips around the back and the thumbs over the middle to lower third of the sternum, 1 cm below the internipple line (Fig. 30.7). The sternum should be depressed about 1.5–2.0 cm 90 times/min. Every third depression should be followed by a lung inflation.

2 Constantly check the effectiveness of massage by observing colour, perfusion and pulses, and briefly stop massage every so often to auscultate the heart.

Drainage of a pneumothorax

If there is a sudden deterioration in an infant with respiratory distress, whether he or she is receiving mechanical ventilation or not, a pneumothorax should be considered and the following carried out.

1 Auscultate. Is air entry different between the two sides?

2 Transilluminate the chest using a cold fibreoptic light source. A pneumothorax will cause the affected hemithorax to glow. In very tiny babies the whole chest may transilluminate normally because of the thin chest wall, and this requires careful interpretation.

3 If the baby is not *in extremis*, perform an urgent chest X-ray.

4 If the condition is critical and a pneumothorax is strongly suspected, a therapeutic thoracocentesis is performed by placing a 19G butterfly needle into the second intercostal space in the midclavicular line. It is essential that the other end of the butterfly tube is attached to a three-way stopcock (turned off) and to a 20-mL syringe. Remember that blindly needling the chest may itself produce a pneumothorax.

5 Once the infant's condition is stable, an intercostal catheter is inserted using aseptic precautions (see below).

6 After securing the catheter do a check X-ray to ensure adequate evacuation of air.

Placement of a pneumothorax drain

There are two positions for drainage insertion:

1 anteriorly in the second intercostal space in the midclavicular line (Fig. 30.8a);

2 laterally in the fifth or sixth intercostal space in the anterior axillary line (Fig. 30.8b).

The anterior position appears to be the most successful in draining pneumothoraces, but it is important to avoid trauma to the infant's nipples and unsightly scarring. The procedure is described below.

1 The skin is cleansed with alcohol, prepared with povidone-iodine and infiltrated with local anaesthetic (1% Xylocaine).

2 A deep incision is made in the second intercostal space in the midclavicular line on the affected side. The intercostal muscle should be breached by the scalpel blade.

3 A size 10-Fr pleural catheter (size 12-Fr is better for larger infants) with trocar is introduced through the chest wall and pleura. The catheter and trocar should be cross-clamped with a pair of forceps 2 cm from the tip to prevent overinsertion. The catheter is introduced in the direction of the lung apex for a distance of 3–5 cm. Once the tip is in the pleural cavity about 2 cm, the trocar is withdrawn and quickly attached to the Heimlich valve. The catheter is then advanced a further 1–2 cm.

4 The catheter is secured with a pursestring suture and strapped to the chest wall with a bridge of Micropore tape or plastic adhesive dressing such as Tegaderm.

(a)

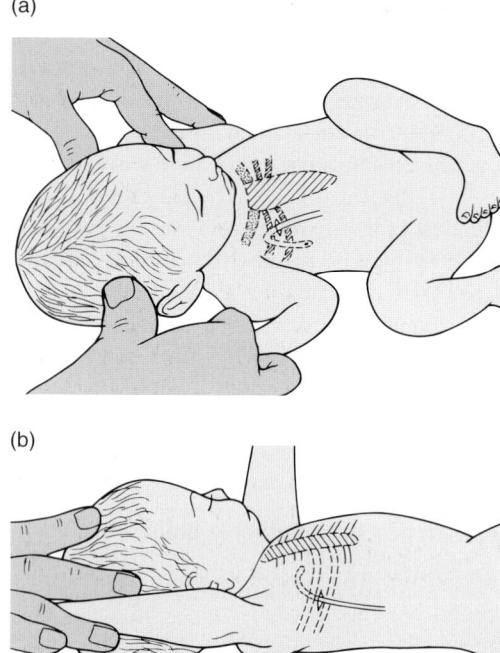

(b)

Figure 30.8 Pneumothorax drainage. (a) Insertion of a pleural drain anteriorly through the second intercostal space in the midclavicular line. (b) Insertion of a pleural drain through the fifth intercostal space in the anterior axillary line.

A flutter valve is very useful instead of an underwater seal if the pneumothorax occurs before transportation of the infant. However, if the flutter valve becomes wet with blood or moisture, the surface tension between the two rubber leaves will significantly increase the pressure required to open the valve. For this reason, it is preferable to attach the tube to an underwater seal under low −10 to −20 continuous suction to prevent obstruction, especially if blood is present in the chest. For a more laterally sited catheter it is important that the catheter be angled anteriorly, as posteriorly positioned catheters are more likely to obstruct.

An alternative and less traumatic Seldinger-like technique is now available that appears to be as effective as the above method and is easier for inexperienced staff to master.

Removal of intercostal catheter

The chest tube is clamped when there has been no bubbling for 24 h, and it is removed after a further 12–24 h if there is no deterioration clinically or reaccumulation of the pneumothorax on chest X-ray. Take care that air is not sucked into the chest after catheter removal. The intercostal catheter is removed slowly and pressure applied to the site. The skin edges can be closed with Steri-strips and an adhesive dressing applied to the site. Pursestring sutures can leave unsightly scars.

Abdominal paracentesis

Approaches may be midline or lateral. The bladder should be empty for this procedure.
1 Midline: a 21G needle is inserted vertically through the abdominal wall 1–2 cm below the umbilicus.
2 Lateral: the needle is inserted into right or left iliac fossa lateral to the rectus abdominis, taking care to avoid a grossly enlarged liver and spleen and inferior epigastric artery.

Large collections will drain freely but may be enhanced by dependent positions.

Pericardial aspiration

This procedure is indicated for cardiac tamponade due to pneumopericardium or a large pericardial effusion or haemorrhage.
1 Use a 23G needle connected to a three-way stopcock and a 10-mL syringe.
2 Enter under the thorax to the left of the xiphisternum and advance upwards and to the left at 45° to vertical and 45° to the midline while applying gentle suction.
3 The pericardium is entered to a depth of 1 cm and air or fluid withdrawn.

Umbilical vessel catheterization

Umbilical arterial catheterization

Umbilical arterial catheterization is performed for intermittent sampling of arterial blood and continuous monitoring of arterial Po_2 and blood pressure. The following catheter sizes are used:

- 3.5FG for infants weighing less than 1500 g;
- 5FG if greater than 1500 g.

There are two common positions for placement of the tip of the umbilical artery catheter:

1 High: in the aorta at the level of the diaphragm (T10).
2 Low: below the level of the renal arteries (L4–L5). This position has a greater risk of thrombosis (Wesstrom *et al.* 1979).

An estimate can be made of how far to pass the catheters on the basis of the distance in centimetres between the umbilicus and the shoulder tip. The length to be inserted can then be read directly from Fig. 30.9.

Technique

1 Measure the shoulder-to-umbilicus distance and estimate the distance to pass the catheter from Fig. 30.9. The calculated distance is for placement in the aorta at T10.
2 Use full surgical scrub technique with gloves, gown and mask. Cleanse cord and abdominal wall with alcohol and povidone-iodine.
3 Apply a piece of ribbon gauze around the cord before cutting the cord with a scalpel. Cut cord horizontally about 1 cm above the abdominal wall. Identify the three cord vessels and dilate the mouth

of one of the arteries with a pair of fine iris forceps or dilator.
4 Attach a three-way stopcock and a syringe of normal saline to the catheter and flush it with heparinized saline solution. Cannulate the artery and introduce the catheter the calculated distance. Check position of catheter radiologically.
5 The catheter is secured *in situ* using a pursestring suture (3–4 bites) and taped to the abdominal wall using a 'bridge' or 'goalposts' (Fig. 30.10).
6 The catheter is connected to an infusion pump and to a pressure transducer for blood pressure monitoring. Circulation to the lower limbs is closely observed.
7 An A—P abdominal X-ray is taken to locate the catheter tip. If the catheter is sited too low for high position it should not be advanced to avoid the risk of introducing infection and instead should be withdrawn to the lower position.

Umbilical venous catheterization

Umbilical venous catheterization is useful in very low birthweight (VLBW) infants for a number of reasons:
1 Urgent resuscitation in the labour ward.
2 Venous access for fluid administration in VLBW infants.
3 Exchange transfusion. A 5FG catheter is used and should be placed in the inferior vena cava (IVC) if possible (although only 70% will pass through the ductus venosus). The location of the catheter tip should always be checked radiographically.

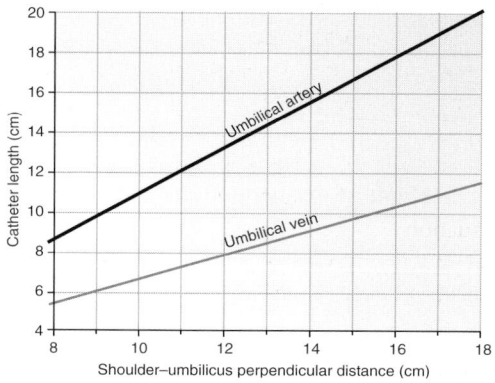

Figure 30.9 Chart showing the distance to insert umbilical artery catheter (high position in aorta at or above diaphragm) and umbilical vein catheter based on the infant's shoulder-to-umbilicus distance. (Adapted from Dunn 1966.).

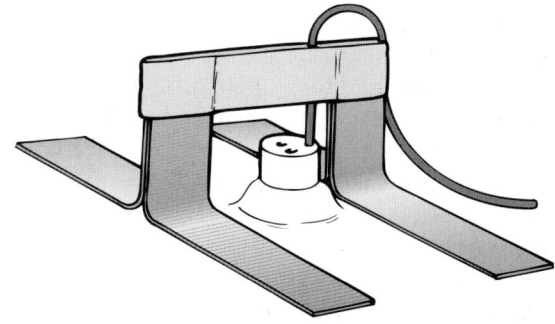

Figure 30.10 Securing the umbilical catheter using Micropore tape.

4 Lack of venous access, e.g. hydrops fetalis.
5 Central venous pressure (CVP) monitoring.
6 Performance of balloon septostomy for transposition of the great arteries (TGA).
7 Administration of drugs and total parenteral nutrition (TPN).

Technique

Emergency resuscitation

1 Secure a cord tie snugly at the base of the umbilical cord (do not pull tight).
2 Make an incision halfway through the superior aspect of the cord 0.5 cm from its base to expose the umbilical vein but avoiding the arteries.
3 Insert a 5FG umbilical catheter or double-lumen catheter into the vein. The distance to be passed for position in IVC is calculated from Fig. 30.9 after measuring the acromioclavicular–umbilical distance. If it is not possible to withdraw blood, then the site of the catheter should be checked after injecting 2 mL of normal saline.
4 Tighten cord tie and tape catheter to the baby's abdomen.

Elective insertion

1 Preparation as for umbilical artery.
2 Distance inserted is calculated from graph.
3 Umbilical vein must be clearly distinguished from two umbilical arteries. Rarely is it necessary to spend much time on dilatation, but clot may need to be removed.
4 Check position before suturing pursestring as catheter can easily slip out.

Exchange transfusion

Exchange transfusion is practised much less frequently these days than formerly, and many units have lost the knowhow. Hence, the operator must be fully acquainted with the technique before embarking on it as this may lead to serious complications. The only real indication for exchange transfusion is unconjugated hyperbilirubinaemia; the technique has been tried in a number of other conditions (see below) but without strong scientific evidence:

1 septicaemia – it may be useful in the early overwhelming variety, e.g. group B β-haemolytic streptococcus;
2 disseminated intravascular coagulation;
3 inborn errors of metabolism;
4 intoxications;
5 to correct anaemia (especially hydrops fetalis).

The blood should be less than 48 h old, ABO compatible with mother and infant and rhesus negative. If the baby is critically ill, blood may be buffered with trishydroxyaminomethane (THAM) 3.5% to correct the pH. The volume to be exchanged is usually 180 mL/kg for a double-volume exchange.

Techniques

1 *Isovolaemic.* Blood is removed from the umbilical artery and given via the umbilical vein.
2 *Single catheter.* Preferably umbilical vein, but the artery may be used.
3 *Peripheral vessels.* A peripheral artery catheter and venous cannula are used.

Donor blood is warmed via a heating coil in a water bath. Generally, 10-mL aliquots are used. The first 10-mL aliquot is sent for serum bilirubin (SRR), haematocrit (Hct), full blood count Full blood count (FBC), electrolytes, proteins, glucose-6-phosphate dehydrogenase (G6PD), liver enzymes, serology, etc. The heart rate, blood pressure, temperature and respirations should be monitored continuously throughout the exchange transfusion. A careful record is kept of all blood sampled and transfused. At the end of the exchange transfusion, blood is sent to the laboratory for haemoglobin, total and direct bilirubin, electrolytes, calcium, sugar and blood culture.

Do not feed the infant for at least 2 h before and at least 4 h after exchange transfusion. Instead give maintenance i.v. fluids.

Complications of exchange transfusion

The possible complications can be summarized in several categories:
- *Vascular:* air/clot embolization, thrombosis.
- *Cardiac:* dysrhythmia, volume overload, arrest.
- *Electrolyte:* hyperkalaemia, hypernatraemia, hypocalcaemia, acidosis.
- *Infective:* bacteraemia, hepatitis B, cytomegalovirus (CMV).
- *Other:* hypoglycaemia, necrotizing enterocolitis (NEC).

Dilutional exchange transfusion for polycythaemia (p. 201)

The indications for an isovolaemic dilutional exchange transfusion are:

1 a venous Hct greater than 70% in an asymptomatic baby; and

2 a venous Hct greater than 65% in a symptomatic baby.

Use fresh frozen plasma or 4–5% albumin:

$$\text{Volume to be exchanged} = \frac{\text{infant's Hct} - \text{desired Hct} \times \text{kg body weight} \times 90}{\text{donor Hct}}$$

The exchange transfusion should take about 30 min and must be performed via a blood vessel with a good blood flow (usually an umbilical vein).

Peripheral arterial catheterization

Cannulation of either the radial or the posterior tibial artery is equally effective as cannulation of the umbilical artery, but for some operators it is technically more difficult, especially in very small babies.

Technique

1 Palpate the vessel and visualize it with a fibreoptic cold transillumination light.

2 Collateral circulation is assessed by the Allen test. The wrist is held firmly on the radial side and the blood squeezed out of the hand. If the colour returns rapidly to the hand while pressure is maintained on the radial artery, it is safe to cannulate the radial artery.

3 The wrist is cleansed with alcohol and povidone-iodine. The transillumination light can be held under the wrist while a 22G catheter is advanced slowly in the direction of the radial artery at an angle of about 20° to the skin. Once blood is seen in the clear plastic chamber the catheter is advanced a further 0.5 mm, and then, while advancing the catheter slightly, the stylet is withdrawn. The index finger is placed over the radial artery to prevent blood loss.

4 The catheter is attached to an extension tubing, three-way stopcock with Luer lock adaptors, and connected to an infusion pump with heparinized saline set at 1–2 mL/h (1 U heparin per mL of solution). The catheter should be attached to a pressure transducer. Under no circumstances should drugs, blood or any other solutions except normal saline be infused through this line. The catheter must be firmly strapped and taped to an armboard, which is immobilized. Sometimes N/2 (0.5N) saline is acceptable.

Complications

One of the major complications of peripheral arterial cannulation is ischaemia of the limb, which presents as discoloration and poor perfusion. This should be recognized straight away and dealt with by immediate removal of the cannula and infusion of saline or low molecular weight dextran to facilitate reperfusion.

Regular close observation of the limb must be maintained for as long as the cannula remains in the artery. Any loss of colour or perfusion should prompt immediate removal of the cannula to prevent severe vascular injury with a risk of losing the hand or limb.

Intermittent arterial sampling

This may be performed most safely from the radial or posterior tibial arteries, as a one-off sampling procedure where arterial blood gas assessment is required. The brachial and femoral arteries are less acceptable because limb ischaemia may occur. Femoral artery puncture is particularly hazardous as it is done blindly and carries a risk of haemorrhage and infection.

Technique

1 Palpate the vessel.

2 Prepare either a 25G needle with a clear barrel or a 25G short butterfly and attach to a millilitre syringe that has been lightly coated with heparin (1000 U/mL).

3 Cleanse skin with an alcohol/chlorhexidine swab and insert the needle at an angle of 30° to the skin surface (Fig. 30.11). The landmark at the wrist is just proximal to the proximal crease and lateral to the flexor carpi radialis tendon. Transfix the artery and then withdraw the needle slowly until blood spurts into the syringe.

4 Remove 0.3 mL of blood and then withdraw the needle. Apply pressure over the artery for at least 3–4 min.

Blood sampling

Venepuncture

The antecubital fossa vein is the first choice for venepuncture, followed by peripheral veins. Giving oral sucrose to baby prior to the procedure reduces pain and is recommended.

1 Visualize and palpate the vessel. Apply a tourniquet (usually a tight finger grip) proximal to the vessel. Cleanse the skin with alcohol/chlorhexidine swab.

2 Use a 21 or 23G needle with a 2-mL syringe but avoid using excessive suction. Blood will usually drip fully from the needle into a specimen container. It is always safer for the operator to use gloves when dealing with blood sampling, and he or she should be conversant with the local procedure for dealing with any inadvertent needle injury.

Heel-prick capillary blood sampling

Most laboratory tests can be carried out readily on small quantities of blood. In newborn infants capillary blood obtained from a heel prick is usually the method of choice. Up to 1 mL of blood can be sampled by this method.

1 Wash hands carefully and clean the heel with a 70% alcohol Mediswab.

2 Hold the leg around the ankle with thumb and fingers (do not hold the leg around the calf or shin as this may cause extensive bruising) (Fig. 30.12).

3 Prick the heel with a disposable lancet or autolet, on the most medial or lateral portion of the plantar surface (see hatched areas on Fig. 30.13). Heel punctures should be performed on the plantar surface of the heel, but beyond the lines defined by the lateral and medial limits of the calcaneus (Fig. 30.13). The heel prick should not be deeper than 2 mm, and should not be on the posterior curvature of the heel, nor at previous sites that may be infected.).

4 Collect the blood into a capillary tube held horizontally.

It may be necessary to squeeze the foot beforehand to get a good flow of blood. Warming the foot using a warm wrap may improve the blood supply. Prior administration of oral sucrose to the baby alleviates pain.

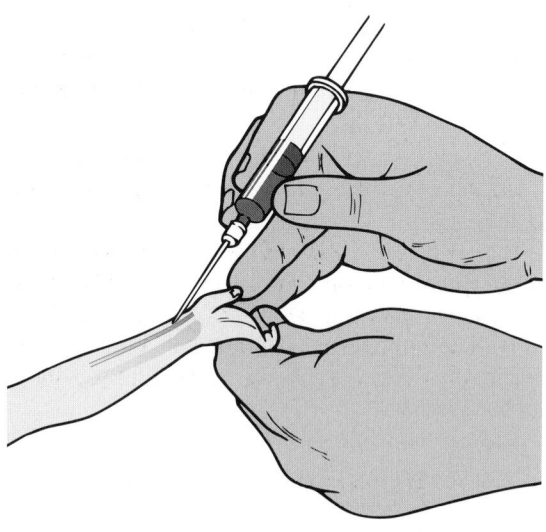

Figure 30.11 Technique for radial artery sampling. The needle transects the artery and is then withdrawn whilst aspirating the syringe.

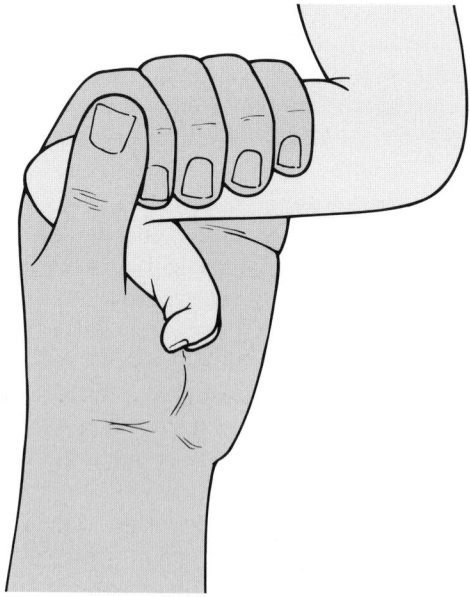

Figure 30.12 Method for holding the heel prior to blood sampling.

Blood culture

It is always helpful to have a nurse in attendance for this procedure. Use a full aseptic technique. Avoid drawing blood from indwelling catheters: it is preferable to take blood from a peripheral vein.

Technique

1 Wash hands before undertaking any invasive procedure such as blood collection, and use gloves.
2 When a blood culture is drawn by venepuncture, a peripheral arterial stab, etc., strict aseptic technique must be adhered to.
3 Swab skin with 70% alcohol and allow to dry, or wait 1 min. This is to remove surface grease and dead skin cells. Repeat procedure with another 70% alcohol swab. This is to disinfect the skin. It is essential to use two separate swabs and allow the skin to dry (or wait 1 min) after each.
4 After removing the covering cap on the blood culture bottle, the rubber bung should be swabbed with 70% alcohol and then allowed to dry, as the rubber bung is not sterile. The same procedure should be used if a yellow-top isolator blood tube is being used in the intensive care nursery (ICN).
5 After skin preparation with 70% alcohol, every effort must be made to prevent contamination by examining fingers. Use a sterile glove or swab the fingertip with 70% alcohol.
6 After obtaining the sample of blood, the needle must be removed and a new needle used to inoculate the blood equally into each blood culture bottle (or yellow-topped isolator tube if in ICN).
7 Volumes of blood to collect are indicated in Table 30.2.
8 Record the site from where the blood was collected (i.e. venous, arterial, central line, arterial catheter, etc.).
9 To avoid contamination, blood culture bottle inoculation must occur *before* blood is placed into any other tubes or into a blood-gas analyser.

Insertion of a silastic long line

This is a useful technique and is not difficult to perform. The following equipment is required (Fig 13.4):
1 a 19G butterfly needle with the plastic tubing cut off close to the needle;
2 a 30-cm length of fine 2FG silastic catheter; and
3 a 25G butterfly needle with its plastic tube intact.

This procedure must be carried out using strict aseptic precautions and the operator should be fully masked and gowned. The veins in the antecubital fossa, long saphenous or superficial temporal veins are the most suitable for cannulation. The area is

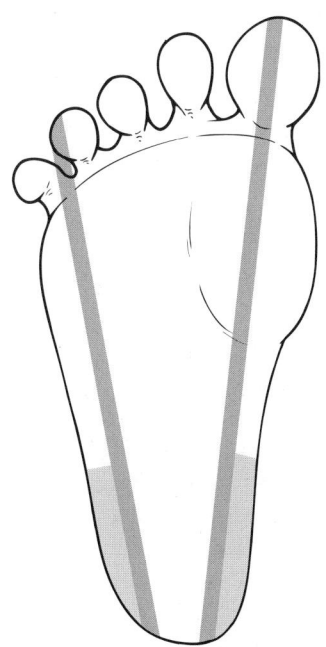

Figure 30.13 Heel-prick specimens should only be taken from the areas of the foot that are shaded in this drawing.

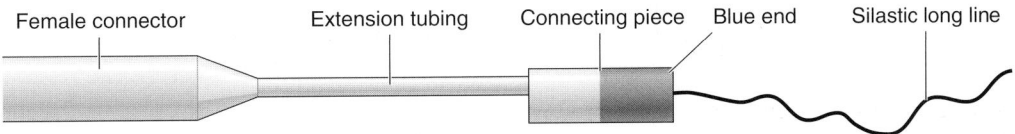

Figure 30.14 Silastic catheter for long peripheral intravenous line insertion.

Table 30.2 Tubes and blood volumes required for culture

Patient category	Adult aerobic (grey top)	Paediatric aerobic (pink top)	Anaerobic (orange top)	Isolator (yellow top)
Neonates (ICN/SCN)	N/A	0.5–3 mL	N/A	0.5–1.5 mL
Babies (nurseries)	N/A	1–3 mL	1–3 mL	N/A
mothers	10 mL	N/A	10 mL	N/A

ICN/SCN, intensive care nursery/special care nursery.

exposed and thoroughly cleansed with alcohol. Before inserting the 19G butterfly, the length of silastic tubing necessary to place the tip in the right atrium is estimated and a mark made on the tube at the required length. The 19G butterfly is inserted into the vein as for venepuncture. When blood is seen to drip out of the needle, the silastic catheter is threaded through the inside of the 19G butterfly until the mark is reached. The 19G butterfly is then removed from the catheter and a 25G needle carefully inserted into the lumen of the catheter. The whole line should then be gently flushed with heparinized saline. Occasionally, the connector needle perforates the fine catheter tubing at the join and the dressing becomes moist. To avoid this complication great care must be taken to prevent movement at this connection site by using a wooden spatula and carefully taping the connector and three-way stopcock. The entry site is then scrubbed with povidone-iodine, secured firmly with sterile adhesive strips, and covered with a sterile transparent dressing (e.g. OpSite). The site of the catheter tip in the peripheral vein is marked on the skin for monitoring purposes. If a limb vein is used, the limb is immobilized by splinting.

Before commencing the infusion the position of the catheter tip should be checked to ensure t is in a central vein, by using contrast X-ray or newer digital X-ray techniques which reduces the need for repeated X-ray exposures. If the tip is in too far it may be pulled back to a more suitable position. Ensure that an X-ray confirms that the catheter tip is not within the heart.

Possible complications

The following observations, indicative of possible complications, should be made following insertion of a long line:

1 Site – blood loss/leakage.
2 Redness.
3 Exudate.
4 Temperature instability.
5 Oedema.
6 Induration.
7 Reduced perfusion of limb.

Lumbar puncture

The indications for lumbar puncture (LP) may be diagnostic (e.g. suspected meningitis, metabolic screen, differentiating between communicating and non-communicating hydrocephalus) or therapeutic (progressive ventricular dilatation).

Technique

1 A full surgical scrub technique is necessary with gloves, gown and mask.
2 An experienced nurse needs to hold the baby in the left lateral position with the head, hips and knees well flexed. The back needs to be completely parallel to the edge of the table. Make sure the airway is not obstructed.
3 The skin is cleansed with povidone-iodine and alcohol. Generally a 22G LP needle with stylet is used. Some operators prefer a 23G butterfly needle, but this does not possess a stylet and there is a greater risk of a dermoid cyst developing at the site in later years.
4 Use lumbar spaces L3–L4 or L4–L5. Ideally the skin should be infiltrated with 1% Xylocaine as local anaesthetic, but this may make the procedure somewhat difficult because of loss of intervertebral space. The lumbar puncture needle is then inserted and directed towards the umbilicus. Once the subarachnoid space is penetrated, the stylet is removed and cerebrospinal fluid (CSF) is allowed to drip into

each of three bottles (Fig. 30.15). Sometimes the needle needs to be gently rotated to check for CSF flow. It is easy to push the needle too far into the anterior vertebral venous plexus.

5 Measurement of lumbar CSF pressure may be necessary in infants with posthaemorrhagic ventricular dilatation (see p. 214). This can be done by attaching a Luer locking pressure transducer directly to the hub of the needle or by using a manometer tube. Pressure measurements are only valid if the infant is breathing quietly and not crying. The head and trunk must be flat and in the same plane, and the infant not too tightly curled up.

6 CSF should always be sent for cell count, Gram stain and culture and glucose and protein estimations. Other tests may include viral studies, syphilis serology, fluorescein staining and counterimmune electrophoresis.

Ventricular tap

Rarely, a ventricular tap will be needed to diagnose ventriculitis or intraventricular haemorrhage, or to instil antibiotics. Generally, the procedure will be performed by a neurosurgeon or other experienced staff.

1 The baby is placed in a supine position with the nose upwards and the neck and face parallel to the mattress.

2 After the scalp has been shaved a full aseptic technique should be used. A long 20G or 22G LP needle with stylet is gently inserted at the lateral angle of the anterior fontanelle and angled towards the medial canthus of the eye on the same side (Fig. 30.16).

3 Once the skin and dura have been pierced, the stylet may be removed and the needle gently advanced until CSF wells up from the needle.

4 CSF from the ventricles should be collected by allowing it to drip into sterile bottles.

Subdural tap

In the past this was a common diagnostic procedure, but with the advent of better computed tomography (CT) and ultrasound scanning it should generally be reserved for therapy and not diagnosis.

1 Full aseptic technique should be used after scalp shaving. The baby lies on his or her back and the operator stands at the baby's head.

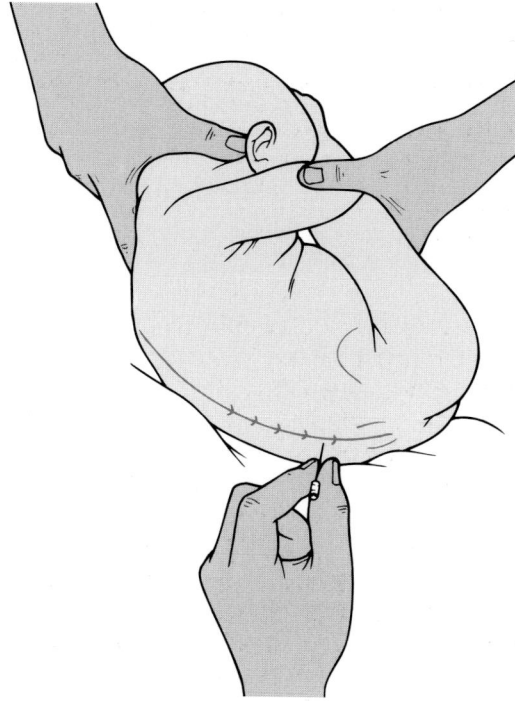

Figure 30.15 Technique for lumbar puncture in the newborn.

2 A 20G or 22G subdural needle with stylet is inserted at the lateral angle of the anterior fontanelle and pushed in a distance of 5–7 mm at right angles to the skin.

3 After the needle has passed through the dura (a slight change in resistance is felt), remove the stylet and wait for fluid to emerge. Normally only a few drops will be obtained. If serous fluid is present, probably not more than 10 mL should be withdrawn at one time. If pure blood is obtained from a subdural haematoma, leave the needle *in situ* until the blood stops dripping.

4 Do not attach a syringe and aspirate subdural fluid.

5 When collection is complete withdraw the needle and apply pressure over the puncture site.

Frequently the procedure will need to be repeated on the other side with a new needle.

Urine collection

This may be performed by a 'clean-catch' bag method, suprapubic aspiration or urethral catheter.

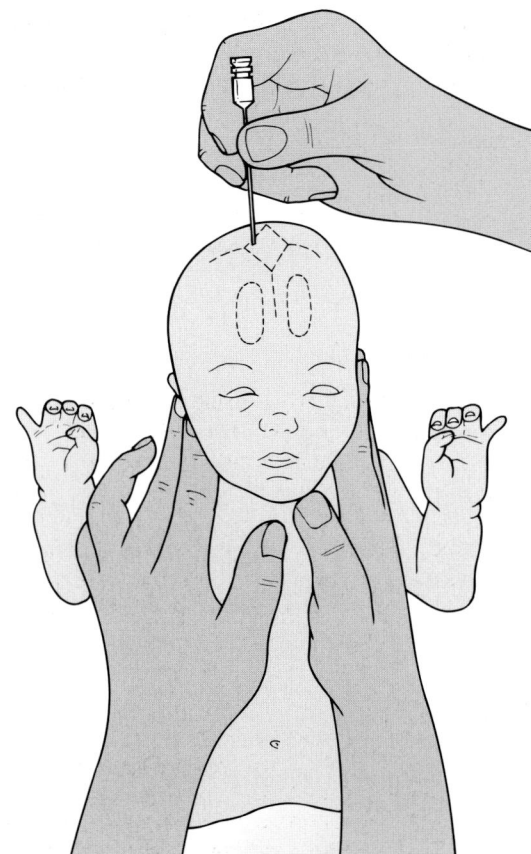

Figure 30.16 Ventricular tap through the anterior fontanelle using a styletted needle.

Suprapubic puncture is a relatively painful procedure and should be discouraged.

Bag collection

A clean-catch bag sample of urine may provide useful information. However, an inexpertly collected sample provides confusing or misleading information.

1 Cleanse a wide area of the perineum and penis with sterile saline-soaked swabs using a no-touch technique. In females the vulva will need to be separated, but the foreskin must not be retracted in males although it needs to be cleaned.

2 Wait for the perineum to dry before attaching a sterile urine-collecting bag. Sometimes the application of tincture of benzoin enhances the adhesion of bag to skin.

3 Inspect the bag periodically, and as soon as the baby has voided remove the bag and immediately pour the urine into a universal sterile container.

4 Send the sample to the laboratory immediately. If there is any delay in transporting the sample, refrigerate it.

5 If no urine has been obtained after 1 h, the skin should be cleansed again and a fresh collecting bag applied.

A suitable alternative to bag collection in babies and small children is to put a pad inside the nappy and when wet, to suck out the urine using a small syringe. This is considered to be as sterile as a bag sample, and widely practised in many centres.

Suprapubic aspiration

The indications for this procedure are an inconclusive culture from a bag specimen, a critically ill child or the presence of vulvovaginitis or balanitis when urinary tract infection is suspected.

1 The bladder must be full prior to commencing the procedure.

2 A wide area of skin over the lower abdomen is prepared with povidone-iodine solution and alcohol.

3 A 21G needle attached to a 10-mL syringe is used to puncture the skin 1 cm above the pubic symphysis in the midline.

4 The needle is advanced into the bladder, angled slightly upwards to the perpendicular. As the needle is slowly advanced gentle suction is applied. The needle usually only needs to be advanced 1.5–2.0 cm below the skin surface (Fig. 30.17).

Peritoneal dialysis (PD)

The indications for PD in the newborn include:

1 uraemia (plasma urea >40 mmol/L);

2 hyperkalaemia (serum potassium >7.5 mmol/L);

3 severe metabolic acidosis due to renal failure;

4 inborn errors of metabolism (see p. 171);

5 inadvertent drug overdose;

6 water overload.

PD can be attempted in infants without major abdominal pathology such as NEC or recent laparotomy. A urinary catheter should be inserted to empty the bladder. A 19G intravenous cannula is

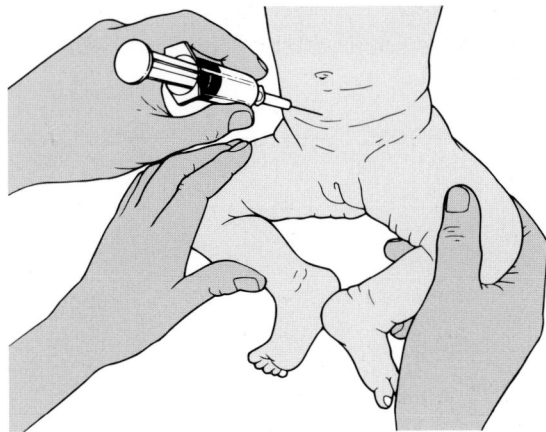

Figure 30.17 Suprapubic aspiration of urine from the bladder. The needle should be aimed slightly superiorly in the midline and 0.5 cm above the pubis.

inserted through the right iliac fossa into the peritoneal cavity, and warmed dialysis fluid is instilled to fill the cavity. This allows the PD catheter to be more safely introduced, with a lower risk of damaging the bowel.

The PD cannula is then inserted at a point midway between the umbilicus and the left anterior superior iliac crest, and secured with a pursestring suture. An isotonic dialysis solution (1.36% glucose) is used for biochemical and metabolic indications. A hypertonic solution (3.86% glucose) is used for fluid overload, but hyperglycaemia is a risk when this solution is used.

Dialysis is undertaken in the following sequence:
1 allow the fluid to drain from the peritoneal cavity;
2 for each cycle, run in 20–30 mL/kg of prewarmed dialysis fluid over 10 min;
3 allow this to remain in the cavity for 20–30 min so that dialysis occurs;
4 let fluid drain out under gravity for 20 min; each cycle therefore lasts about 1 h;
5 accurately record the volumes in and out; and
6 perform microscopy of the dialysate every 24 h to detect infection.

References

Dunn PM. Localisation of the umbilical catheter by post mortem measurement. *Arch Dis Child* 1966;**41**:69–74.

Palme C, Nystrom B, Tunnell R. An evaluation of face masks in the resuscitation of newborn infants. *Lancet* 1985;**i**:207–210.

Wesstrom G, Finnstrom O, Stenport G. Umbilical artery catheterization in newborns. 1. Thromboses in relation to catheter type and position. *Acta Paediatr Scand* 1979;**68**:575–581.

Further reading

Barr P. *Newborn Intensive Care*. Sydney: Royal Alexandra Hospital for Children, 1992.

Fleming PJ, Speidel BD, Marlow N, Dunn PM (eds) *A Neonatal Vade-Mecum*, 2nd edn. London: Edward Arnold, 1991.

Halliday HL, McClure G, Reid M (eds) *Neonatal Intensive Care*, 3rd edn. London: Baillière Tindall, 1989.

Robertson NRC. *A Manual of Neonatal Intensive Care*, 3rd edn. London: Edward Arnold, 1993.

Index